Substance Abuse Education in Nursing
Volume II
Curriculum Modules

Substance Abuse Education in Nursing

Volume II

Curriculum Modules

Madeline A. Naegle, Editor

National League for Nursing Press • New York
Pub. No. 15-2463

Copyright © 1992
National League for Nursing
350 Hudson Street, New York, NY 10014

All rights reserved. No part of this book may be reproduced in print, or by photostatic means, or in any other manner, without the express written permission of the publisher.

ISBN 0-88737-545-6

> The views expressed in this book reflect those of the authors and do not necessarily reflect the official views of the National League for Nursing.

This book was set in Caledonia by Publications Development Company. The editor and designer was Allan Graubard. Northeastern Press was the printer and binder. The cover was designed by Lillian Welsh.

Printed in the United States of America.

CONTENTS

Acknowledgements		vii
Preface		ix
Foreword		xi
II.1	Fetal Effects of Maternal Alcohol and Drug Use *Eileen Gigliotti*	1
	Instructor's Guide	13
II.2	Impaired Practice by Health Professionals *Madeline A. Naegle*	117
	Instructor's Guide	127
II.3	Addictions: Nursing Diagnosis and Treatment *Janet S. D'Arcangelo* *Thomas Adamski*	221
	Instructor's Guide	255
II.4	Nursing Care in Acute Intoxication *Margaret Compton*	347
	Instructor's Guide	359
II.5	Nursing Care in Withdrawal *Margaret Compton*	409
	Instructor's Guide	421
II.6	Drug Misuse and Dependence in the Elderly *Gean Mathwig* *Janet S. D'Arcangelo*	463
	Instructor's Guide	477
II.7	Drug and Alcohol Problems in Special Populations *Aileen H. Clucas* *Vivian P. J. Clarke*	531
	Instructor's Guide	549
II.8	Nursing Care of Drug and Alcohol Problems in Special Populations *Aileen H. Clucas* *Vivian P. J. Clarke*	603
	Instructor's Guide	617

CONTRIBUTORS

Thomas Adamski, MEd, MSN, RNC, CRNA, is Assistant Clinical Professor of Nursing, Division of Nursing, School of Education, Health, Nursing and Arts Professions, New York University.

Vivian P. J. Clarke, EdD, CHES, is Associate Professor and Chair, Department of Health Studies, School of Education, Health, Nursing and Arts Professions, New York University.

Aileen H. Clucas, MSN, RN, CCDN, is Nursing Clinical Coordinator, Smithers Alcoholism Treatment Center, New York, New York.

Margaret Compton, MS, RN, is Research Nurse Clinician, Legion Avenue Methadone Clinic, The APT Foundation, and Assistant Clinical Professor, Yale University School of Nursing.

Janet S. D'Arcangelo, MA, RN, C, is Clinical Instructor of Community Health at New York University, and is a practicing psychotherapist and community health educator in Darien, Connecticut.

Eileen Gigliotti, MA, RN, is Clinical Instructor, Division of Nursing, New York University.

Gean Mathwig, PhD, RN, is Professor Emerita, Division of Nursing, New York University.

Madeline A. Naegle, PhD, RN, FAAN, is Associate Professor and Principal Investigator, Faculty Development Program in Alcohol and Other Drug Abuse Education, Division of Nursing, New York University.

ACKNOWLEDGMENTS

The development of a model curriculum in substance abuse education for nursing was supported by the NIDA-NIAAA contract number 88-008. The award and successful completion of this contract was greatly facilitated by the guidance of contract officers Frances Cotter, MPH, and Dorynne Czechowicz, MD, and project officers Claire Callahan, MSW, and Donna English, RN, MPH. We thank them for their consistent support of substance abuse education in nursing and their efforts to make the curriculum project a reality.

Throughout the development and implementation of Project SAEN, the project coordinator, Janet D'Arcangelo, RN, MA, C, has demonstrated exceptional commitment and effort to this task in a variety of ways. From the completion of administrative details to the authorship, careful refinement of modules and study guides, Ms. D'Arcangelo has performed every assignment professionally and in a manner supportive of working committee members, authors and the project director. As assistant editor of this publication, she has demonstrated a broad knowledge of nursing and substance abuse education for professionals.

Members of the working committee of Project SAEN, Margret Wolf, EdD, RN, Gean Mathwig, PhD, RN, Cassie Greeley, MA, RN, Eileen Wolkstein, PhD, Joanne Griffin, PhD, RN, Beth Duthie, BSN, MA, RN, and Vivian Clarke, EdD, were the architects of the curriculum as well as authors of several modules. Their careful assessment of curricular issues and their recommendations for module development was comprehensive and visionary. The project evaluator, Sharon Weinberg, PhD, assisted greatly with the project design and evaluation. The support of the Division of Nursing, New York University, in particular, its head, Diane O'Neill McGivern, PhD, RN, FAAN, was essential to the implementation of the modules in the standing curriculum and the acceptance of the content in the core curriculum.

The expertise of several consultants enriched the contents and scope of the modules. It is because of their suggestions and guidance that the project reflects not only the thinking of the members of the Project SAEN but current educational trends in substance abuse education today. They were Rothlyn Zahourek, MS, RN, CS, Sandra Jaffe-Johnson, EdD, RN, Marc Galanter, MD, John Morgan, MD, and Richard Frances, MD.

The modules were authored by faculty members at the School of Education, Health, Nursing and Arts Professions in the Division of Nursing and other departments, New York University, and nurses specializing in treatment of clients with drug and alcohol problems. Special thanks are extended to the authors who generously shared their thinking and clinical expertise.

Ms. Bonnie Johnson, Ms. Maureen Doyle, and Ms. Linda Patterson rotated as Research Assistants to the project, and were unable to remain with the project due to curricular demands of the doctoral programs in which they were enrolled. Research assistants were responsible for identifying resources and establishing a data base of over 500 entries.

Acknowledgments

Central to the final form and high quality of these final products has been the assistance of the New York University **SEHNAP** Office of Research and Development. Mr. Charles Sprague, Director, and his staff have contributed many hours to the organization of content, formatting and final production of the learning modules. Special thanks are extended to him and to Leslie Anndeherz for her skillful reproduction of many graphics as well as key modules.

These volumes are dedicated to advancing the knowledge of health professionals, especially nurses, about alcohol and other drug abuse, and to the many health professionals recovering from the personal experience of the addictions and their devastating consequences.

Madeline A. Naegle, PhD, RN, FAAN
Project Director, Project SAEN
Associate Professor
Division of Nursing
New York University

PREFACE

New York University Division of Nursing, under the leadership of Dr. Madeline A. Naegle and with the support of a curriculum development grant from the National Institute on Alcohol Abuse and Alcoholism (NIAAA) and the National Institute on Drug Abuse (NIDA), has prepared an extensive and well-developed set of materials appropriate for use in nursing and other health care professional programs. The curriculum has been designed in modules for three levels of instruction: beginning baccalaureate (Volume I); advanced baccalaureate (Volume II); and master's degree level (Volume III). The materials include a content outline for each topic and an instructor's guide presenting learner objectives, audiovisual resources, overhead and handout masters, recommended teaching strategies, test questions and answers, and a faculty and student reading list.

A comprehensive substance abuse education curriculum for both baccalaureate and master's nursing and other health care professional education is provided. Baccalaureate level modules specifically include physiological consequences, pharmacology, psychological manifestations, specific nursing care, care of special populations, and attitudes regarding drug and alcohol use. Master's level modules cover nursing intervention in client populations, advanced practice in addictions nursing, alcohol and drug research, and management of impaired practice. Alternative course placement in the nursing curriculum are presented with each module. Thus, the materials may be used in any program's specific curricular arrangement.

The extent of alcohol and drug abuse problems in the population, and the absence of a concerted effort to provide education content on the topic to health professions' students in the past, increases the importance of providing relevant and extensive information to nursing students. NIAAA has estimated that at least 30 percent of acute care patients have a health problem directly or indirectly related to alcohol or drug use or abuse. While recipients of nursing care are frequently suffering from alcohol or drug related problems, most nurse (and other health care providers) ignore both symptomatology and intervention with these problems. The primary reason for ignoring an obvious health problem is the health professionals' lack of educational preparation regarding addictions. If medical and nursing schools have included alcohol or drug content, it usually has been concerned with the pharmacology of alcohol and drugs or pathology caused by substance use. Recent initiatives by NIAAA and NIDA have targeted nursing and medical schools to support and improve alcohol and drug abuse education.

The strengths of this project include its breadth and depth. The scope of this work is extensive, exhaustive, and comprehensive. It is scientifically sound, including essential and current findings, and integrating the body of knowledge into useful

Preface

materials. These materials provide an invaluable resource to the nursing and other health care professional educator and curriculum planner in offering current and complete information about alcohol and drug abuse relevant to nursing and other health care practice.

Eleanor J. Sullivan, PhD, RN, FAAN
Dean, School of Nursing,
University of Kansas

FOREWORD

This volume on substance abuse education in nursing represents an important step in the development of sophisticated health care for addicted people in the United States. The nursing profession is, at the very least, the body of health professionals who work most closely and intimately with our hospitalized ill. More broadly, however, it is the profession that organizes care, provides bedside treatment, and serves as the primary health provider for millions of Americans. Because of this, the establishment of effective treatment options in addiction for nursing is a *sine qua non* for such care nationwide.

The issues dealt with here represent a particularly important perspective on the role that nurses play in the addiction treatment system. "Dysfunctional Patterns in Families with Drug and Alcohol Problems," for example, lays out the basic issues in which the social context of addiction is played out outside the health care system. It suggest the systemic changes that will be necessary to stabilize abstinence. A section on "Special Populations" deals with the increasing importance of subgroups within the addiction patient population whose special needs must be attended to. Women, minorities, and the psychiatrically ill have unique needs which cannot be merged into a homogeneous body of care. Finally, the "Fetal Effects of Maternal Alcohol and Drug Use" is an area of grave concern within the medical context, and one that must be addressed in pre-natal care, as well as in the public health context.

In order to understand the importance of these nursing initiatives, it is useful to look at some of the background of the development of medical care in this field.

The magnitude of the alcohol and drug abuse problem today is well-documented, with the cost to the public calculated at over $125 billion per year in health care and lost work. In general medical facilities alone, on average 20 percent of patients present with such problems, many of which go undiagnosed. Only when the sequelae of addiction, such as cirrhosis, trauma, and infection present, may such patients receive proper medical attention. Nonetheless, the patients' primary addictive problems go untreated. Furthermore, the rate of substance abuse among general psychiatric patients with non-addictive disorders has been found to be 25 to 60 percent, depending on the region and clinical setting. Despite this, medical education has been seriously lacking in the addictions until recently. For example, training in this area was not formally required of psychiatrists until 1985, and is not required in other medical specialties.

Clearly we need to assure greater medical sophistication in substance abuse. Where, however, do we stand in developing the needed teaching faculty and specialists in the field? In 1972, the federal government initiated a program of three-year grants for Career Teachers in Alcoholism and Drug Abuse, but in 1981, after only one grantee had been funded in each of 55 of the 124 eligible schools, the program was terminated. Subsequently, modest grants have addressed nursing and curriculum development, but have failed to provide meaningful support for training positions. Recent federal faculty development awards have provided partial support for training faculty, but none for residents or fellows.

Foreword

    Given this perspective on the evolution of nursing and medical care in the field, it is clear that the development of this nursing curriculum package represents an important stage in our growing sophistication of care for addictive illness. Further evolution in this regard will provide an important assurance for effective treatment of addicted patients across the country.

Marc Galanter, MD
Professor of Psychiatry
Director of the Division of Alcoholism and
   Drug Abuse
New York University School of Medicine

MODULE II.1
FETAL EFFECTS OF MATERNAL ALCOHOL AND DRUG USE

Eileen Gigliotti, MA, RN

Madeline A. Naegle, PhD, RN, FAAN
Project Director
Janet S. D'Arcangelo, MA, RN, C
Project Coordinator

Project SAEN
SUBSTANCE ABUSE
EDUCATION IN NURSING

CONTENT OUTLINE

I. Maternal Drug Use During Pregnancy and the Postpartum Period
   A. Drugs Used During Pregnancy
   B. Incidence and Prevalence of Drug-Related Fetal Effects
   C. Factors Associated with Drug-Related Fetal Effects in Newborns and Children

II. Patterns of the Neonate Indicating Presence of Drug Effects, Dependence, or Withdrawal
   A. Fetal Alcohol Effects and Fetal Alcohol Syndrome
      1. Effects
      2. Fetal alcohol syndrome
      3. Corroborative maternal alcohol/drug history
      4. Lab data
      5. Implications for the immediate neonatal period
      6. Nursing strategies
   B. Effects of Maternal Cocaine Use
      1. Patterns manifested by the mother
      2. Cocaine effects on the neonate
      3. Corroborative maternal alcohol/drug use history
      4. Implications for the immediate neonatal period
      5. Nursing strategies for care of the cocaine-affected infant
   C. Heroin Dependence and Withdrawal
   D. Methadone Maintenance During Pregnancy
   E. Effects of Maternal Use of Nicotine, Caffeine, Marijuana, and Other Drugs on Fetal Development
      1. Nicotine
      2. Caffeine
      3. Marijuana
      4. Polydrug use and other drugs

III. Nursing Strategies Related to Fetal Drug Effects
   A. Assessment
      1. Comprehensive nursing assessment, including drug and alcohol history
      2. Neonatal assessment scales
      3. Nurse-client relationship
   B. Prenatal Care
      1. Screening for alcohol abuse
      2. Suspicion of alcohol abuse
      3. Prenatal teaching
   C. Parent Education
      1. Breast-feeding
      2. Family life-style
      3. Other abusive behaviors
      4. Parenting patterns
   D. Planning and Referral
      1. Referral for childbirth education
      2. Postpartal and infant care
      3. Mother and infant care referral
      4. Inpatient treatment
      5. Psychiatric treatment
      6. Counseling, psychotherapy, and substance abuse therapy
      7. Social agencies
      8. Community agencies

CONTENTS

I. **MATERNAL DRUG USE DURING PREGNANCY AND THE POSTPARTUM PERIOD**

   A. **Drug Used During Pregnancy**

   1. Drug metabolites have been identified in as high as 11% of births nationwide (NAACOG, 1989).
   2. In the past, alcohol, nicotine, and caffeine were the drugs most commonly used by women.
   3. Heroin, methadone, and PCP use and their effects have been studied in populations of mothers and infants.
   4. Use of drugs with teratogenic effects which may or may not be drugs which are abused/addictive has been studied in the past also. Examples of these drugs are tetracycline, thalidomide, diethylstilbestrol (DES), and certain anti-convulsants (such as dilantin). (Effects of therapeutic and abused drugs may be similarly teratogenic.)
   5. The availability of cocaine and its derivative crack and their highly addictive quality have resulted in rapid escalation of cocaine use in women of child-bearing age and pregnant women.
   6. The use of ampthetamines and other amphetamine-like drugs is also of concern during pregnancy.

   B. **Incidence and Prevalence of Drug-Related Fetal Effects**

   1. Fetal alcohol syndrome (FAS) is estimated to affect 1.9 infants/1,000 (Abel & Sokol, 1986).
   2. Fetal alcohol effects (FAE) occur in an unknown number of children.
   3. Approximately 22 million adults have ever used cocaine. Of these 9 million are estimated to be female users of child-bearing age (NIDA, 1990 National Household Survey on Drug Abuse).
   4. A significant number of women bearing children are users of cocaine, heroin, and alcohol.
   5. Several researchers believe that spontaneous abortion during first trimester is related to significant substance abuse prior to and during early pregnancy.
   6. Substance abuse is significantly correlated with VLBW (very low birth weight) infants.

   C. **Factors Associated with Drug-Related Effects in Newborns and Children**

   1. Overall nutritional status.
   2. Number of drugs used.
   3. Period of gestation during which the drug is used.
   4. Amount of drug used.

Module II.1

5. The child-rearing environment.
6. The individual sensitivity of the fetus.

II. PATTERNS OF THE NEONATE INDICATING PRESENCE OF DRUG EFFECTS, DEPENDENCE, OR WITHDRAWAL

A. Fetal Alcohol Effects and Fetal Alcohol Syndrome

1. Fetal alcohol effects.
   a. Patterns of alcohol effects without clear manifestations of fetal alcohol syndrome are observed in children of women who drank regularly during pregnancy (Streissguth & LaDue, 1985).
   b. The relationships between effects in humans and the amount of alcohol consumed, timing of its consumption and other factors are unclear.
   c. Effects include:
      (1) Attention deficits in childhood, leading to decreased learning ability.
      (2) Mild to severe cognitive deficits, leading to decreased learning.
      (3) Fine and gross motor behavioral effects.
      (4) Neurobehavioral effects including hyperactivity, decreased learning ability, poor locomotion, developmental delays, response inhibition, and sucking and feeding difficulties (Streissguth & LaDue, 1985).
   d. Conclusions from animal research on prenatal alcohol effects include the following:
      (1) There is a relationship between the magnitude of the dose and the severity of the response.
      (2) Behavioral effects are observed at levels of exposure too low to produce malformation and growth deficiency (Boggan & Randall, 1980; Abel, Sachs, Tracy, & Wise, 1983).
      (3) Vulnerability to damage from a given dose of alcohol differs radically from individual to individual.
2. Fetal alcohol syndrome.
   a. Manifestations of fetal alcohol syndrome include:
      (1) Mental retardation.
      (2) Heart defects, including Tetralogy of Fallot, septal defects, and patent ductus arteriosus (Clarran & Smith, 1978).
      (3) Craniofacial anomalies: epicanthal folds, minor ear anomalies, short nose, micrognathia, low nasal bridge, thin upper lip, indistinct philtrum, flat midface, and short palpebral fissures (Streissguth, 1982).
      (4) Growth deficiency.
      (5) Central nervous system (CNS) dysfunction.
      (6) Low APGAR scores.
      (7) Behavioral manifestations.
         (a) Infants are tremulous, irritable, fail to thrive, overreact to sounds, and have problems sucking and feeding, and diminished muscle tone.

Fetal Effects of Maternal Alcohol and Drug Use

   - (b) Preschool children often are hyperactive, inattentive, impulsive, fearless, and demonstrate poor motor function.
   - (c) Adolescents continue to manifest borderline or retarded mental functioning, poor social judgment, and growth deficiencies.
  - (8) Signs of physical dependence and withdrawal are manifested in post-partal tremulousness, irritability, sleep disturbance, and feeding problems.
 3. Corroborative maternal alcohol/drug history.
    a. Most drinkers underestimate their consumption. Pregnant women who are addicted are ambivalent and may be guilty about their alcohol use.
    b. Corroborative evidence about drinking patterns can often be gleaned by a discussion of their social life and their partners' drug-using behaviors.
    c. Sexual history (use of sex for drugs) can give evidence of patterns of abuse.
    d. Questions about alcohol use should be asked even if the drug of choice is some other substance; alcohol is frequently combined with or substituted for other drugs.
 4. Lab data.
    Urine screens during early labor may give evidence of recent drug metabolites, especially if there is cocaine or crack history.
 5. Implications for the immediate neonatal period.
    a. Special care and attention to feeding and handling of the infant.
    b. Comprehensive physical exam by pediatrician and/or nurse practitioner.
    c. Problems with parental acceptance of the infant with multiple anomalies.
    d. Toxicology evaluation of maternal and infant blood and urine.
    e. Consultation with nurse or physician specializing in alcohol and other drug problems to determine indications for referrals to treatment.
    f. Evaluation with/by social worker regarding referrals to social service agencies.
 6. Nursing strategies.
    a. Comprehensive nursing assessment of infant.
    b. Identification of nursing diagnoses.
    c. Psychosocial assessment of mother and other family members.
    d. Nursing assessment of mother/infant interaction.
    e. Short-form drug-use history.
    f. Emotional support to parents/families regarding infant problems or evident abnormalities.
    g. Counseling regarding alcohol consumption, breast feeding, and parenting patterns.

B. **Effects of Maternal Cocaine Use (In general, effects appear to be dose related.)**

 1. Patterns manifested by the mother. Use of cocaine and its derivative crack is manifested in pathological outcomes for mother and infant. The mother may experience:

Module II.1

   a. Life threatening severe bleeding associated with abruptio placentae or a stillbirth.
   b. Emergency cesarean section delivery.
   c. Premature labor or spontaneous abortion.
   d. Sleep disturbances, including insomnia.
   e. Seizures.
   f. Respiratory problems including shortness of breath and damage to nasal mucosa and lungs.
   g. Cardiovascular problems including hypertension, arrhythmias, tachycardia, and cerebrovascular accident.
   h. Gastrointestinal problems including anorexia leading to weight loss and malnutrition.
   i. Seropositive for HIV.
2. Cocaine effects on the neonate.
   a. Neurological signs including increased irritability, jitteriness, inconsolableness, tremors, and an increased startle response.
   b. Respiratory difficulties including increased respiratory rate, abnormal ventilatory patterns, and a higher than normal incidence of SIDS (Sudden Infant Death Syndrome).
   c. Cardiovascular signs including intrauterine growth retardation, tachycardia, and cerebral hemorrhage.
   d. Gastrointestinal signs including diarrhea, and poor tolerance for feeding.
   e. Impairment of neonatal interactive and organizational abilities.
   f. Low birth weight.
   g. Meconium staining.
3. Corroborative maternal alcohol/drug history is basic to understanding implications of drug use for mother and infant. Informants other than the mother should be asked to corroborate patterns of use and related dysfunctional behaviors.
4. Implications for the immediate neonatal period.
   a. Infants experience some discomfort related to abstinence from cocaine (Chasnoff, Hunt, Kletter, & Kaplan, 1989).
   b. Assistance is needed regarding the handling and feeding difficulties of the neonate.
   c. Interpretation of infant distress to family is necessary.
   d. Toxicologic evaluation of infant's body fluids is indicated.
   e. Vulnerability of mother during periods of labor, delivery and post partum offers potential to change—for example: kicking a drug habit or learning new parenting skills.
   f. Another source of motivation to change habits at this time is the legal sanctions imposed on pregnant women to protect the child—for example: jailing pregnant women to keep them away from drugs and placing infants in foster care until mothers can demonstrate the ability to parent.

Fetal Effects of Maternal Alcohol and Drug Use

5. Nursing strategies for care of the cocaine-affected infant.
   a. Comprehensive assessment of the infant.
   b. Assessment of maternal-infant interaction.
   c. Short-form drug-use history.
   d. Assistance with parenting skills.
   e. Interpretation of infant's dysfunctional responses.
   f. Assistance to infant regarding comfort and organizational patterns.
   g. Counseling regarding drug use and potential referral for treatment.

C. Heroin Dependence and Withdrawal

1. Patterns manifested by the neonate.
   a. Infants of mothers dependent on heroin manifest symptoms of neonatal abstinence syndrome.
   b. This syndrome is characterized by behaviors associated with central and autonomic nervous system hyperarousal such as:
      (1) Tremors.
      (2) Hypertonus.
      (3) Hyperactive reflexes.
      (4) High-pitched cries.
      (5) Feeding difficulties.
      (6) Sleep disturbances.
      (7) Fever.
      (8) Rapid respirations.
   c. Neonatal abstinence syndrome generally subsides within one week.
   d. These infants may manifest:
      (1) Low birth weight.
      (2) Poor response to comforting measures.
      (3) Excessive crying.
   e. Nursing measures during withdrawal.
      (1) Quiet, darkened environment—cover top of incubator with cloth.
      (2) Pacifiers.
      (3) Swaddling.
      (4) Holding and rocking.
      (5) Hydrotherapy.
      (6) Therapeutic touch.
      (7) Protection of skin abrasions.
         (a) Soft linen.
         (b) Ointment applied liberally to knees, buttocks, and chin.
      (8) Monitor fluid intake and output.
         (a) Small, frequent feedings.

(b) Holding upright after feedings.

(c) Use of premature nipple to improve poor sucking ability.

(9) Liberal visiting by family.

(10) Crisis intervention for parents.

D. Methadone Maintenance During Pregnancy

1. Results in physiologic dependence in the fetus.
2. Provided in the context of a comprehensive program, does not appear to impair the developmental and cognitive functioning of the fetus. (Kaltenbach & Finnegan, 1989).
3. Is less traumatic to the fetus than systematic withdrawl during fetal life.

E. Effects of Maternal Use of Nicotine, Caffeine, and Marijuana on Fetal Development

1. Nicotine.
    a. When other contributing variables are controlled, nicotine use has been observed to result in:
        (1) Low birth weight.
        (2) Low neonatal APGAR scores.
        (3) Suggested behavioral trends, including:
            (a) Deficits in cognitive development and educational achievement.
            (b) Frequent problems of temperament, adjustment, and behavior.
            (c) Abnormally high levels of activity and inattention.
    b. Research findings on nicotine must be considered in relation to social and environmental influences.
2. Caffeine.
    a. Ingested in doses greater than 5–10 mg./kg. (moderate to excessive consumption) has been associated with anxiety, tension, headache, disturbed sleep, irritability, and decrease in hand steadiness.
    b. Pregnancy changes the metabolism of caffeine, extending its half-life to 16 times longer than that of non-pregnant adults. Within 6–7 months after birth, this reverts to normal adult levels.
    c. Pregnancy slows the metabolism of caffeine.
    d. Animal study findings suggest that caffeine in doses in excess of 20–30 mg./kg. daily result in subtle alterations in physical, behavioral, and neurochemical development.
3. Marijuana.
    Neonates exposed to marijuana have demonstrated fine tremors, tremors associated with the Moro reflex, and moderately increased irritability (Fried, Barnes and Drake 1985).
4. Infants exposed to more than one drug, for example, cocaine and opiates, and drugs in combination, have a higher incidence of low birth weight, and neurological problems, and have greater needs for intensive care as well as longer

hospital stays following delivery than infants who have not been exposed to drugs.

III. **NURSING STRATEGIES RELATED TO FETAL DRUG EFFECTS**

   A. **Assessment**

   1. Comprehensive nursing assessment should be conducted with mother and infant, including drug and alcohol history, psychosocial history, and history of treatment (if any).
   2. Neonatal assessment should include the use of an instrument to evaluate neonatal status such as Kron's "Behavior of Infants Born to Drug Dependent Mothers" (1977) or Lipsitz's "Neonatal Drug Withdrawal Scoring System" (1975). Other commonly employed neonatal assessment systems regarding APGAR, are Bubowitz and Ballard scales.
   3. The nurse-client relationship should be initiated during assessment.
      a. The nurse must self-assess to be aware of personal biases and negative feelings regarding maternal drug use during pregnancy.
      b. A relationship characterized by credibility and concern for the mother's well-being as well as that of the infant is essential. Emotional support of the mother is key.

   B. **Prenatal Care**

   1. Screening for alcohol abuse (Sokol, Miller, & Martier, 1983).
      a. The nurse should be alert to indications that drinking is interfering with the woman's physical, social, work, or family life as the nursing assessment, history, and physical are implemented.
      b. A nonjudgmental, accepting, and concerned attitude is essential in gaining the client's cooperation.
      c. Explain urine screen procedure if it is part of the protocol.
   2. If alcohol abuse is suspected:
      a. Suggest limited drinking: taking an occasional drink and avoidance of binge drinking.
      b. Refer to a special program, if necessary.
      c. Stress healthier outcomes for mother and infant if intake is stopped or limited.
      d. Maintain contact with the client.
      e. Document the diagnosis and referral.
   3. Prenatal and family planning teaching for all women should include the information that:
      a. Avoidance of alcohol or other drugs is most desirable.
      b. Smoking should be avoided.
      c. Caffeine intake should be limited.
      d. Only prescribed drugs should be used.
      e. Review specific potential effects of OTC and recreational drugs.

Module II.1

C. Parent Education

1. In breast-feeding, mother's alcohol and other drug metabolites are transferred in breast milk.
2. The life-style of the family may support or advocate the social and/or regular use of alcohol and other drugs.
3. Parental drug use appears to coincide with a higher incidence of marital conflict, domestic violence, and neglect of children.
4. Parenting patterns are affected by the active use of drugs by mother and father.
   a. Income is directed toward the purchase of drugs and away from domestic needs.
   b. Drug use is a major preoccupation of the addicted client.
   c. Cognitive and affective changes secondary to drug ingestion interfere with nurturing behaviors and communication.

D. Planning and Referral

1. Referral for childbirth education as necessary.
2. Planning for postpartal and infant care beyond hospitalization should be addressed with the client.
3. Mother and infant need primary care and should be referred to independent providers or clinics.
4. Referrals for inpatient treatment of the drug dependent mother is most desirable; when resources are limited, ambulatory treatment is preferable to no treatment at all.
5. The patient/client who is addicted to a substance or substances and has a psychiatric diagnosis should be referred for psychiatric treatment with a physician, psychiatric nurse, or social worker.
6. Counseling, psychotherapy, and substance abuse treatment can prevent the resumption or continuation of drug use, thereby preventing associated ill effects on the physical and mental heath of family members.
7. Social agencies can provide an extended supportive network for the infant, mother, and other family members.
8. Other community agencies can be utilized to provide additional social assistance and education.

MODULE II.1
FETAL EFFECTS OF MATERNAL ALCOHOL AND DRUG USE

INSTRUCTOR'S GUIDE

Eileen Gigliotti, MA, RN

Madeline A. Naegle, PhD, RN, FAAN
Project Director
Janet S. D'Arcangelo, MA, RN, C
Project Coordinator

Project SAEN
SUBSTANCE ABUSE
EDUCATION IN NURSING

CONTENTS

Component	Page
Module Description	16
Time Frame	16
Placement	16
Learner Objectives	17
Recommended Readings	18
Faculty Readings	18
Student Readings	18
Recommended Audiovisual and Other Resources	19
Overhead Masters	24
Handout Masters	77
Recommended Teaching Strategies and Sample Assignments	102
Test Questions and Answers	109
Bibliography	112

Module II.1

MODULE DESCRIPTION

This module will help the student of maternal-child health nursing to develop an understanding of maternal-fetal interaction associated with drug and alcohol use and to formulate intervention strategies. Content on fetal drug effects and their identification in the neonate and nursing activities to address drug effects, dependence, and withdrawal will be presented. Strategies to address the health needs of mother and infant will be described and demonstrated.

TIME FRAME

3 hours

PLACEMENT

Maternal-Child Health, Family Development, Community Health

Instructor's Guide

LEARNER OBJECTIVES

Upon successful completion of this module, the learner will:

1. Identify common licit and illicit drugs that, when used during pregnancy, may affect fetal development.
2. Describe the impact of factors associating nicotine, cocaine, heroin, and alcohol use with potential fetal effects.
3. Identify patterns in the neonate that suggest dependence on, or withdrawal from, alcohol or heroin.
4. Identify physical/psychological effects of maternal cocaine use on the fetus.
5. Implement nursing strategies to restore health in the drug-dependent neonate.
6. Implement health teaching directed toward prevention of fetal anomalies related to maternal drug use.
7. Implement nursing strategies with mother and infant to diminish drug-related effects.
8. Implement health teaching on parenting that will promote infant and family needs.
9. Evaluate nursing strategies implemented with mother and infant in relation to maternal drug use.

Module II.1

RECOMMENDED READINGS

FACULTY READINGS

Abel, E. L. (1984). Pharmacology of alcohol relating to pregnancy and lactation. In *Fetal Alcohol Syndrome and Fetal Alcohol Effects.* (pp. 29–45). New York: Plenum Press.

Howard, J., Beckwith, L., Rodning, C., & Kropenske, V. (1989). The development of young children of substance-abusing parents: Insights from seven years of intervention research. *Zero to Three,* 9(5), 8–12.

Minkoff, H., Nanda, D., Menez, R., & Fikrig, S. (1987). Pregnancies resulting in infants with acquired immunodeficiency syndrome or AIDS-related Complex. *Obstetrics and Gynecology,* 69(3), 285–287.

Russell, M. (1985). Alcohol abuse and alcoholism in the pregnant woman: Identification and intervention. *Alcohol Health and Research World,* 10(1), 28–31, 74.

STUDENT READINGS

Bennett, K. (1987). AIDS: A generation of children at risk. *Journal of Psychosocial Nursing and Mental Health Services,* 25(12), 32–34.

Busch, D., McBride, A. B., & Benaventura, L. M. (1986). Chemical dependency in women: The link to OB/GYN problems. *Journal of Psychosocial Nursing and Mental Health Services,* 24(4), 26–30.

Streissguth, A., & LaDue, R. (1985). Psychological and behavioral effects in children prenatally exposed to alcohol. *Alcohol Health and Research World,* 10(1), 6–12, 71–72.

Streissguth, A. P., Clarren, S. K., & Jones, D. L. (1985). Natural history of the fetal alcohol syndrome: A ten-year follow-up of eleven patients. *Alcohol Health and Research World,* 10(1), 13–19, 70, 73.

Weiner, L., Rossett, H., & Mason, E. (1985). Training professionals to identify and treat pregnant women who drink heavily. *Alcohol Health and Research World,* 10(1), 32–38, 71.

Instructor's Guide

RECOMMENDED AUDIOVISUAL AND OTHER RESOURCES

AUDIOVISUAL RESOURCES

1. **A Challenge to Care**

   Examines all aspects of chemical dependency and pregnancy. This film provides specific strategies for the comfort and care of the drug-exposed newborn. **Available from Vida Health Communications, 6 Bigelow Street, Cambridge, Massachusetts 02139.**

2. **Born Hooked**

   Views complex medical, social, and ethical problems related to the pregnant drug addict and to the newborn suffering from narcotic withdrawal. 13:30 minutes Videocassette. Film 16mm. **Available from March of Dimes, Supply Division, 1275 Mamaroneck Avenue, White Plains, New York 10605.**

3. **Born with a Habit**

   Describes the pregnant addict, prenatal care, delivery problems and treatment of the addicted neonate. For rental or sale. **Available from Harvard Medical School, Mental Health Training Film Program, 58 Fenwood Road, Boston, Massachusetts 02115.**

4. **Death of the High Risk Infant**

   Outlines stages of grieving and provides guidelines for assisting parents in their grief. Thirty minutes. Videocassette rental ($60) or sale ($250). **Available from the American Journal of Nursing Company, Educational Services Division, 555 West 57th Street, New York, New York 10019-2961. Phone: 1-800-223-2282 or (212) 582-8820.**

5. **Fetal Alcohol Syndrome**

   Discusses effects of alcohol on the fetus and fetal alcohol syndrome. Reviews techniques for diagnosis, detection, and prevention. **Available from Addiction Research Foundation, 33 Russell Street, Toronto, Canada M5S 2S1.**

6. **One for My Baby**

   Symptoms of FAS are reviewed as well as risk to unborn infants when mothers drink. Two families with children with the disorder are interviewed. Twenty-seven minutes. Film 16mm. **Available from WHA-TV Marketing Department, 821 University Avenue, Madison, Wisconsin 53706.**

7. **Pregnancy: Caring for Your Unborn Baby**

   This film identifies the benefits of making the right choices—and the consequences of making some wrong choices. Filmed case studies and interviews. Videocassette or 16mm film. Twenty minutes, #9788. Sale ($445 16mm) or ($380 video). Rental ($50). **Available from AIMS Media, 6901 Woodley Avenue, Van Nuys, California 91406-4878. Phone: 1-800-267-2467 or (818) 785-4111.**

8. **Pregnancy on the Rocks: The Fetal Alcohol Syndrome**

   This film delineates the major causes and effects of FAS including amount ingested, nutrition habits, use of tobacco and other drugs as well as manifestations of FAS in infants and children. 52 minutes. Film 16mm. **Available from Peter Glaws Productions, 138 B Avenue, Coronado, California 92118.**

9. **Taking a Drinking History and Counseling and Referral**

   These two films were developed to stimulate group discussion, and help health professionals become aware of their own feelings about alcohol and pregnancy. Interview segments are designed so that clinicians imagine themselves as interviewers and approach the situations in their own styles. Two films on either a 16mm reel ($195) or videocassette ($95). Rental ($30) per day. **Available from, Documentaries for Learning, 74 Fernwood Road, Boston, Massachusetts 02115.**

BOOKLETS/PAMPHLETS/BOOKS

1. **American Council for Drug Education**

   204 Monroe Street, Suite 110
   Rockville, Maryland 20852
   (301) 294-0600

2. **Healthy Mothers, Healthy Babies Coalition**

   409 12th Street, SW, Room 309
   Washington, D.C. 20024
   (202) 638-5577 or (202) 863-2458
   Information and education to improve maternal/infant health.

3. **March of Dimes Birth Defects Foundation**

   1275 Mamaroneck Avenue
   White Plains, New York 10605
   (914) 428-7100

Instructor's Guide

Materials on prenatal care, drugs, and pregnancy. Copies of some pamphlets and other materials available in Spanish.

4. **National Clearinghouse for Alcohol and Drug Information**

   Information Services
   P.O. Box 2345
   Rockville, Maryland 20852
   (301) 468-2600
   Publications catalogue contains material for educators, health care providers, and clients on alcohol and drug abuse.

5. **National Council on Alcoholism and Drug Dependence, Inc.**

   12 West 21st Street, Eighth Floor
   New York, New York 10010
   1-800-NCA-CALL or (212) 206-6770
   Materials on alcoholism, FAS, and FAE.

6. **National Head Start Association**

   1220 King Street, Suite 200
   Alexandria, Virginia 22314
   (703) 739-0875
   Materials and support for preschool education and parenting.

7. **National Sudden Infant Death Syndrome Clearinghouse**

   8201 Greensboro Drive, Suite 600
   McLean, Virginia 22102
   (703) 821-8955
   Materials to explain this serious risk associated with drug use during pregnancy.

8. **Teratology Society**

   9650 Rockville Pike
   Bethesda, Maryland 20814
   (301) 571-1841
   Information on specific teratogenic agents.

9. **National Association for Perinatal Addiction Research and Education (NAPARE)**

   11 East Hubbard Street, Suite 200
   Chicago, Illinois 60611
   (302) 329-2512

Module II.1

RESOURCE GUIDES

1. The National Maternal and Child Health Clearinghouse

38th and R Streets, NW
Washington, DC 20057
(202) 625-8410
Starting Early: A Guide to Federal Resources in Maternal and Child Health (November 1988).

2. WIC Supplemental Food Program

Food and Nutrition Service
U.S. Department of Agriculture
(202) 756-3730
Drug Abuse Information and Referrals in the Special Supplemental Food Program for Women, Infants and Children: A Resource Manual for Program Development (March 1990). Annotated bibliography of written and audiovisual materials to educate staff and low literacy clients about the hazards of drug use during pregnancy and breast feeding.

SPECIFIC PUBLICATIONS

Alcohol and Pregnancy

1. NCADI

P.O. Box 2345
Rockville, Maryland 20852
(301) 468-2600 or 1-800 729-6686
My Baby . . . Strong and Healthy, 1988 DHHS Publication No. (ADM) 86-1436. An illustrated 16-page booklet that describes the risks and potential effects of drinking on the unborn baby. Discusses dangerous interactive risks when drinking is mixed with smoking and other drug use. (Spanish: *Mi Bebe . . . Fuerto y Sano*).

2. Health and Nutrition Service of Racine, Inc.

2316 Rapids Drive
Racine, Wisconsin 53404
(414) 637-7750
Fact sheet suitable for low literacy clients that discusses how alcohol can damage unborn babies, FAS, and some suggestions for abstaining. Single copies are free and can be duplicated.

3. March of Dimes Birth Defects Foundation

1275 Mamaroneck Avenue
White Plains, New York 10605
(914) 428-7100
Will Drinking Hurt My Baby? (1986). An easy-to-read 2-page pamphlet that summarizes the dangers of drinking during pregnancy and defines FAS. Single copies are free and can be duplicated.

Instructor's Guide

Drugs and Pregnancy

1. **March of Dimes Birth Defects Foundation**

   1275 Mamaroneck Avenue
   White Plains, New York 10605
   (914) 428-7100
   Drugs, Alcohol, and Tobacco Abuse During Pregnancy (1987). A 2-page booklet with basic facts about the effects on the fetus and newborn of exposure to tobacco, alcohol, prescription drugs, antacids, aspirin, laxatives, vitamins, caffeine, uppers, downers, and street drugs. Single copies are free and can be duplicated.

2. **Trish Magyari**

   Georgetown University Child Development Center
   3800 Reservoir Road, NW
   Washington, D.C. 20008
   (202) 687-8635
   I Want to Have a Healthy, Happy Baby (1988). A 6-page pamphlet describing the dangers of alcohol, cigarettes, and other drugs during pregnancy. Also discusses risks for AIDS. Developed for a primarily black, inner-city audience in the District of Columbia. Single copies are free and can be duplicated.

Tobacco and Pregnancy

1. **March of Dimes Birth Defects Foundation**

   1275 Mamaroneck Avenue
   White Plains, New York 10605
   (914) 428-7100
   Babies Don't Thrive in Smoke-Filled Rooms (1986). A 4-page pamphlet that highlights risks of smoking during pregnancy.

2. **American Lung Association**

   1740 Broadway
   New York, New York 10019
   (212) 315-8700
   Freedom from Smoking for You and Your Baby (1986). A 10-day self-help guide for mothers to stop smoking. Includes a progress record. Copies are $1.40 each.

3. **National Institute of Health**

   NHLBI Smoking Educational Program Information Center
   4733 Bethesda Avenue, Suite 530
   Bethesda, Maryland 20814
   (301) 951-3260
   Pregnant? That's Two Good Reasons to Quit Smoking (1983). An 8-page booklet that describes risks and encourages mothers to quit smoking. There is an accompanying poster. Single copies free.

Module II.1

OVERHEAD MASTERS

MODULE II.1 FETAL EFFECTS OF MATERNAL ALCOHOL AND DRUG USE

1. Characteristics of Drugs and the Fetus that Affect Risk
2. Effects of Maternal Cocaine Use on the Fetus
3. Effects of Maternal Cocaine Use on Mother and Fetus
4. Effects of Alcohol
5. Manifestations of Fetal Alcohol Syndrome
6. Effects of Nicotine on the Fetus
7. Effects of Marijuana on the Fetus
8. Effects of Heroin and Methadone on the Fetus
9. Atypical Behavior Patterns in Infants Affected by Cocaine
10. Items Used to Score Neonatal Withdrawal Symptoms in the Nursery
11. Neonatal Drug Withdrawal Scoring System
12. Assessment of Substance Abuse
13. Nursing Measures During Withdrawal
14. Nursing Interventions for Specific Behaviors of Infants Prenatally Exposed to Drugs
15. Broussard's Maternal Perception Inventory
16. Brazelton Neonatal Behavioral Assessment Scale

Module II.1—Overhead #1

CHARACTERISTICS OF DRUGS AND THE FETUS THAT AFFECT RISK

- Genetic Vulnerability of the Fetus.
- Timing of Drug Exposure.
  - Embryonic Phase (2–8 weeks after conception).
    Spontaneous abortion.
    Malformed limbs.
    Malformed organs.
  - Fetal Stage (8 weeks–birth).
    Impaired neurological development.
    Intrauterine Growth Retardation (IUGR).
    Subtle mental and behavioral deficits.
    Prematurity.
  - Delivery.
    Abruptio placenta.
    ↑ Uterine contractions.
    ↑ Fetal distress.
- Dosage and Patterns of Consumption.
- Chemical Properties of the Drug.
  - Alcohol—full range of dose-related effects.
  - Illicit drugs—deficits and delays in neurobehavioral functioning.

Module II.1—Overhead #2

EFFECTS OF MATERNAL COCAINE USE ON THE FETUS

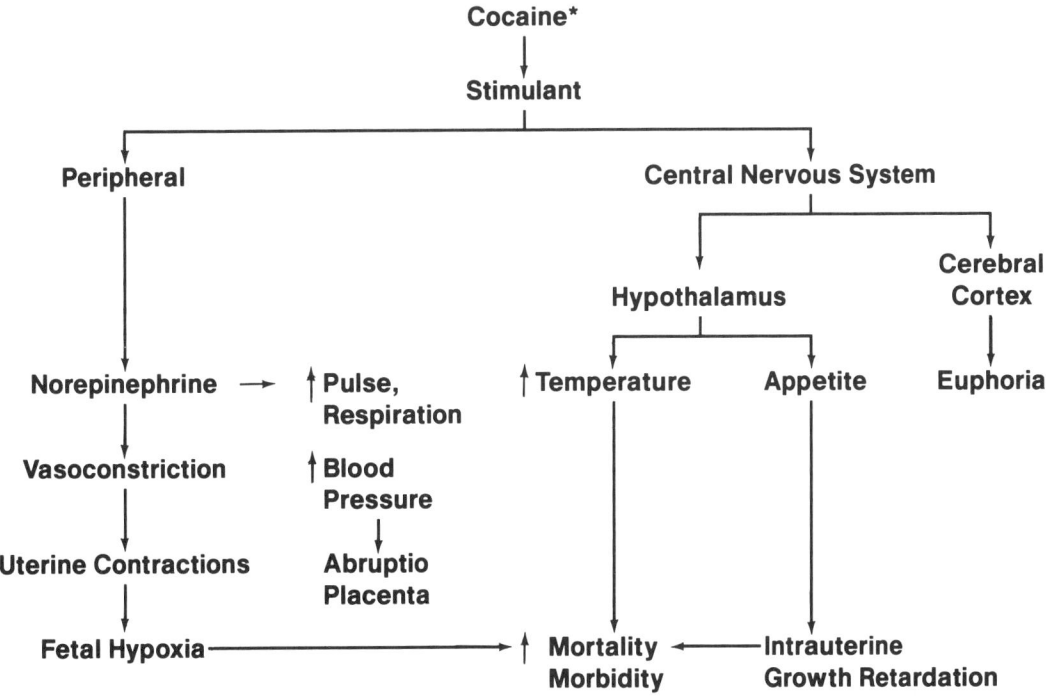

*Passes readily into breast milk and remains for up to 60 hours after maternal use.

Effects on the Breast-Feeding Infant

- Sweating
- Dilated Pupils
- Vomiting
- Diarrhea
- Extreme Irritability
- Hypertension
- Apnea

From: Lynch, M., & McKeon, V. A. (1990). Cocaine use during pregnancy: Research findings and clinical implications. *Journal of Obstetric, Gynecologic and Neonatal Nursing, 19*(4), 285–292.

Instructor's Guide

Module II.1—Overhead #3

EFFECTS OF MATERNAL COCAINE USE ON MOTHER AND FETUS

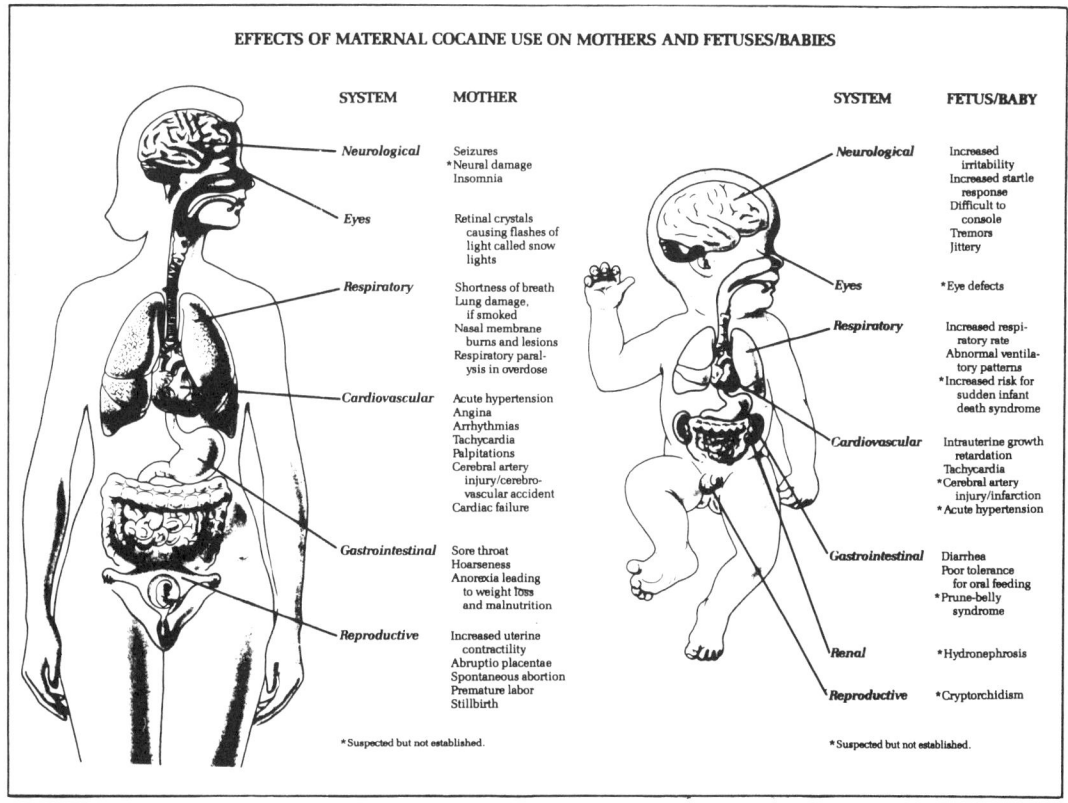

From: Smith, J. (1988). The dangers of prenatal cocaine use. *American Journal of Maternal Child Nursing, 13,* 175–179.

Instructor's Guide

Module II.1—Overhead #4

EFFECTS OF ALCOHOL

- Alcohol and its primary metabolite acetaldehyde are directly toxic to developing embryo and fetus.
- Exact etiology is unclear.
- Appears to produce wider range, systemic effects.
- May decrease delivery of maternal nutrients.
  — Impair fetal oxygenation.
  — Derange protein synthesis/metabolism.
  — Stimulate excess production of prostaglandins that modulate cellular function.
- Effects appear to be dose related.
- May be complicated by:
  — Poor nutrition.
  — Low socioeconomic status.
  — Cigarette smoking.
  — Other drug use.

From: Rementeria, J. L. (1977). *Drug abuse in pregnancy and neonatal effects.* St. Louis, MO: C.V. Mosby Co.

Module II.1—Overhead #5

MANIFESTATIONS OF FETAL ALCOHOL SYNDROME

Perinatal Problems

- Intrauterine growth retardation: birth weight, length, and head circumference below the third percentile for gestational age.
- Irritability or tremulousness.
- Hypotonic (poor muscle tone).

Craniofacial Abnormalities

- Short palpebral fissures (short eyeslits).
- Short upturned nose.
- Midface hypoplasia (underdeveloped, small midface).
- Indistinct philtrum (absence of, or minimal ridges between, nose and mouth).
- Hypoplastic maxilla.
- Thin upper vermillion border of lip.
- Retrognathia in infancy.
- Micrognathia or relative prognathia in adolescence.

Postnatal Growth

- Height and weight continue to be below third percentile for age (despite adequate caloric intake).
- Small head circumference.

Module II.1—Overhead #5 *(continued)*

Central Nervous System Dysfunction

- Mental retardation, from mild to severe levels.
- Poor motor coordination, including abnormal fine motor functioning.
- Delays in gross motor development.
- Microcephaly (small brain size).

Skeletal Abnormalities

- Aberrant palmar creases.

From: Landesman-Dwyer, S. (1982). Drinking during pregnancy: Effects on human developments. *Biomedical processes and consequences of alcohol use.* Rockville, MD: National Institute on Alcohol Abuse and Alcoholism.

Module II.1—Overhead #6

EFFECTS OF NICOTINE ON THE FETUS

Nicotine
↓
Sympathomimetic response
↓
Vasoconstriction
↓
Intermittent reduction
of uterine blood flow
↓
Fetal hypoxia
(↑ by carbon monoxide interfering
with body's ability to distribute O_2)
↓
↓ Fetal breathing movements
IUGR

(Average 7 oz. lighter than non-smokers, smaller head and chest circumference, smaller in length)

Breast-Feeding: Transmitted in breast milk and seems to inhibit milk production, as well as reduce the level of vitamin C found in breast milk.

Module II.1—Overhead #7

EFFECTS OF MARIJUANA ON THE FETUS

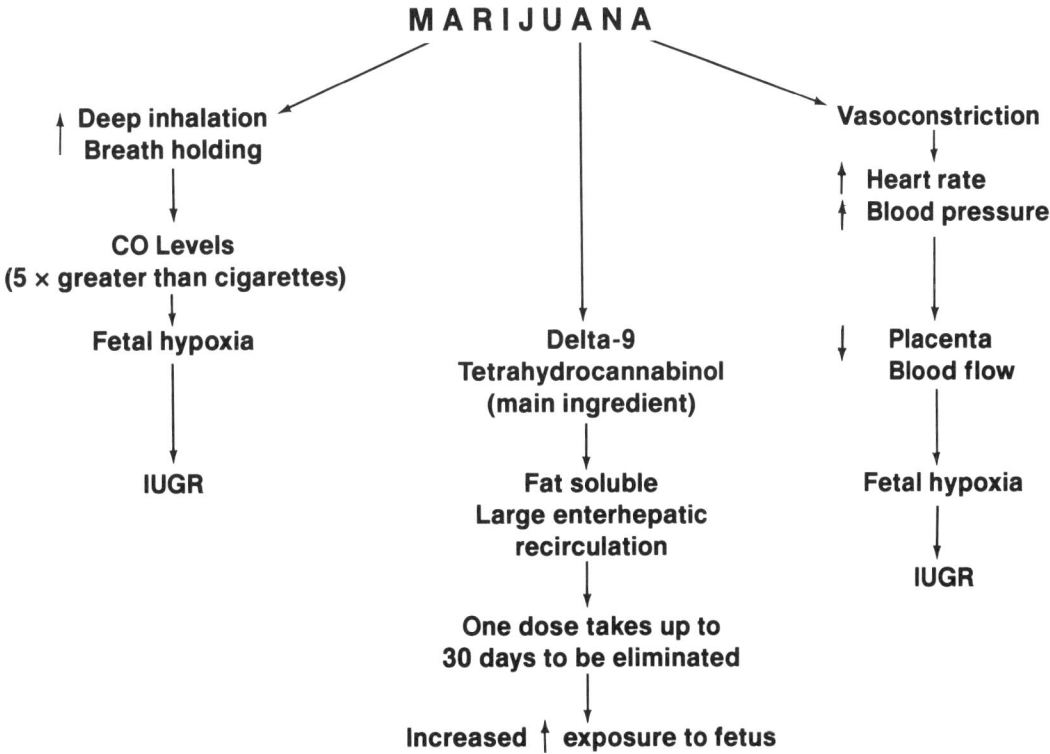

Breast-Feeding: Rapidly transmitted to breast milk and remains there for a long time.

Module II.1—Overhead #8

EFFECTS OF HEROIN AND METHADONE ON THE FETUS

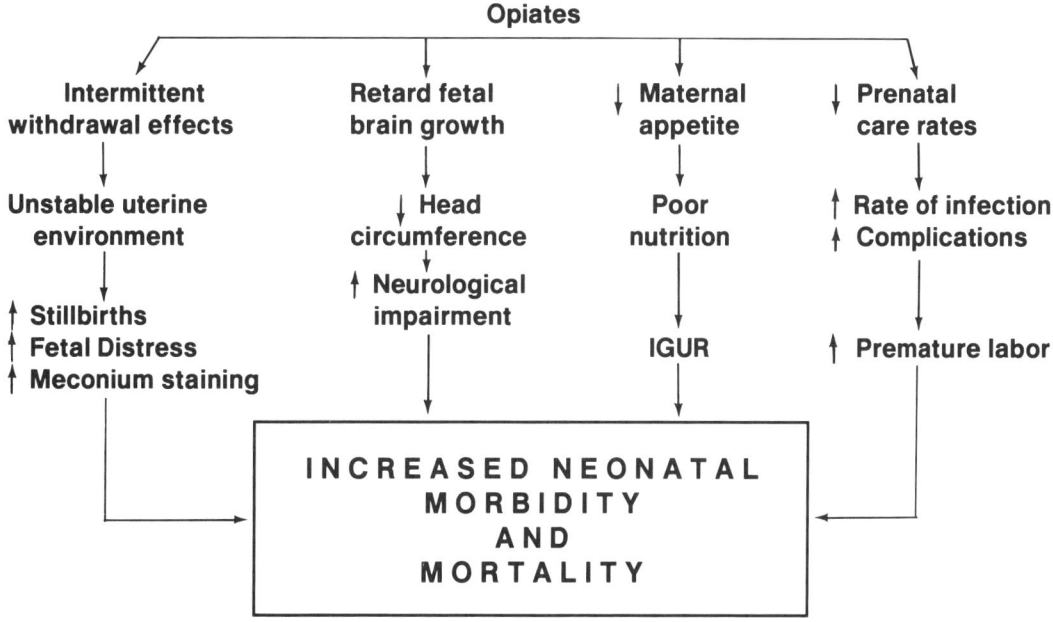

Methadone is more lipid soluble than heroin; therefore, it crosses the placenta more readily.

Breast-Feeding: Transmitted in breast milk. Baby could become opiate dependent from breast feeding.

Module II.1—Overhead #9

ATYPICAL BEHAVIOR PATTERNS IN INFANTS AFFECTED BY COCAINE

CHARACTERISTICS	Occurrence				
	Seldom				Frequent
	1	2	3	4	5
Vomiting					✓
Poor feeding				✓	✓
Uncoordinated sucking and swallowing				✓	✓
Weak pull-to-sit					✓
Irritability					✓
Difficulty sleeping					✓
Tremors/trembling					✓
Constant extraneous movement				✓	✓
Stiffness/rigidity					✓
Arms held in "W" position					✓
Passivity				✓	✓
Visual concerns					✓
Poor muscle tone				✓	✓
Fluctuating muscle tone				✓	✓
Uncoordinated movements					✓
Intolerance to cuddling					✓
Difficult to comfort					✓
Frequent state changes				✓	

- Intensity varies
- Frequency and intensity decrease with age

From: Lewis, K. D., Bennett, B., & Schmeder, N. H. (1989). The care of infants menaced by cocaine abuse. *American Journal of Maternal Child Nursing, 14,* 324–329. Reprinted with permission.

Module II.1—Overhead #10

ITEMS USED TO SCORE NEONATAL WITHDRAWAL SYMPTOMS IN THE NURSERY

Symptoms	Score Value
High-pitched cry	2
Continuous high-pitched cry	3
Sleeps less than 1 hr after feeding	3
Sleeps less than 2 hr after feeding	2
Sleeps less than 3 hr after feeding	1
Hyperactive Moro reflex	2
Markedly hyperactive Moro reflex	3
Mild tremors when disturbed	1
Marked tremors when disturbed	2
Mild tremors when undisturbed	3
Marked tremors when undisturbed	4
Increased muscle tone	2
Generalized convulsion	5
Frantic sucking of fists	1
Poor feeding	2
Regurgitation	2
Projectile vomiting	3
Loose stools	2
Watery stools	3
Dehydration	2
Frequent yawning	1
Sneezing	1
Nasal stuffiness	1
Sweating	1
Mottling	1
Fever less than 101°F	1
Fever greater than 101°F	1
Respiratory rate over 60/min	1
Respiratory rate over 60/min with retractions	1
Excoriation of nose	1
Excoriation of knees	1
Excoriation of toes	1

Module II.1—Overhead #10 *(continued)*

Phenobarbital Dosage Schedule as Prescribed According to Abstinence Score

Score	Phenobarbital
8–10	6.6 mg/(kg)(24 hr) in three divided doses
11–13	8.8 mg/(kg)(24 hr) in three divided doses
14–16	11.0 mg/(kg)(24 hr) in three divided doses
17 or above	13.2 mg/(kg)(24 hr) in three divided doses

Withdrawal Symptoms in the Nursery

Rated

Hourly—1st day
q2h —2nd day
q4h —thereafter

- **No pharmacologic treatment if score is 7 or less.**
- **Phenobarbital is used to control irritability and insomnia.**
- **Sucking *improves* with less pharmacologic support therefore:**

    Nursing measures are critical.

From: Kron, R. E., et al. (1977). Behavior of infants born to drug dependent mothers: Effects of prenatal and postnatal drugs. In *Drug abuse in pregnancy and neonatal effects.* St. Louis, MO: C.V. Mosby Co.

Module II.1—Overhead #11

NEONATAL DRUG WITHDRAWAL SCORING SYSTEM

Signs	Score 0	1	2	3
Tremors (muscle activity of limbs)	Normal	Minimally ↑ when hungry or disturbed	Moderate or marked ↑ when undisturbed, subside when fed or held snugly	Marked even when undisturbed, going on to seizure-like movements
Irritability (excessive crying)	None	Slightly ↑	Moderate to severe when disturbed or hungry	Marked even when undisturbed
Reflexes	Normal	Increased	Markedly increased	
Stools	Normal	Explosive, but normal frequency	Explosive, more than 8/day	
Muscle tone	Normal	Increased	Rigidity	
Skin abrasions	No	Redness of knees and elbows	Breaking of skin	
Respiratory rate/min.	<55	55–75	76–95	
Repetitive sneezing	No	Yes		
Repetitive yawning	No	Yes		
Vomiting	No	Yes		
Fever	No	Yes		

Identification of Newborn Infant with Narcotic Withdrawal When Score 74 (77% probability).

From: Lipsitz, P. J. (1975). A proposed narcotic withdrawal score for use with newborn infants: A pragmatic evaluation of its efficacy. *Clinical Pediatrics, 14,* 592.

Instructor's Guide

Module II.1—Overhead #12

ASSESSMENT OF SUBSTANCE ABUSE

Identifying the Substance Abuser

Physical appearance and demeanor.
- Patient looks physically exhausted.
- Pupils are extremely dilated or constricted.
- Appearance of pregnancy fails to coincide with stated gestational age.
- Track marks, abscesses, or edema are visible in upper or lower extremities.
- Nasal mucosae are inflamed or indurated.
- Patient is not well-oriented.

Medical history.
- Acquired Immunodeficiency Syndrome.
- Cellulitis.
- Cirrhosis.
- Endocarditis.
- Hepatitis.
- Pancreatitis.
- Pneumonia.

Obstetric history in prior pregnancies.
- Abruptio placentae.
- Fetal death.
- Low-birth-weight infant.
- Meconium staining.
- Premature labor.
- Premature rupture of membranes.
- Sexually transmitted disease.
- Spontaneous abortion.

Module II.1—Overhead #12 *(continued)*

Identifying the Substance Abuser*

In current pregnancy.

- History or evidence of early contractions.
- Inactive or hyperactive fetus.
- Poor weight gain.
- Sexually transmitted disease.
- Spotting or vaginal bleeding.

Other guidelines.[†]

- Develop relationship of trust.
- Be nonjudgmental.
- Start with less threatening questions:
  — Cigarette smoking.
  — Caffeine.
  — Over the counter and prescription drugs.
- Follow with questions concerning alcohol consumption.
- End with questions concerning past and present use of illicit drugs.

---

*From: Chasnoff, I. J., Burnes, W. J., Schroll, S. H., & Burns, K. A. (1985). Cocaine use in pregnancy. *The New England Journal of Medicine, 313*(11), 666–669.

[†]*From:* Lynch, M., & McKeon, V. A. (1990). Cocaine use during pregnancy: Research findings and clinical implications. *Journal of Obstetric, Gynecologic and Neonatal Nursing, 19*(4), 285–292.

Module II.1—Overhead #13

NURSING MEASURES DURING WITHDRAWAL

- Quiet, darkened environment.
  - Cover top of incubator with cloth.
- Pacifiers.
- Swaddling.
- Holding and rocking.
- Hydrotherapy.
- Therapeutic touch.
- Protection of skin abrasions.
  - Soft linen.
  - Ointment applied liberally to knees, buttocks, chin.
- Monitor fluid intake and output.
  - Small, frequent feedings.
  - Holding upright after feedings.
  - Use of premature nipple for poor suck.
- Liberal visiting by family.
- Crisis intervention for parents.

Module II.1—Overhead #14

NURSING INTERVENTIONS FOR SPECIFIC BEHAVIORS OF INFANTS PRENATALLY EXPOSED TO DRUGS

Infant Behavior	Behavior Description	Strategies
Vomiting or poor feeding	Infants frequently display gastrointestinal difficulties throughout their first year of life. Vomiting is frequent during the first six to nine months, as are intermittent constipation and diarrhea. These difficulties tend to increase irritability and discomfort. If allowed to, some infants sleep up to 20 hours per day during the first six months of life and miss feedings. They are, therefore, at risk for inadequate nutrition and failure to thrive.	• If necessary, wake infant for feeding. • Give small quantities of food. • Allow infant to rest frequently during feeding. • Have infant upright for feeding. After feeding, place infant in side-lying or prone position to prevent aspiration of milk. • If infant vomits, clean skin immediately to prevent irritation from stomach acid.
Uncoordinated sucking and swallowing	A variety of abnormal oral-motor behaviors have been observed, including a preemie-like suck pattern, poorly coordinated suck/swallow patterns, inability to stabilize tongue in midline, and occasionally, tongue thrusting and tongue tremors. These abnormal patterns increase feeding time. Consequently, a great deal of infant energy is required, and stress and frustration may occur in mother and infant.	• Hold infant in sitting position with arms forward in slight trunk flexion (curve) during feeding. • Keep infant's chin tucked downward. Infants prenatally exposed to drugs often push head back, which causes an abnormal swallow pattern. • If sucking is difficult for infant, support the infant's chin, or chin and cheeks with your hand. • Play soft, rhythmic music to help infant relax and facilitate rhythmic sucking.

Module II.1—Overhead #14 *(continued)*

Infant Behavior	Behavior Description	Strategies
Weak pull-to-sit development	Infants often are slow learning to pull-to-sit; frequently it is accomplished with head lag or excessive effort after six months of age. (Infants normally pull-to-sit with no head lag by four months.) Some prenatally exposed to drugs who are able to pull-to-sit with no head lag may compensate by pulling their arms back into a strong "W" position. Usually pull-to-sit is accomplished with arms forward and some trunk flexion. The skill is a developmental milestone that indicates abdominal and neck muscle strength, and later affects the quality and endurance of balance, sitting, walking, and protective reflexes.	• Move infant from supine to sitting position, supporting the head so that it does not lag. • While moving infant into sitting position, support shoulders close to infant's body with head forward (neck flexion). With infant semireclined (45° angle), encourage infant to assist with pull-to-sit. Give additional head support if needed to prevent head lag, and bring infant's arms forward into midline position. • Place infant in supported sitting position and move infant slowly backward within the range of head control. Then slowly rock or move infant back and forth to strengthen neck and abdominal muscles.
Irritability and difficulty sleeping	Exposure to drugs in utero can cause an infant's state to vary from highly irritable to very passive. Most of these infants, however, are highly irritable and often have difficulty sleeping. Irritable infants can reach a frantic-cry state, which needs to be avoided. If an infant is passive, interaction needs to take place during quiet alert, not hyperalert, states. Caregivers need to monitor their interactions by being alert to infant behavioral and psychological cues that indicate stress, and adjust interactions appropriately. Caregivers will be affected by infant irritability, resulting in frustration and feelings of inadequacy in the mothering role and in infant/caregiver attachment.	• Reduce noise in environment. • Turn down lights. • Swaddle infant in a cotton blanket in flexed position with arms close to body. • Hold swaddled infant close. • Put infant in bunting-type wrapper and carry close to body. • Rock infant slowly and rhythmically, either horizontally or with head supported vertically, whichever soothes. • Place in a front-pack carrier. • Walk with infant. • Give child pacifier. • Provide hydrotherapy (warm bath). • Respond to stress cues by stopping activity with infant. This response will give the infant a "time-out."

Module II.1—Overhead #14 *(continued)*

Infant Behavior	Behavior Description	Strategies
Irritability and difficulty sleeping (continued)	The caregiver needs to be made aware of behavior typical in infants prenatally exposed to drugs. Subsequently, the quality of their relationship will improve, negative judgments about the infant will be reduced, and the likelihood of child abuse will be decreased.	• Provide firm, calm touch to the mid-chest, back, or soles of the infant's feet. • Play soft music or sing or hum quietly. • Provide background noise (for example, a hair dryer or vacuum cleaner), often called white noise, which may calm the infant. • If all else fails, place infant in a quiet, darkened room with no outside stimulation. (Caregivers report this works with both premature and full-term infants exposed prenatally to drugs.)
Tremors, trembling, and extraneous movement	Tremors of the hands, arms, legs, chin, and tongue are commonly observed in infants prenatally exposed to drugs, although usually more pronounced and intense in a younger infant. We have observed tremors and tremulousness of movements in infants older than one year, but the intensity is diminished. In younger infants, tremors are primarily observed when infants are at rest. As they get older, fewer and less intense at-rest tremors occur, and intention tremors emerge. They tend to increase as the infant tires. Intention tremors occur when the infant is actively attempting a specific motor movement, for example, reaching for a toy. Intervention is often successful with intention tremors of arms and hands. Signs of stress often occur after persisting with an activity that elicits intention tremors, because physical movements are difficult and more energy and time are required to accomplish a task.	• Swaddling and holding infant close may be helpful for early at-rest tremors and extraneous movement. • Hold infant semireclined (almost sitting) with arms and shoulders forward to reduce the effort exerted by infant to maintain arm at midline while reaching for, holding, or manipulating toys. • Touch tremulous area firmly and calmly. Touch chest firmly and calmly.

Module II.1—Overhead #14 *(continued)*

Infant Behavior	Behavior Description	Strategies
Tremors, trembling, and extraneous movement (continued)	Fine-motor development is at risk. Some infants prenatally exposed to drugs exhibit constant extraneous movements that make it difficult for them to soothe themselves. These extraneous movements slow acquisition of organized intentional motor control and visual-motor skills.	
Stiffness and rigidity	Stiffness and rigidity, or increased extensor tone, are often seen in infants prenatally exposed to drugs. The increased muscle tone, which causes these infants to frequently rollover at a few weeks of age, interferes with normal motor development, ability to cuddle, and pull-to-sit, and delays control of arms at midline. We have observed many infants with increased extensor tone that tends to diminish slowly. By one year of age, some degree of increased tone usually remains, and diminishes the quality and smoothness of gross-motor patterns, as well as balance and protective reactions. These infants often arch their backs when held in a variety of positions, or when being fed. Arching occurs up to 12 months of age. More energy is used to accomplish fine and gross motor tasks, thus some level of frustration is created.	• Bathe infant in warm water. • Try gentle, calming massage. • Swaddle in flexion with shoulders and arms close to body. • Place infant in baby hammock to help ease rigidity, to maintain infant in slight spinal flexion, and to inhibit abnormal extension pattern. • Do not leave these infants supine if the position maintains or increases stiffness, for example, spinal extension, head pushing back with scapular retraction (shoulder blades pinching together), or arms pushing into "W" position. Instead, put infant in cloth, sling-type seat, as this position inhibits abnormal extension pattern. • Discourage the use of baby walkers, as they are known to further increase extensor tone.

Instructor's Guide

Module II.1—Overhead #14 *(continued)*

Infant Behavior	Behavior Description	Strategies
Arms in "W" position	A large majority of infants prenatally exposed to drugs exhibit scapular retraction and/or resistance or weakness when attempting to bring arms to midline. When supine, arms are typically widespread and in a "W" position or one arm is in a unilateral "W" position. As these infants develop, difficulty continues in bringing arms to midline or sustaining a midline position. Younger infants compensate by locking their hands together, but when they release them, their arms snap backward into a "W" position, much like a rubber-band effect. When the infants are older, they can use their arms against increased extensor tone and, thus, use large amounts of active energy to maintain control. Fine-motor performance is compromised and development of bimanual skills is difficult. Maintaining hands at midline is an important developmental step in acquiring fine-motor skills.	• Swaddle infant with arms in midline position. • Carry or hold infant in a semireclining position with shoulders forward so that infant will experience arms at midline without excessive effort. • Place infant in cloth, sling-style infant seat. • Use reverse figure-eight strap to sustain arms in forward position while infant is in cloth, sling-style seat or in prone or sitting position. Infant can have successful experience without struggling for control. • Use a foam rubber Tumble Form™ infant feeder chair to position child and assist in keeping arms at midline. This strategy can be used for infants who **cannot tolerate** the reverse figure-eight strap.

From: Lewis, K. D., Bennett, B., & Schmeder, N. H. (1989). The care of infants **menaced by cocaine abuse.** *American Journal of Maternal Child Nursing, 14,* 324–329.

Module II.1—Overhead #15

BROUSSARD'S MATERNAL PERCEPTION INVENTORY

Neonatal Perception Inventory I

Average Baby

How much crying do you think the average baby does?

☐ a great deal   ☐ a good bit   ☐ moderate amount   ☐ very little   ☐ none

How much trouble do you think the average baby has in feeding?

☐ a great deal   ☐ a good bit   ☐ moderate amount   ☐ very little   ☐ none

How much spitting up or vomiting do you think the average baby does?

☐ a great deal   ☐ a good bit   ☐ moderate amount   ☐ very little   ☐ none

How much difficulty do you think the average baby has in sleeping?

☐ a great deal   ☐ a good bit   ☐ moderate amount   ☐ very little   ☐ none

How much difficulty does the average baby have with bowel movements?

☐ a great deal   ☐ a good bit   ☐ moderate amount   ☐ very little   ☐ none

How much trouble do you think the average baby has in settling down to a predictable pattern of eating and sleeping?

☐ a great deal   ☐ a good bit   ☐ moderate amount   ☐ very little   ☐ none

Instructor's Guide

Module II.1—Overhead #15 *(continued)*

Neonatal Perception Inventory I

Average Baby

How much crying do you think your baby will do?

☐ a great deal ☐ a good bit ☐ moderate amount ☐ very little ☐ none

How much trouble do you think your baby will have in feeding?

☐ a great deal ☐ a good bit ☐ moderate amount ☐ very little ☐ none

How much spitting up or vomiting do you think your baby will do?

☐ a great deal ☐ a good bit ☐ moderate amount ☐ very little ☐ none

How much difficulty do you think your baby will have in sleeping?

☐ a great deal ☐ a good bit ☐ moderate amount ☐ very little ☐ none

How much difficulty does your baby to have with bowel movements?

☐ a great deal ☐ a good bit ☐ moderate amount ☐ very little ☐ none

How much trouble do you think your baby will have settling down to a predictable pattern of eating and sleeping?

☐ a great deal ☐ a good bit ☐ moderate amount ☐ very little ☐ none

Module II.1—Overhead #15 *(continued)*

Degree of Bother Inventory

Crying	☐ a great deal	☐ somewhat	☐ very little	☐ none
Spitting up or vomiting	☐ a great deal	☐ somewhat	☐ very little	☐ none
Sleeping	☐ a great deal	☐ somewhat	☐ very little	☐ none
Feeding	☐ a great deal	☐ somewhat	☐ very little	☐ none
Elimination	☐ a great deal	☐ somewhat	☐ very little	☐ none
Lack of predictable schedule	☐ a great deal	☐ somewhat	☐ very little	☐ none
Other (Specify):				
_____	☐ a great deal	☐ somewhat	☐ very little	☐ none
_____	☐ a great deal	☐ somewhat	☐ very little	☐ none
_____	☐ a great deal	☐ somewhat	☐ very little	☐ none
_____	☐ a great deal	☐ somewhat	☐ very little	☐ none

From: Broussard, E. R., & Hartner, M. S. (1971). Further considerations regarding maternal perception of firstborns. In J. Hellmuth (Ed.), *Exceptional infants: Studies in abnormalities* (Vol. 2). New York: Brunner Mazel, Inc.

Instructor's Guide

Module II.1—Overhead #16

BRAZELTON NEONATAL BEHAVIORAL ASSESSMENT SCALE

- 27 items.
- Scored on a scale of 1–9.
- Based on infant's best, rather than average, performance.
- Lengthy exam.
- Requires trained examiner.
- Useful to guide your demonstration of the infant's individuality.

Brazelton Scale Criteria

1. Response decrement to light
2. Response decrement to rattle
3. Response decrement to bell
4. Response decrement to pinprick
5. Orientation response—inanimate visual
6. Orientation response—inanimate auditory
7. Orientation—animate visual
8. Orientation—animate auditory
9. Orientation—animate visual and auditory
10. Alertness
11. General tonus
12. Motor maturity
13. Pull-to-sit
14. Cuddliness
15. Defensive movements
16. Consolability with intervention
17. Peak of excitement
18. Rapidity of buildup

Module II.1—Overhead #16 *(continued)*

> 19. Irritability (to aversive stimuli-uncover, undress, pull-to-sit, prone, pinprick, Tonic Neck Response, Moro, defensive reaction)
> 20. Activity
> 21. Tremulousness
> 22. Amount of startle during exam
> 23. Lability of skin color
> 24. Lability of states
> 25. Self-quieting activity
> 26. Hand to mouth facility
> 27. Smiles

Babies vary greatly in the amount of time they spend in various states (quiet, alert, crying, etc.) and in the ease or difficulty with which they make the transition from one state to another. If parents can learn to recognize the various states and the individuality of their infant, they can interact better with him or her.

From: Brazelton, T. B. (1973). *Neonatal behavioral assessment scale.* Philadelphia: J.B. Lippincott Co.

Instructor's Guide

HANDOUT MASTERS

MODULE II.1   FETAL EFFECTS OF MATERNAL ALCOHOL AND DRUG USE

1. Characteristics of Drugs and the Fetus that Affect Risk
2. Effects of Maternal Cocaine Use on the Fetus
3. Effects of Maternal Cocaine Use on Mother and Fetus
4. Effects of Alcohol
5. Manifestations of Fetal Alcohol Syndrome
6. Effects of Nicotine on the Fetus
7. Effects of Marijuana on the Fetus
8. Effects of Heroin and Methadone on the Fetus
9. Atypical Behavior Patterns in Infants Affected by Cocaine
10. Items Used to Score Neonatal Withdrawal Symptoms in the Nursery
11. Neonatal Drug Withdrawal Scoring System
12. Assessment of Substance Abuse
13. Nursing Measures During Withdrawal
14. Nursing Interventions for Specific Behaviors of Infants Prenatally Exposed to Drugs
15. Broussard's Maternal Perception Inventory
16. Brazelton Neonatal Behavioral Assessment Scale

Module II.1

Module II.1—Handout #1

CHARACTERISTICS OF DRUGS AND THE FETUS THAT AFFECT RISK

- Genetic Vulnerability of the Fetus.
- Timing of Drug Exposure.
  — Embryonic Phase (2–8 weeks after conception).
    Spontaneous abortion.
    Malformed limbs.
    Malformed organs.
  — Fetal Stage (8 weeks–birth).
    Impaired neurological development.
    Intrauterine Growth Retardation (IUGR)
    Subtle mental and behavioral deficits.
    Prematurity.
  — Delivery.
    Abruptio placenta.
    ↑ Uterine contractions.
    ↑ Fetal distress.
- Dosage and Patterns of Consumption.
- Chemical Properties of the Drug.
  — Alcohol—full range of dose-related effects.
  — Illicit drugs—deficits and delays in neurobehavioral functioning.

Instructor's Guide

Module II.1—Handout #2

EFFECTS OF MATERNAL COCAINE USE ON THE FETUS

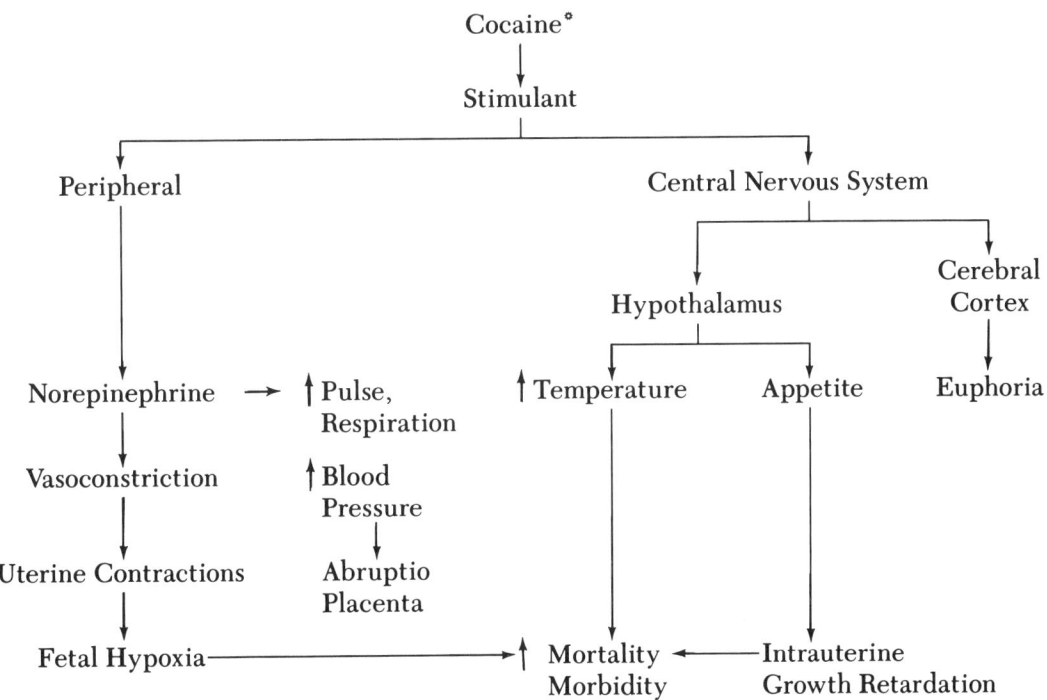

*Passes readily into breast milk and remains for up to 60 hours after maternal use.

Effects on the Breast-Feeding Infant

- Sweating
- Dilated Pupils
- Vomiting
- Diarrhea
- Extreme Irritability
- Hypertension
- Apnea

From: Lynch, M., & McKeon, V. A. (1990). Cocaine use during pregnancy: Research findings and clinical implications. *Journal of Obstetric, Gynecologic and Neonatal Nursing, 19*(4), 285–292.

Module II.1—Handout #3

EFFECTS OF MATERNAL COCAINE USE ON MOTHER AND FETUS

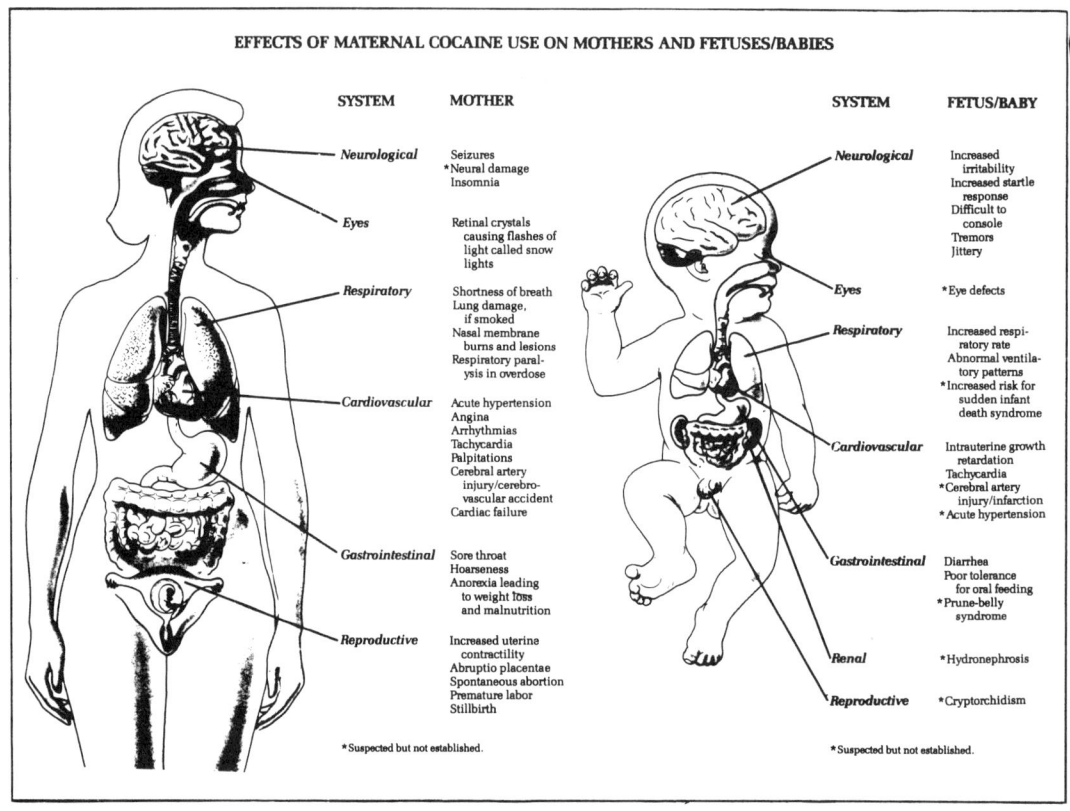

From: Smith, J. (1988). The dangers of prenatal cocaine use. *American Journal of Maternal Child Nursing, 13,* 175–179.

Instructor's Guide

Module II.1—Handout #4

EFFECTS OF ALCOHOL

- Alcohol and its primary metabolite acetaldehyde are directly toxic to developing embryo and fetus.
- Exact etiology is unclear.
- Appears to produce wider range, systemic effects.
- May decrease delivery of maternal nutrients.
  — Impair fetal oxygenation.
  — Derange protein synthesis/metabolism.
  — Stimulate excess production of prostaglandins that modulate cellular function.
- Effects appear to be dose related.
- May be complicated by:
  — Poor nutrition.
  — Low socioeconomic status.
  — Cigarette smoking.
  — Other drug use.

From: Rementeria, J. L. (1977). *Drug abuse in pregnancy and neonatal effects.* St. Louis, MO: C.V. Mosby Co.

Module II.1

Module II.1—Handout #5

MANIFESTATIONS OF FETAL ALCOHOL SYNDROME

The conditions listed represent features observed in the majority of cases of fetal alcohol syndrome (FAS). There are numerous other abnormalities associated with FAS. For a comprehensive list, write to the National Clearinghouse for Alcohol Information, Box 2345, Rockville, MD 20852.

Perinatal Problems

- Intrauterine growth retardation: birth weight, length, and head circumference below the third percentile for gestational age.
- Irritability, tremulousness.
- Hypotonic (poor muscle tone).

Craniofacial Abnormalities

- Short palpebral fissures (short eyeslits).
- Short upturned nose.
- Midface hypoplasia (underdeveloped, small midface).
- Indistinct philtrum (absence of, or minimal ridges between, nose and mouth).
- Hypoplastic maxilla.
- Thin upper vermillion border of lip.
- Retrognathia in infancy.
- Micrognathia or relative prognathia in adolescence.

Postnatal Growth

- Height and weight continue to be below third percentile for age (despite adequate caloric intake).
- Small head circumference.

Central Nervous System Dysfunction

- Mental retardation, from mild to severe levels.
- Poor motor coordination, including abnormal fine motor functioning.
- Delays in gross motor development.
- Microcephaly (small brain size).

Skeletal Abnormalities

- Aberrant palmar creases.

From: Landesman-Dwyer, S. (1982). Drinking during pregnancy: Effects on human development. In *Biomedical processes and consequences of alcohol use.* Rockville, MD: National Institute on Alcohol Abuse and Alcoholism.

Instructor's Guide

Module II.1—Handout #6

EFFECTS OF NICOTINE ON THE FETUS

Nicotine
↓
Sympathomimetic response
↓
Vasoconstriction
↓
Intermittent reduction
of uterine blood flow
↓
Fetal hypoxia
(↑ by carbon monoxide interfering
with body's ability to distribute O_2)
↓
↓ Fetal breathing movements
IUGR

(Average 7 oz. lighter than non-smokers, smaller head and chest circumference, smaller in length)

Breast-Feeding: Transmitted in breast milk and seems to inhibit milk production, as well as reduce the level of vitamin C found in breast milk.

Module II.1

Module II.1—Handout #7

EFFECTS OF MARIJUANA ON THE FETUS

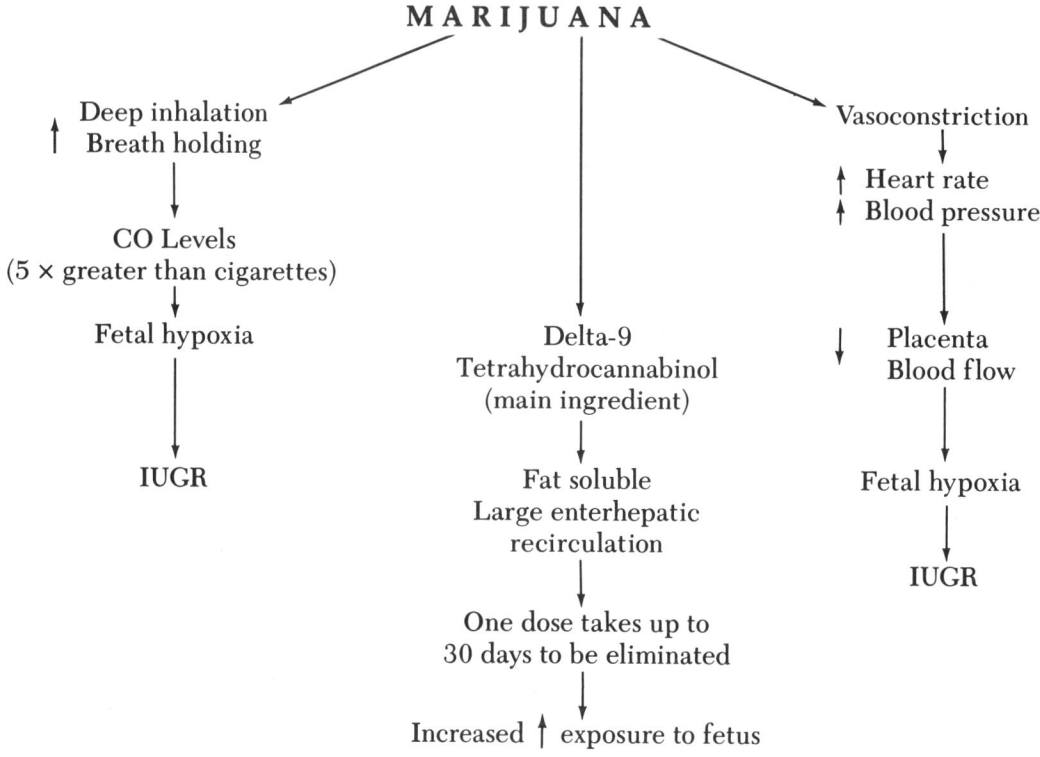

Breast-Feeding: Rapidly transmitted to breast milk and remains there for a long time.

Module II.1—Handout #8

EFFECTS OF HEROIN AND METHADONE ON THE FETUS

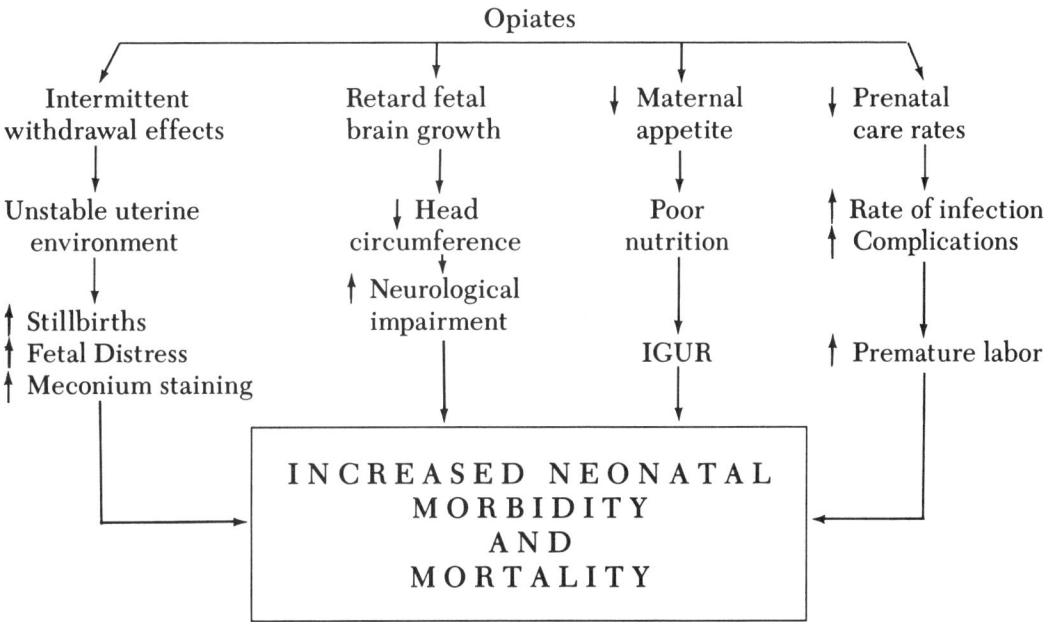

Methadone is more lipid soluble than heroin; therefore, it crosses the placenta more readily.

Breast-Feeding: Transmitted in breast milk. Baby could become opiate dependent from breast feeding.

Module II.1

Module II.1—Handout #9

ATYPICAL BEHAVIOR PATTERNS IN INFANTS AFFECTED BY COCAINE

CHARACTERISTICS	Seldom 1	2	Occurrence 3	4	Frequent 5
Vomiting					X
Poor feeding				X	X
Uncoordinated sucking and swallowing				X	
Weak pull-to-sit					X
Irritability					X
Difficulty sleeping					X
Tremors/trembling					X
Constant extraneous movement			X	X	X
Stiffness/rigidity				X	X
Arms held in "W" position					X
Passivity				X	
Visual concerns					X
Poor muscle tone			X	X	X
Fluctuating muscle tone				X	X
Uncoordinated movements					X
Intolerance to cuddling					X
Difficult to comfort					X
Frequent state changes				X	

- Intensity varies
- Frequency and intensity decrease with age

From: Lewis, K. D., & Schmeder, N. H. (1989). The care of infants menaced by cocaine abuse. *American Journal of Maternal Child Nursing, 14,* 324–329. Copyright 1989 by *MCN.* Reprinted with permission.

Instructor's Guide

Module II.1—Handout #10

ITEMS USED TO SCORE NEONATAL WITHDRAWAL SYMPTOMS IN THE NURSERY

Symptoms	Score Value
High-pitched cry	2
Continuous high-pitched cry	3
Sleeps less than 1 hr after feeding	3
Sleeps less than 2 hr after feeding	2
Sleeps less than 3 hr after feeding	1
Hyperactive Moro reflex	2
Markedly hyperactive Moro reflex	3
Mild tremors when disturbed	1
Marked tremors when disturbed	2
Mild tremors when undisturbed	3
Marked tremors when undisturbed	4
Increased muscle tone	2
Generalized convulsion	5
Frantic sucking of fists	1
Poor feeding	2
Regurgitation	2
Projectile vomiting	3
Loose stools	2
Watery stools	3
Dehydration	2
Frequent yawning	1
Sneezing	1
Nasal stuffiness	1
Sweating	1
Mottling	1
Fever less than 101°F	1
Fever greater than 101°F	1
Respiratory rate over 60/min	1
Respiratory rate over 60/min with retractions	1
Excoriation of nose	1
Excoriation of knees	1
Excoriation of toes	1

Module II.1—Handout #10 *(continued)*

Phenobarbital Dosage Schedule as Prescribed
According to Abstinence Score

Score	Phenobarbital
8–10	6.6 mg/(kg)(24 hr) in three divided doses
11–13	8.8 mg/(kg)(24 hr) in three divided doses
14–16	11.0 mg/(kg)(24 hr) in three divided doses
17 or above	13.2 mg/(kg)(24 hr) in three divided doses

Withdrawal Symptoms in the Nursery

Rated

Hourly—1st day
q2h —2nd day
q4h —thereafter

- No pharmacologic treatment if score is 7 or less.
- Phenobarbital is used to control irritability and insomnia.
- Sucking *improves* with less pharmacologic support therefore:

Nursing measures are critical.

From: Kron, R. E., et al. (1977). Behavior of infants born to drug dependent mothers: Effects of prenatal and postnatal drugs. In *Drug abuse in pregnancy and neonatal effects.* St. Louis, MO: C.V. Mosby Co.

Instructor's Guide

Module II.1—Handout #11

NEONATAL DRUG WITHDRAWAL SCORING SYSTEM

Signs	Score 0	1	2	3
Tremors (muscle activity of limbs)	Normal	Minimally ↑ when hungry or disturbed	Moderate or marked ↑ when undisturbed, subside when fed or held snugly	Marked even when undisturbed, going on to seizure-like movements
Irritability (excessive crying)	None	Slightly ↑	Moderate to severe when disturbed or hungry	Marked even when undisturbed
Reflexes	Normal	Increased	Markedly increased	
Stools	Normal	Explosive, but normal frequency	Explosive, more than 8/day	
Muscle tone	Normal	Increased	Rigidity	
Skin abrasions	No	Redness of knees and elbows	Breaking of skin	
Respiratory rate/min	<55	55–75	76–95	
Repetitive sneezing	No	Yes		
Repetitive yawning	No	Yes		
Vomiting	No	Yes		
Fever	No	Yes		

Identification of Newborn Infant with Narcotic Withdrawal When Score 74 (77% probability).

From: Lipsitz, P. J. (1975). A proposed narcotic withdrawal score for use with newborn infants: A pragmatic evaluation of its efficacy. *Clinical Pediatrics, 14,* 592.

Module II.1—Handout #12

ASSESSMENT OF SUBSTANCE ABUSE

Identifying the Substance Abuser*

Physical appearance and demeanor.
- Patient looks physically exhausted.
- Pupils are extremely dilated or constricted.
- Appearance of pregnancy fails to coincide with stated gestational age.
- Track marks, abscesses, or edema are visible in upper or lower extremities.
- Nasal mucosae are inflamed or indurated.
- Patient is not well-oriented.

Medical history.
- Acquired Immunodeficiency Syndrome.
- Cellulitis.
- Cirrhosis.
- Endocarditis.
- Hepatitis.
- Pancreatitis.
- Pneumonia.

Obstetric history in prior pregnancies.
- Abruptio placentae.
- Fetal death.
- Low-birth-weight infant.
- Meconium staining.
- Premature labor.
- Premature rupture of membranes.
- Sexually transmitted disease.
- Spontaneous abortion.

In current pregnancy.
- History or evidence of early contractions.
- Inactive or hyperactive fetus.
- Poor weight gain.
- Sexually transmitted disease.
- Spotting or vaginal bleeding.

Other guidelines.[†]
- Develop relationship of trust.
- Be nonjudgmental.
- Start with less threatening questions:
  - Cigarette smoking.
  - Caffeine.
  - Over the counter and prescription drugs.
- Follow with questions concerning alcohol consumption.
- End with questions concerning past and present use of illicit drugs.

From: Chasnoff, I. J., Burnes, W. J., Schroll, S. H., & Burns, K. A. (1985). Cocaine use in pregnancy. *The New England Journal of Medicine, 313*(11), 666–669.

[†]*From:* Lynch, M., & McKeon, V. A. (1990). Cocaine use during pregnancy: Research findings and clinical implications. *Journal of Obstetric, Gynecologic and Neonatal Nursing, 19*(4), 285–292.

Instructor's Guide

Module II.1—Handout #13

NURSING MEASURES DURING WITHDRAWAL

- Quiet, darkened environment.
  - Cover top of incubator with cloth.
- Pacifiers.
- Swaddling.
- Holding and rocking.
- Hydrotherapy.
- Therapeutic touch.
- Protection of skin abrasions.
  - Soft linen.
  - Ointment applied liberally to knees, buttocks, chin.
- Monitor fluid intake and output.
  - Small, frequent feedings.
  - Holding upright after feedings.
  - Use of premature nipple for poor suck.
- Liberal visiting by family.
- Crisis intervention for parents.

Module II.1

Module II.1—Handout #14

NURSING INTERVENTIONS FOR SPECIFIC BEHAVIORS OF INFANTS PRENATALLY EXPOSED TO DRUGS

Infant Behavior	Behavior Description	Strategies
Vomiting or poor feeding	Infants frequently display gastrointestinal difficulties throughout their first year of life. Vomiting is frequent during the first six to nine months, as are intermittent constipation and diarrhea. These difficulties tend to increase irritability and discomfort. If allowed to, some infants sleep up to 20 hours per day during the first six months of life and miss feedings. They are, therefore, at risk for inadequate nutrition and failure to thrive.	• If necessary, wake infant for feeding. • Give small quantities of food. • Allow infant to rest frequently during feeding. • Have infant upright for feeding. After feeding, place infant in side-lying or prone position to prevent aspiration of milk. • If infant vomits, clean skin immediately to prevent irritation from stomach acid.
Uncoordinated sucking and swallowing	A variety of abnormal oral-motor behaviors have been observed, including a preemie-like suck pattern, poorly coordinated suck/swallow patterns, inability to stabilize tongue in midline, and occasionally, tongue thrusting and tongue tremors. These abnormal patterns increase feeding time. Consequently, a great deal of infant energy is required, and stress and frustration may occur in mother and infant.	• Hold infant in sitting position with arms forward in slight trunk flexion (curve) during feeding. • Keep infant's chin tucked downward. Infants prenatally exposed to drugs often push head back, which causes an abnormal swallow pattern. • If sucking is difficult for infant, support the infant's chin, or chin and cheeks with your hand. • Play soft, rhythmic music to help infant relax and facilitate rhythmic sucking.
Weak pull-to-sit development	Infants often are slow learning to pull-to-sit; frequently it is accomplished with head lag or excessive effort after six months of age. (Infants normally pull-to-sit with no head lag by four months.)	• Move infant from supine to sitting position, supporting the head so that it does not lag. • While moving infant into sitting position, support shoulders close to infant's body with head forward (neck flexion).

Instructor's Guide

Module II.1—Handout #14 *(continued)*

Infant Behavior	Behavior Description	Strategies
Weak pull-to-sit development (continued)	Some prenatally exposed to drugs who are able to pull-to-sit with no head lag may compensate by pulling their arms back into a strong "W" position. Usually pull-to-sit is accomplished with arms forward and some trunk flexion. The skill is a developmental milestone that indicates abdominal and neck muscle strength, and later affects the quality and endurance of balance, sitting, walking, and protective reflexes.	With infant semireclined (45° angle), encourage infant to assist with pull-to-sit. Give additional head support if needed to prevent head lag, and bring infant's arms forward into midline position. • Place infant in supported sitting position and move infant slowly backward within the range of head control. Then slowly rock or move infant back and forth to strengthen neck and abdominal muscles.
Irritability and difficulty sleeping	Exposure to drugs in utero can cause an infant's state to vary from highly irritable to very passive. Most of these infants, however, are highly irritable and often have difficulty sleeping. Irritable infants can reach a frantic-cry state, which needs to be avoided. If an infant is passive, interaction needs to take place during quiet alert, not hyper-alert, states. Caregivers need to monitor their interactions by being alert to infant behavioral and psychological cues that indicate stress, and adjust interactions appropriately. Caregivers will be affected by infant irritability, resulting in frustration and feelings of inadequacy in the mothering role and in infant/caregiver attachment. The caregiver needs to be made aware of behavior typical in infants prenatally exposed to drugs. Subsequently, the quality of their relationship will improve, negative judgments about the infant will be reduced, and the likelihood of child abuse will be decreased.	• Reduce noise in environment. • Turn down lights. • Swaddle infant in a cotton blanket in flexed position with arms close to body. • Hold swaddled infant close. • Put infant in bunting-type wrapper and carry close to body. • Rock infant slowly and rhythmically, either horizontally or with head supported vertically, whichever soothes. • Place in a front-pack carrier. • Walk with infant. • Give child pacifier. • Provide hydrotherapy (warm bath). • Respond to stress cues by stopping activity with infant. This response will give the infant a "time-out." • Provide firm, calm touch to the mid-chest, back, or sole of the infant's feet. • Play soft music or sing or hum quietly. • Provide background noise (for example, a hair dryer or vacuum cleaner), often called white noise, which may calm the infant.

Module II.1

Module II.1—Handout #14 *(continued)*

Infant Behavior	Behavior Description	Strategies
Irritability and difficulty sleeping (continued)		• If all else fails, place infant in a quiet, darkened room with no outside stimulation. (Caregivers report this works with both premature and full-term infants exposed prenatally to drugs.)
Tremors, trembling, and extraneous movement	Tremors of the hands, arms, legs, chin, and tongue are commonly observed in infants prenatally exposed to drugs, although usually more pronounced and intense in a younger infant. We have observed tremors and tremulousness of movements in infants older than one year, but the intensity is diminished. In younger infants, tremors are primarily observed when infants are at rest. As they get older, fewer and less intense at-rest tremors occur, and intention tremors emerge. They tend to increase as the infant tires. Intention tremors occur when the infant is actively attempting a specific motor movement, for example, reaching for a toy. Intervention is often successful with intention tremors of arms and hands. Signs of stress often occur after persisting with an activity that elicits intention tremors, because physical movements are difficult and more energy and time are required to accomplish a task. Fine-motor development is at risk. Some infants prenatally exposed to drugs exhibit constant extraneous movements that make it difficult for them to soothe themselves. These extraneous movements slow acquisition of organized intentional motor control and visual-motor skills.	• Swaddling and holding infant close may be helpful for early at-rest tremors and extraneous movement. • Hold infant semireclined (almost sitting) with arms and shoulders forward to reduce the effort exerted by infant to maintain arm at midline while reaching for, holding, or manipulating toys. • Touch tremulous area firmly and calmly. Touch chest firmly and calmly.

Instructor's Guide

Module II.1—Handout #14 *(continued)*

Infant Behavior	Behavior Description	Strategies
Stiffness and rigidity	Stiffness and rigidity, or increased extensor tone, are often seen in infants prenatally exposed to drugs. The increased muscle tone, which causes these infants to frequently rollover at a few weeks of age, interferes with normal motor development, ability to cuddle, and pull-to-sit, and delays control of arms at midline. We have observed many infants with increased extensor tone that tends to diminish slowly. By one year of age, some degree of increased tone usually remains, and diminishes the quality and smoothness of gross-motor patterns, as well as balance and protective reactions. These infants often arch their backs when held in a variety of positions, or when being fed. Arching occurs up to 12 months of age. More energy is used to accomplish fine and gross motor tasks, thus some level of frustration is created.	• Bathe infant in warm water. • Try gentle, calming massage. • Swaddle in flexion with shoulders and arms close to body. • Place infant in baby hammock to help ease rigidity, to maintain infant in slight spinal flexion, and to inhibit abnormal extension pattern. • Do not leave these infants supine if the position maintains or increases stiffness, for example, spinal extension, head pushing back with scapular retraction (shoulder blades pinching together), or arms pushing into "W" position. Instead, put infant in cloth, sling-type seat, as this position inhibits abnormal extension pattern. • Discourage the use of baby walkers, as they are known to further increase extensor tone.

Module II.1—Handout #14 *(continued)*

Infant Behavior	Behavior Description	Strategies
Arms in "W" position	A large majority of infants prenatally exposed to drugs exhibit scapular retraction and/or resistance or weakness when attempting to bring arms to midline. When supine, arms are typically widespread and in a "W" position or one arm is in a unilateral "W" position. As these infants develop, difficulty continues in bringing arms to midline or sustaining a midline position. Younger infants compensate by locking their hands together, but when they release them, their arms snap backward into a "W" position, much like a rubber-band effect. When the infants are older, they can use their arms against increased extensor tone and, thus, use large amounts of active energy to maintain control. Fine-motor performance is compromised and development of bimanual skills is difficult. Maintaining hands at midline is an important developmental step in acquiring fine-motor skills.	• Swaddle infant with arms in midline position. • Carry or hold infant in a semireclining position with shoulders forward so that infant will experience arms at midline without excessive effort. • Place infant in cloth, sling-style infant seat. • Use reverse figure-eight strap to sustain arms in forward position while infant is in cloth, sling-style seat or in prone or sitting position. Infant can have successful experience without struggling for control. • Use a foam rubber Tumble Form™ infant feeder chair to position child and assist in keeping arms at midline. This strategy can be used for infants who cannot tolerate the reverse figure-eight strap.

From: Lewis, K. D., Bennett, B., & Schmeder, N. H. (1989). The care of infants menaced by cocaine abuse. *American Journal of Maternal Child Nursing, 14,* 324–329.

Instructor's Guide

Module II.1—Handout #15

BROUSSARD'S MATERNAL PERCEPTION INVENTORY

Neonatal Perception Inventory I

Average Baby

How much crying do you think the average baby does?

☐ a great deal ☐ a good bit ☐ moderate amount ☐ very little ☐ none

How much trouble do you think the average baby has in feeding?

☐ a great deal ☐ a good bit ☐ moderate amount ☐ very little ☐ none

How much spitting up or vomiting do you think the average baby does?

☐ a great deal ☐ a good bit ☐ moderate amount ☐ very little ☐ none

How much difficulty do you think the average baby has in sleeping?

☐ a great deal ☐ a good bit ☐ moderate amount ☐ very little ☐ none

How much difficulty does the average baby have with bowel movements?

☐ a great deal ☐ a good bit ☐ moderate amount ☐ very little ☐ none

How much trouble do you think the average baby has in settling down to a predictable pattern of eating and sleeping?

☐ a great deal ☐ a good bit ☐ moderate amount ☐ very little ☐ none

Module II.1

Module II.1—Handout #15 *(continued)*

Neonatal Perception Inventory I

Average Baby

How much crying do you think your baby will do?

☐ a great deal ☐ a good bit ☐ moderate amount ☐ very little ☐ none

How much trouble do you think your baby will have in feeding?

☐ a great deal ☐ a good bit ☐ moderate amount ☐ very little ☐ none

How much spitting up or vomiting do you think your baby will do?

☐ a great deal ☐ a good bit ☐ moderate amount ☐ very little ☐ none

How much difficulty do you think your baby will have in sleeping?

☐ a great deal ☐ a good bit ☐ moderate amount ☐ very little ☐ none

How much difficulty do you expect your baby to have with bowel movements?

☐ a great deal ☐ a good bit ☐ moderate amount ☐ very little ☐ none

How much trouble do you think your baby will have settling down to a predictable pattern of eating and sleeping?

☐ a great deal ☐ a good bit ☐ moderate amount ☐ very little ☐ none

Instructor's Guide

Module II.1—Handout #15 *(continued)*

Degree of Bother Inventory

Crying	☐ a great deal	☐ somewhat	☐ very little	☐ none
Spitting up or vomiting	☐ a great deal	☐ somewhat	☐ very little	☐ none
Sleeping	☐ a great deal	☐ somewhat	☐ very little	☐ none
Feeding	☐ a great deal	☐ somewhat	☐ very little	☐ none
Elimination	☐ a great deal	☐ somewhat	☐ very little	☐ none
Lack of predictable schedule	☐ a great deal	☐ somewhat	☐ very little	☐ none
Other (Specify):				
_____	☐ a great deal	☐ somewhat	☐ very little	☐ none
_____	☐ a great deal	☐ somewhat	☐ very little	☐ none
_____	☐ a great deal	☐ somewhat	☐ very little	☐ none
_____	☐ a great deal	☐ somewhat	☐ very little	☐ none

From: Broussard, E. R., & Hartner, M. S. (1971). Further considerations regarding maternal perception of firstborns. In Hellmuth, J. (Ed.), *Exceptional infants: Studies in abnormalities* (Vol. 2). New York: Brunner Mazel, Inc.

Module II.1

Module II.1—Handout #16

BRAZELTON NEONATAL BEHAVIORAL ASSESSMENT SCALE

- 27 items.
- Scored on a scale of 1–9.
- Based on infant's best, rather than average, performance.
- Lengthy exam.
- Requires trained examiner.
- Useful to guide your demonstration of the infant's individuality.

Brazelton Scale Criteria

1. Response decrement to light
2. Response decrement to rattle
3. Response decrement to bell
4. Response decrement to pinprick
5. Orientation response—inanimate visual
6. Orientation response—inanimate auditory
7. Orientation—animate visual
8. Orientation—animate auditory
9. Orientation—animate visual and auditory
10. Alertness
11. General tonus
12. Motor maturity
13. Pull-to-sit
14. Cuddliness
15. Defensive movements
16. Consolability with intervention
17. Peak of excitement
18. Rapidity of buildup
19. Irritability (to aversive stimuli-uncover, undress, pull-to-sit, prone, pinprick, Tonic Neck Response, Moro, defensive reaction)
20. Activity
21. Tremulousness
22. Amount of startle during exam

Instructor's Guide

Module II.1—Handout #16 *(continued)*

23. Lability of skin color
24. Lability of states
25. Self-quieting activity
26. Hand to mouth facility
27. Smiles

Babies vary greatly in the amount of time they spend in various states (quiet, alert, crying, etc.) and in the ease or difficulty with which they make the transition from one state to another. If parents can learn to recognize the various states and the individuality of their infant, they can interact better with him or her.

From: Brazelton, T. B. (1973). *Neonatal behavioral assessment scale.* Philadelphia: J.B. Lippincott Co.

Module II.1

RECOMMENDED TEACHING STRATEGIES AND SAMPLE ASSIGNMENTS

SUGGESTED CLINICAL EXPERIENCES

1. Prenatal Clinics
2. Visiting Nurse Service Field Trip
3. Transition/Observation Nursery
4. Hale House
5. Foundling Hospital

RECOMMENDED TEACHING STRATEGIES (SAMPLES ATTACHED)

1. Values Clarification Exercise
2. Values Clarification Exercise—Group
3. Nursing Process—Designing a Plan of Care
4. Role Plays

TEACHING STRATEGY #1

VALUES CLARIFICATION EXERCISE

Objectives:

1. To help the student identify personal attitudes concerning substance abuse during pregnancy.
2. To assist the student in clarifying how personal attitudes influence nursing care.
3. To promote acknowledgement and open discussion of these attitudes.

Directions:

Please answer these questions as honestly as possible. It will assist you in explaining your very real feelings and concern regarding substance abuse during pregnancy. There are no right answers.

1. A woman who would abuse a substance during pregnancy:
   a. Probably doesn't know the harmful effects.
   b. Probably knows the harmful effects but doesn't care about anyone but herself.
   c. Probably knows the harmful effects and is worried about her baby.

Instructor's Guide

2. A woman who has delivered two addicted babies 13 months apart should:
   a. Be sterilized.
   b. Have both infants taken from her and put in foster care.
   c. Undergo voluntary drug detoxification and be allowed to keep both babies.

3. Baby J. is a two-day-old infant who is experiencing severe drug withdrawal. He is hyperirritable, sweating, crying furiously, has diarrhea, and won't suck. You have been taking care of Baby J. (as well as 12 other infants all day). At 3:00 p.m., Mrs. J. comes into the nursery for the first time and says "Why is he acting like that?"

   Write a statement that best describes your *thoughts*. (This is not what you would actually say but only what you probably think.)

   _____
   _____
   _____
   _____
   _____
   _____

4. How would you rate your chance of succeeding in making a real difference in this woman's life?
   a. None
   b. 25%
   c. 50%
   d. 100%

5. How do you think that your chance of success will affect your nursing care?

   _____
   _____
   _____
   _____
   _____
   _____

6. Baby L. is a 2 lb. infant born to parents who have a history of infertility. Baby M. is a 5 lb. infant born to a substance-addicted mother. They both need a respirator immediately, and you have only one respirator available. Who should get the respirator?

   _____
   _____
   _____
   _____
   _____
   _____

Module II.1

TEACHING STRATEGY #2

VALUES CLARIFICATION EXERCISE—GROUP

Questions for Small Group Discussion:

1. Do you think it is natural to feel uncomfortable toward a woman who would knowingly cause her infant to be at risk?
2. Is it possible to intervene effectively if you feel that the mother is totally responsible for the baby's condition?
3. How do you think your perceived chance of success would influence your plan of care?
4. How would you define a "real difference" in a woman's life?
5. Given that small bit of information in question 6—what factors influenced your choice?
6. What clinical principles might influence your actions?

TEACHING STRATEGY #3

THE NURSING PROCESS: DESIGNING A PLAN OF CARE FOR MOTHERS AND INFANTS AFFECTED BY MATERNAL DRUG USE

Objectives:

1. To assist the student in the assessment, diagnosis, planning, implementation, and evaluation of Mothers/Infants affected by maternal drug use.
2. To promote the synthesis of material presented.
3. To guide the student in the creative process of developing nursing interventions.

Directions:

1. Students will design their own plan of care using the nursing process.
2. The following material entitled "A Nursing Care Plan" may serve as a guide for you.
3. Students should be encouraged to develop creative interventions such as music-therapy, use of movement, and so forth.
4. "A Nursing Care Plan" may also be used as a handout.

A NURSING CARE PLAN

A. Assessment.
   1. Follow guidelines suggested in Handouts #12A–12B: Assessment of Substance Abuse.
   2. Be alert for distinctive manifestations of FAS in neonate. (Handouts #4 & 5)
   3. Be alert for manifestations of drug withdrawal in neonatal period. (Handouts #2, 3, 6, 7, 8)
   4. Evaluate laboratory data to determine mother's last drug intake and dosage.

B. Possible Nursing Diagnoses.
   1. Maternal:
      a. Sensory perceptual alteration.
      b. Alteration in nutrition: Less than body requirements.
      c. Knowledge deficit.
      d. Alteration in thought processes.
      e. Impaired communication.
      f. Ineffective individual coping.
      g. Alteration in self-concept.
      h. Anxiety.
      i. Fear.
      j. Social isolation.
      k. Altered parenting.
      l. Grief.
   2. Infant:
      a. Altered nutrition: Less than body requirements related to decreased food intake and hyperirritability.
      b. Potential for injury related to seizure activity secondary to CNS dysfunction or chemical dependence.
      c. Pain related to skin excoriation over bony prominence secondary to constant activity.
      d. Alteration in sensory perception related to CNS dysfunction and/or chemical dependence.
   3. Mother-Infant Dyad:
      a. Altered parenting related to hyperirritability.
      b. Ineffective family coping related to potential developmental delay and/or guilt over diagnosis.
C. Planning.
   1. Promotion of physical well-being of mother and infant.
   2. Promotion of emotional well-being of mother and infant.
   3. Promotion of effective parent-child relationship.
D. Implementation.
   1. Mother:
      a. Provide factual information.
      b. Use nonjudgmental manner.
      c. Encourage drug treatment program.
      d. Encourage support group.
      e. Encourage visiting in nursery.
      f. Evaluate mother's perception of infant (Broussard's Perception Inventory—Handout #15).

Module II.1

   g. Evaluate infant's temperament (Brazelton's infant temperament scale—Handout #16).

   h. Provide role modeling to teach mother to care for her infant's special needs.

   i. Foster extended family's relationship with mother and infant.

  2. Infant:

   a. Provide for physical well-being using nursing interventions (Handouts #13, 14, and 17).

   b. Evaluate temperament (Brazelton's infant temperament scale).

   c. Role supplementation in nursery until mother is able to assume mothering role.

  3. Mother-Infant:

   a. Role modeling to foster mother-child relationship.

   b. Teach specific techniques to quiet the infant.

   c. Encourage interaction through extended visits to nursery.

E. Evaluation.

  1. The infant tolerates feedings and gains weight.

  2. The infant's hyperirritability is controlled.

  3. The infant has suffered no physical injury.

  4. The mother is able to identify the special needs of the infant.

  5. The mother is able to use quieting techniques that ensure effective feeding and control hyperirritability.

  6. The mother has specific plans to eliminate substance abuse.

  7. The mother is able to cope with her frustrations and begin to use outside resources as needed.

TEACHING STRATEGY #4

FETAL EFFECTS OF MATERNAL DRUG AND ALCOHOL USE—ROLE PLAY #1

Time: About 15 minutes

Objectives:

1. Recall the manifestations of substance withdrawal in the neonate.

2. Recall the manifestations of fetal alcohol syndrome.

3. Help the student identify with the role of therapeutic caregiver.

4. Help the student to gain new perceptions and insights into this difficult situation.

Instructor's Guide

CASE VIGNETTE

Baby Tommy and His Mother

Tommy was born four weeks prematurely to a mother who is addicted to cocaine and alcohol. He had a high-pitched cry, racing heart rate, and hyperexcitability at birth. He is now three weeks old and appears to have successfully withdrawn from the cocaine; however, his pediatrician is concerned about possible fetal alcohol syndrome as his head is unusually small and he has very short eye slits. Tommy's mother adamantly denies that her use of alcohol and cocaine was excessive throughout her pregnancy and has little motivation to maintain her sobriety. She claims that she never had nose bleeds like some of her friends, never went into exorbitant financial debt, and lives a "respectable, hard-working life." She believes that Tommy was born prematurely because she was over-worked and tired and that his physical symptoms are related to Tommy's father's family history of epilepsy.

Note: Only willing players should be selected. Players should be given ample preparation time.

Role-Play—Baby Tommy and His Mother

Nurses' Script:

1. Identify patterns in the neonate that suggest withdrawal of chemical dependence.
2. Inform the mother of the diagnosis as evidenced by:
    a. Documented withdrawal signs.
    b. Urine toxicology report.
    c. Physical manifestations of FAS.
3. Through mutual process, discuss:
    a. The benefits of ceasing alcohol and drug use.
    b. The effects of alcohol and drug use on Tommy.
    c. Her immediate plans for detoxification—if any.
    d. Possible long range plans—support groups.
    e. The possible benefits of early intervention programs for Tommy.

FETAL EFFECTS OF MATERNAL DRUG AND ALCOHOL USE—ROLE PLAY #2

Time: About 15 minutes (maybe longer)

Objectives:

1. Recall the effects of maternal cocaine use on the neonate.
2. Recall the atypical behavior patterns in infants exposed to cocaine prenatally.
3. Conduct an assessment of withdrawal symptoms.

Module II.1

4. Teach a mother to assess her infant's temperament.
5. Synthesize content by establishing an effective plan to enhance mother/infant interaction.
6. Assist the student to identify with the role of therapeutic caregiver.
7. Assist the student to gain new perception and insights.

Items Needed: Baby doll, bottle, rocking chair, blanket, and pacifier.

CASE VIGNETTE

Teaching Mrs. F to Care for Baby F

Baby F is a 3-day-old infant born at 38 weeks gestation to a mother who has admitted to using cocaine sporadically throughout her pregnancy. He is exhibiting many signs of cocaine withdrawal. Mrs. F arrives at the Transitional Nursery where you are a staff nurse. She begins to feed Baby F but he arches his back and pulls away. When she finally forces the nipple into his mouth, he sucks slowly, then vomits. Mrs. F is overheard to say "You are bad, just like your father, don't you go acting bad with me!"

Your role as Baby F's nurse is to:

1. Assess Mrs. F's perception of her baby's temperament.
2. Demonstrate effective interventions.
3. Help Mrs. F to carry out these interventions.
4. Help Mrs. F and Baby F to begin to establish a mutually rewarding relationship.
5. Foster a sense of accomplishment in Mrs. F.

Note: Only willing players should be selected. Players should be given ample preparation time.

Instructor's Guide

TEST QUESTIONS AND ANSWERS

TEST QUESTIONS

1. You are admitting Mrs. Jones, whom you suspect is abusing alcohol. She is in early labor. Which of the following assessment inquiries is likely to elicit accurate information from Mrs. Jones regarding use of alcohol:

    a. "You don't drink, do you?" asked during pelvic exam.

    b. "How much do you drink?" asked between contractions.

    c. "Your baby seems very small, do you drink?" asked while palpating her abdomen.

    d. "How much alcohol are you drinking now?" asked while taking a general health history.

2. Baby Jones is delivered vaginally weighing 2,200 gms. at 40 weeks gestation. When assessing Baby Jones for fetal alcohol syndrome, you should know that:

    a. 7–10 infants per 1,000 are affected by FAS.

    b. Alcohol effects are found in children with normal facial features as well as typical FAS facial features.

    c. A thin upper lip is the most common problem associated with FAS.

    d. Baby Jones is likely to be underweight in relation to his length.

3. When conducting your physical assessment of Baby Jones you should look for the signs of FAS which include:

    a. CNS dysfunction, sensorineural hearing loss, macrosomia, and hydrocephalus.

    b. CNS dysfunction, midfacial hypoplasia, dysmorphia, and microencephaly.

    c. Seizure, cleft lip/palate, dysmorphia, and respiratory distress syndrome.

    d. Dislocated hips, CNS dysfunction, macrosomia, and absent philtrum.

4. One of your nursing diagnoses is: alteration in nutrition—Less than body requirements related to hyperirritability. One nursing intervention you would probably institute would be:

    a. Gavage feed Baby Jones after he sucks for 10 minutes to avoid overtiring him.

    b. Maintain 10 fluids to avoid risk of aspiration.

    c. Feed Baby Jones by propping the bottle in a darkened isolette.

    d. Swaddle Baby Jones and feed using a premature nipple.

5. Baby Jones displays some but not all of the manifestations of FAS. His grandmother visits the nursery and says, "He look so normal, it is hard to believe he will be retarded, how bad will he be?" Your response to her question is based on your knowledge that the most powerful predictor of the severity of FAS is:

a. Severity of diagnosis and malformation at birth.

b. Amount of alcohol consumed by the mother.

c. Interaction between mother/infant.

d. Genetic vulnerability of the fetus.

6. Mrs. Fountain is a 19-year-old woman who is admitted to labor and delivery at 37 weeks gestation in active labor. Her prenatal records indicate that she is suspected of using cocaine. Based on the above information, you know that during the course of her labor, you must be alert for:

    a. Hyperinsulin, hypertension, and placenta previa.

    b. Abruptio placenta, meconium staining, and fetal distress.

    c. Placenta previa, pre-eclampsia, and hypoglycemia.

    d. Hypertension, abruptio placenta, and nausea.

7. Baby Fountain is born weighing 2,200 gms. On the second day after birth, he exhibits a mildly hyperactive Moro reflex, poor sucking, regurgitation and hyperirritability. The doctor has ordered Phenobarbital in order to promote Baby Fountain's optimal functioning and facilitate feeding. Which of these actions, based on your knowledge of Phenobarbital's action, should you take?

    a. Institute nursing measures to facilitate feeding and reduce hyperirritability.

    b. Ask the doctor to order the Phenobarbital A.C.

    c. Request that the Phenobarbital be given in two divided doses.

    d. Plan your nursing care and feedings to occur after Phenobarbital Administration.

8. While feeding Baby Fountain in the transitional nursery, Mrs. Fountain makes all of the following comments. Which comment indicates the need for more discussion:

    a. "I'm glad my friend bought me a baby bath, water seems to relax him."

    b. "I see if I hold him close in a blanket, he eats better."

    c. "He seems so at ease with you, I hope I can do that soon."

    d. "I plan to breast feed because I heard it is better for the baby."

9. In preparing for discharge, the teaching plans should include which of the following information?

    a. It is good to avoid overstimulation, therefore decreased handling is advised.

    b. It will be better for him if you don't treat him differently than another baby.

    c. Pacifiers should never be used because it promotes non-nutritive sucking.

    d. If necessary, wake him for feedings in order to give small, frequent feedings.

10. You administer the Broussard Neonatal Perception Inventory (NPI) to Mrs. Fountain before discharge. Your purpose in doing this is to:

    a. Determine how she rates her baby with the average baby.

    b. Determine what type of temperament Baby Fountain has.

    c. Determine if Ms. Fountain needs in-patient drug rehabilitation.

    d. Determine how Baby Fountain will fit in an early intervention program.

Instructor's Guide

ANSWER KEY

1. d
2. b
3. b
4. d
5. a
6. b
7. a
8. d
9. d
10. a

BIBLIOGRAPHY

MODULE II.1 FETAL EFFECTS OF MATERNAL ALCOHOL AND DRUG USE

Abel, E. L. (1984). Pharmacology of alcohol relating to pregnancy and lactation. *Fetal alcohol syndrome and fetal alcohol effect.* (pp. 29–45). New York: Plenum Press.

Abel, E. L., & Sokol, R. (1986). Fetal alcohol syndrome is now the leading cause of mental retardation. *Lancet, 2,* 1222.

Abel, E. L., & Sokol, R. J. (1987). Incidence of fetal alcohol syndrome and economic import of FAS-related anomalies. *Drug Alcohol Dependency, 19,* 51–70.

Acker, D., Sachs, M. D., Tracy, K. J., & Wise, W. E. (1983). Abruptio placenta associated with cocaine use. *American Journal of Obstetrics and Gynecology, 146*(2), 120–221.

Adams, C., et al. (1990). Nursing interventions with mothers who are substance abusers. *Journal of Perinatal, Neonatal Nursery, 3*(4), 43–52.

American Nurses' Association. (1988). *Standards of addictions nursing practice with selected diagnoses and criteria.* Kansas City, MO: Author.

Barbour, B. (1989). Is fetal alcohol syndrome completely irreversible? *American Journal of Maternal Child Nursing, 14,* 44–46.

Bennett, K. (1987). AIDS: A generation of children at risk. *Journal of Psychosocial Nursing and Mental Health Services, 25*(12), 32–34.

Bingol, N., Schuster, C., & Fuches, M. (1987). The influence of socioeconomic factors on the occurrence of fetal alcohol syndrome. *Advances in Alcohol and Substance Abuse, 6*(4), 105–118.

Boggan, W. O., & Randall, C. L. (1980). Effect of low-dose prenatal alcohol exposure on behavior and the response to alcohol. *Alcohol: Clinical and Experimental Research, 4,* 226.

Brazelton, T. B. (1973). *Neonatal behavioral assessment scale.* Philadelphia, PA: J.B. Lippincott Co.

Brooten, D., Peters, M. A., Glatts, M., & et al. (1987). A survey of nutrition, caffeine, cigarette and alcohol intake in early pregnancy in an urban clinic population. *Journal of Nurse Mid-wifery, 32*(2), 85–90.

Broussard, E. R., & Hartner, M. S. (1971). Further considerations regarding maternal perception of firstborns. In J. Hellmuth (Ed.), *Exceptional infants: Studies in abnormalities* (Vol. 2). New York: Brunner Mazel, Inc.

Bullard, I. D. (1983). Maternal and child nursing. In C. Vourakis & C. Bennett (Eds.), *Substance abuse: Perspectives.* New York: J. Wiley.

Busch, D., McBride, A. B., & Benaventura, L. M. (1986). Chemical dependency in women: The link to OB/GYN problems. *Journal of Psychosocial Nursing and Mental Health Services 24*(4), 26–30.

Chasnoff, I. J., Schnoll, S., Burno, W. I., & Burne, K. (1984). Maternal non-narcotic substance abuse during pregnancy: Effects on infant development. *Neurobehavioral Toxicology and Teratology, 6,* 271–275.

Chasnoff, I. J., Schnoll, S. H., Burns, W. J., & Burns, D. (1984). Maternal non-narcotic substance abuse during pregnancy: Effects on infant development. *Neurobehavioral Toxicology and Teratology, 6*(4), 277–280.

Chasnoff, I. J., Burnes, W. J., Schnoll, S. H., & Burns, K. A. (1985). Cocaine use in pregnancy. *The New England Journal of Medicine, 313*(11), 666–669.

Chasnoff, I. J. (1987). Perinatal effects of cocaine. *Contemporary Obstetrics and Gynecology, 29,* 163–79.

Chasnoff, I. J., & Griffith, D. R. (1989). Cocaine: Clinical studies of pregnancy and the newborn. In D. E. Hutchings (Ed.), *Prenatal abuse of licit & illicit drugs: Annals of the New York Academy of Sciences,* (Vol. 562, pp. 260–266). New York: New York Academy of Sciences.

Chasnoff, I. J., Hunt, C. E., Kletter, R., & Kaplan, D. (1989). Prenatal cocaine exposure is associated with respiratory pattern abnormalities. *AJDC, 143* (May 1989), 583–587.

Chisum, G. M. (1990). Nursing interventions with the antepartum substance abuser. *Journal of Perinatal Neonatal Nursing, 3*(4), 26–33.

Chychula, N. M. (1984). Screening for drug abuse in a primary care setting. *Nurse Practitioner, 9,* 15–24.

Clarren, S. K., & Smith, D. W. (1978). The fetal alcohol syndrome. *New England Journal of Medicine, 298,* 1063–1067.

Cohen, S.(1981). The Fetal Alcohol Syndrome: Alcohol as a teratogen. In *The Substance Abuse Problems* (Vol. 1, pp. 245–250). New York: The Haworth Press.

Coles, C. D., & Smith, I. E. (1984). Neonatal ethanol withdrawal: Characteristics in clinically normal, nondysmorphic neonates. *Journal of Pediatrics, 105*(3), 445–451.

Coles, C. D., Smith, I. E., Lancaster, J. S., & Falek, A. (1987). Persistence over the first month of neurobehavioral differences in infants exposed to alcohol prenatally. *Infant Behavior and Development 10*(1), 23–37.

Dorris, M. (1989). The broken cord. *New Age Journal,* (November, December). 46–49, 101.

Edelir, K. C., et al. (1988). Methadone maintenance in pregnancy: Consequences to care and outcome. *Obstetrics and Gynecology 71*(3), 399–404.

Eliason, M. J., et al. (1990). Fetal alcohol syndrome and the neonate. *Journal of Perinatal Neonatal Nursing, 3*(4), 64–72.

Erickson, M. L. (1976). *Assessment and management of developmental changes in children.* St. Louis, MO: C.V. Mosby Co.

Fost, N. (1989). Maternal-fetal conflicts: Ethical and legal considerations. In D. E. Hutchings (Ed.), *Prenatal abuse of licit and illicit drugs: Annals of the New York Academy of Sciences* (Vol. 562, pp. 248–254). New York: New York Academy of Sciences.

Module II.1

Fox, N. L., Sexton, M. J., & Hebel, R. J. (1987). Alcohol consumption among pregnant smokers: Effects of smoking cessation intervention program. *American Journal of Public Health, 77*(2), 211–213.

Fried, P. A., Buckingham, M., & Von Kuloniz, P. (1983). Marijuana use during pregnancy and perinatal risk factors. *American Journal of Obstetrics and Gynecology, 146*(8), 992–994.

Fried, P. A., Barnes, M. V., & Drake, E. R. (1985). Soft drug use after pregnancy compared to use before and during pregnancy. *American Journal of Obstetrics and Gynecology, 151*(6); 787–792.

Golden, N. L., Kuhnert, B. R., Sokol, R. J., Martier, S., & Bagby, M. S. (1984). Phencyclidine use during pregnancy. *American Journal of Obstetrics and Gynecology, 148*(3), 254–259.

Golden, N. L., Sokol, R. T., Martier, S., & Miller, S. I. (1982). A practical method for identifying angel dust abuse during pregnancy. *American Journal of Obstetrics and Gynecology, 142*(3), 359–361.

Goldstein, D. B. (1983). Note on fetal alcohol syndrome. In D. Goldstein (Ed.), *Pharmacology of alcohol.* New York: Oxford University Press.

Greenlaw, J. L. (1990). Treatment refusal, noncompliance and substance abuse in pregnancy: Legal and ethical issue. *Birth, 17*(3), 152–156.

Hill, L. M., & Kleinberg, F. (1984). Effects of drugs and chemicals on the fetus and newborn. *Mayo Clinic Proceedings, 59,* 707–716; 755–765.

Howard, J., Beckwith, L., Rodning, C., & Kropenske, V. (1989). The development of young children of substance abusing parents: Insights from seven years of intervention research. *Zero to Three, 9*(5), 8–12.

James, J. E., & Paul, I. (1985). Caffeine and human reproduction. *Reviews on Environmental Health, 5*(2), 151–167.

Kaltenback, K., & Finnegan, L. (1984). Developmental outcome of children born to methadone maintained women: A review of longitudinal studies. *Neurobehavioral Toxicology and Teratology, 6,* 271–275.

Kinnard, M. J. (1990). Cocaine use during pregnancy: Fetal and neonatal effects. *Journal of Perinatal Neonatal Nursing, 3*(4), 53–63.

Kron, R. E., et al. (1977). Behavior of infants born to drug dependent mothers: Effects of prenatal and postnatal drugs. In *Drugs abuse in pregnancy and neonatal effects.* St. Louis, MO: C.V. Mosby Co.

Landesman-Dwyer, S. (1982). Drinking during pregnancy: Effects on human developments. In *Biomedical processes and consequences of alcohol use.* Rockville, MD: National Institute on Alcohol Abuse and Alcoholism.

Lee, M. I., Stayker, J. C., & Sokol, R. J. (198—). Perinatal care for narcotic-dependent gravidas. *Perinatology-Neonatology, 9*(6), 135–140.

Leduc, E. (1989). The healing touch. *American Journal of Maternal Child Nursing, 14,* 41–43.

Lewis, K. D., Bennett, B., & Schmeder, N. H. (1989). The care of infants menaced by cocaine abuse. *American Journal of Maternal Child Nursing, 14,* 324–329.

Lipsitz, P. J. (1975). A proposed narcotic withdrawal score for use with newborn infants: A pragmatic evaluation of its efficacy. *Clinical Pediatrics, 14,* 592.

Livesay, S., Chrlich, S., Ryan, L., & Finnegan, L. (1989). Cocaine and pregnancy: Maternal and infant outcome. In D. E. Hutchings (Ed.), *Prenatal abuse of licit and illicit drugs: Annals of the New York Academy of Sciences* (Vol. 562, pp. 358–359). New York: New York Academy of Sciences.

Lynch, M., & McKeon, V. A. (1990). Cocaine use during pregnancy: Research findings and clinical implications. *Journal of Obstetric, Gynecologic and Neonatal Nursing, 19*(4), 285–292.

Madden, J. D., Payne, T. F., & Miller, S. (1986). Maternal cocaine abuse and effect on the newborn. *Pediatrics, 77*(2), 209–211.

Minkoff, H., Nanda, D., Menez, R., & Fikrig, S. (1987). Pregnancies resulting in infants with acquired immunodeficiency syndrome or AIDS-related complex. *Obstetrics and Gynecology, 69*(3), 285–287.

NAACOG (1989, October). Caring for cocaine's mothers and babies. *16*(10).

Ostrea, E. M., Jr., & Rammundo, A. L. (1989). Has cocaine abuse increased perinatal morbidity in maternal drug addiction? In D. E. Hutchings (Ed.), *Prenatal abuse of licit and illicit drugs: Annals of the New York Academy of Sciences* (Vol. 562, p. 376). New York: New York Academy of Sciences.

Rementeria, J. L. (1977). *Drug abuse in pregnancy and neonatal effects.* St. Louis, MO: C.V. Mosby Co.

Rodning, C., Beckwith, L., & Howard, J. (1989). Prenatal exposure to drugs and its influence on attachment. In D. E. Hutchings (Ed.), *Prenatal abuse of licit and illicit drugs: Annals of the New York Academy of Sciences* (Vol. 562, pp. 353–354). New York: New York Academy of Sciences.

Rosett, H. L., & Weiner, L. (1984). *Alcohol and the fetus: A clinical perspective.* New York: Oxford University Press.

Rosett, H. L., Weiner, L., & Edelin, K. (1981). *Obstetrics and Gynecology, 57,* 1–7.

Russell, M. (1985). Alcohol abuse and alcoholism in the pregnant woman: Identification and intervention. *Alcohol Health and Research World, 10*(1), 28–31, 74.

Skinner, K. S. (1990). Drug use: A step by step guide. *Nursing Management, 21*(6), 14–15.

Smith, J. (1988). The dangers of prenatal cocaine use. *American Journal of Maternal Child Nursing, 13,* 174–179.

Sobrian, S. K., Robinson, N. L., Burton, L. E., James, H., Stokes, D. L., & Turner, L. M. (1989). Neurobehavioral effects of prenatal exposure to cocaine. In D. E. Hutchings (Ed.), *Prenatal abuse of licit and illicit drugs: Annals of the New York Academy of Sciences* (Vol. 562, pp. 383–386). New York: New York Academy of Sciences.

Sokol, R. J., Miller, D. I., & Martier, S. (1983). Identifying the alcohol-abusing obstetrics-gynecologic patient: A practical approach. U.S. Department of Health and Human Services, National Institute on Alcohol Abuse and Alcoholism, DHH8 Publication No. (ADH) 81–1162, 1981.

Module II.1

Stimmel, B., Goldberg, J., Reisman, A., Murphy, R., & Teets, K. (1982–83). Fetal outcome in narcotic-dependent women: The importance of the type of maternal narcotic used. *American Journal of Drug and Alcohol Abuse, 9*(4), 383–395.

Stone, M., Salerno, L., & Green, M. (1971). Narcotic addiction in pregnancy. *American Journal of Obstetrics and Gynecology, 109,* 717.

Streissguth, A. P. (1983). Alcohol and pregnancy: An overview on an update. *Journal of Substance and Alcohol Actions/Misuse, 4,* 149–173.

Streissguth, A., & LaDue, R. (1985). Psychological and behavioral effects in children prenatally exposed to alcohol. *Alcohol Health and Research World, 10*(1), 6–12, 71–72.

Streissguth, A. P., Clarren, S. K., & Jones, D. L. (1985). Natural history of the fetal alcohol syndrome: A 10-year follow-up of 11 patients. *Alcohol Health and Research World, 10*(1), 13–19, 70, 73.

Vanderveen, E. (1989). Public Health policy: Maternal substance use and child health. In Hutchings, D. E., (Ed.), *Prenatal abuse of licit and illicit drugs, Annals of the New York Academy of Sciences* (Vol. 562, pp. 255–259). New York: New York Academy of Sciences.

Watson, B., & Fried, P. A. (1985). Maternal caffeine use before, during and after pregnancy and effects upon offspring. *Neurobehavioral Toxicology Teratology, 7*(1), 9–17.

Weiner, L., Rossett, H., & Mason, E. (1985). Training professionals to identify and treat pregnant women who drink heavily. *Alcohol, Health and Research World, 10,* 32.

MODULE II.2
IMPAIRED PRACTICE
BY HEALTH PROFESSIONALS

Madeline A. Naegle, PhD, RN, FAAN

Madeline A. Naegle, PhD, RN, FAAN
Project Director
Janet S. D'Arcangelo, MA, RN, C
Project Coordinator

Project SAEN
SUBSTANCE ABUSE
EDUCATION IN NURSING

CONTENT OUTLINE

I. Drug and Alcohol Use by Health Professionals
   A. Prevalence of the Problem
   B. Issues of Attitude and Accessibility
   C. Behaviors by the Employer and Coworkers Which Perpetuate Substance Abuse
   D. Health Professionals Who Receive Treatment and Return to Practice Have Good Prognoses for Recovery

II. Impaired Practice in the Work Place
   A. Definition and Signs
   B. Interventions with Nurses with Drug, Alcohol, and Psychiatric Problems

III. Legal/Regulatory Action
   A. Disciplinary Action
   B. Infraction of Laws Related to Drug Diversion
   C. Diversion Legislation
   D. Roles of State Boards for Nursing

IV. Ethical Aspects of Impaired Practice
   A. Provisions of Professional Codes
   B. Ethical Implications

V. Professional Organization Activity
   A. Policy Statements and Action by Professional Nursing Organizations
   B. Models of Peer Assistance Programs

VI. Employment-Based Resources to Assist the Practitioner with Drug, Alcohol, and Psychiatric Problems
   A. Employee Assistance Programs
   B. Mechanisms for Consultation and Referral
   C. In-Service Education
   D. Return to Work Contracts

Module II.2

CONTENTS

I. DRUG AND ALCOHOL USE BY HEALTH PROFESSIONALS

A. Prevalence of the Problem

Health professionals experience drug and alcohol dependence with a prevalence that is at least equal to, and may surpass, that of drug and alcohol problems in the general public.

1. Health professionals experience drug and alcohol problems at an incidence of 10–18% over a lifetime of professional practice.
2. Members of male-dominated professions become drug- and/or alcohol-dependent more frequently than women who are health professionals.
3. Health professionals are most frequently addicted to prescription drugs in combination with alcohol and illicit drugs.
4. An estimated 6–12% of nurses are addicted to alcohol and/or other drugs (ANA, 1987).
5. Recovering nurses report one or more drug dependent parents, dysfunctional family patterns, and a high incidence of incest and sexual molestation (Sullivan, 1987).
6. Nurses report a higher prevalence rate of depression than women in the general population (Van Servellen, Soccorso, Palermo & Faude, 1985).

B. Issues of Attitude and Accessibility

Attitudes on the parts of health professionals and the accessibility of drugs appear to support initiation of prescription drug abuse.

1. Nurses and others self-medicate for fatigue, chronic physical pain, or psychic pain.
2. In the education of the health care provider, information that attributes positive healing qualities to drugs is not balanced by an equal emphasis on education for risks of dependence.
3. Prescription availability decreases negative sanctions against misuse and abuse of prescription drugs.
4. In many settings, narcotics and analgesics are not adequately controlled and are therefore readily accessible to the practitioner.
5. Nurses espouse beliefs that emphasize the needs of others over personal needs and self-care.

C. Behaviors by the Employer and Coworkers Which Perpetuate Substance Abuse

1. Poor monitoring of pharmaceutical supplies and dispensation.
2. Infrequent job performance evaluations.
3. Positive peer sanctions for drug use.
4. Reluctance to give peer feedback.
5. Support of the nurse's denial.

Impaired Practice by Health Professionals

D. Health Professionals Who Receive Treatment and Return to Practice Have Good Prognoses for Recovery

1. Family and community support is usually extended to them.
2. When health professionals are able to return to work, financial resources are effective supports.
3. Employee benefits available to health professionals decrease problems of poverty and interruptions in continuation of care.
4. Peer assistance and regulatory agency monitoring provide positive reinforcement for the health professional's recovery efforts.

II. IMPAIRED PRACTICE IN THE WORK PLACE

A. Definition and Signs

1. Definition of impaired practice: Nursing practice is impaired when the individual is unable to meet the requirements of the professional codes of ethics and the standards of practice because cognitive, interpersonal, or psychomotor skills are affected by alcohol or other drug dependencies or psychiatric illness (ANA, 1984).
2. Signs suggesting drug and/or alcohol dependence and/or psychiatric illness commonly observed in the work place:
   a. Excessive and inadequately documented absenteeism.
   b. Lateness or long periods away from the job or unit.
   c. Poor job performance.
   d. Signs of psychomotor responses to drug intoxication or withdrawal; e.g., tremors, gait disturbance, poor handwriting.
   e. Signs of deterioration in personal health and grooming:
      (1) Poor hygiene.
      (2) Unkempt appearance.
      (3) Appearance of fatigue or lethargy.
      (4) Altered nutritional state: Undernourishment or obesity.
   f. Withdrawal or isolation from peers.
   g. Frequent interpersonal conflicts.

B. Interventions with Nurses with Drug, Alcohol, and Psychiatric Problems

1. Nurse administrators and/or other supervisory personnel are responsible for evaluating employee job performance; when questions arise as to the occurrence of impaired nursing practice, the first-line manager (i.e., head nurse or supervisor) should:
   a. Document observations of impaired job performance, episodes of illness, or failure to appear for work.

b. Meet with the employee to review the record of poor job performance.

c. Require that the employee seek consultation with the employee assistance program, private practitioner, health service, or clinic.

d. Require that clearance for readiness to work and positive health status be obtained in a given period of time (e.g., 1–2 weeks) in order for the nurse/health professional to return to work.

e. Evaluate the potential to support a medical leave of absence to seek treatment, if consultation indicates the need.

2. If the nurse/health care provider refuses to comply with administrative requests, an *intervention* may be planned. Intervention is accomplished in the following steps:

a. Organize documentation of impaired practice.

b. Obtain support and participation of peers, supervisors or others who have observed the employee/nurse practicing while impaired.

c. Meet with the nurse and a person he/she identifies as a source of support.

d. Clearly outline actions requested of the nurse.

e. Clearly outline steps which the employing agency is willing to undertake regarding leave of absence, continued benefits, and return to work.

III. LEGAL/REGULATORY ACTION

A. Disciplinary Action

1. Legal provisions which describe and provide for dealing with nurses manifesting drug, alcohol, or psychiatric problems vary from state to state and are prescribed by state law.

2. Such laws designate which state agency will investigate and discipline licensed health care professionals when impaired practice occurs; e.g., rehabilitative versus punitive treatment of nurses with addiction or psychiatric diagnoses.

3. Disciplinary action may result in censure, probation, or license revocation. Some states have developed legislation which allows the licensed professional to voluntarily surrender licensure for a designated period of treatment time. This legislation is called "diversion legislation" because the individual bypasses the usual disciplinary process.

B. Infraction of Laws Related to Drug Diversion

1. Local, state, or federal agencies gather data and investigate drug diversion, and legal charges are brought, dependent on:

a. Extent of loss.

b. Action by institution.

c. Sale of drugs to others.

d. Harm to patients.

Impaired Practice by Health Professionals

C. Diversion Legislation

1. "Diversion legislation" provides for a monitored program whereby the practitioner who is experiencing a drug, alcohol, or psychiatric problem can voluntarily surrender his or her license during the period of time required for treatment and rehabilitation.

    a. The program requires certain components for monitoring, such as body fluids analysis and periodic written reports.

    b. Acceptance by the program means that the practitioner will not have his or her nursing license acted upon in the usual disciplinary process.

    c. Acceptance in a diversion program does not protect the practitioner from prosecution for charges related to drug diversion or patient harm.

2. Diversion legislation has been passed in at least five states.

D. Roles of State Boards for Nursing

1. State Boards for Nursing oversee the conduct of investigations of charges of impaired nursing practice.

    a. Charges are filed with the State Board for Nursing.

    b. Members of the board hold hearings and organize data.

    c. The state board may be responsible for decisions regarding censure, suspension, or revocation of the nurse's license, or may forward recommendations to a higher authority in the state.

    d. State boards maintain data on disciplinary action which is available for statistical purposes and is often communicated to the National Council of State Boards for Nursing for use when nurses apply for licensure in other states.

2. Some State Boards for Nursing maintain programs through which they monitor recovering nurses on their compliance with prescribed treatment regimens and restrictions on work activities.

IV. ETHICAL ASPECTS OF IMPAIRED PRACTICE

A. Provisions of Professional Codes

1. Ethical codes of professions and professional organizations, including the ANA Code, mandate that health professionals seek to do good, prevent harm, and protect the public from incompetent or unsafe practitioners.

B. Ethical Implications

1. Ethical guidelines identify the rights of the impaired practitioner (ANA, 1984).

2. Ethical obligations are met when the practitioner utilizes available resources to assist in the solution of a problem, thereby protecting the consumer as well as halting the deterioration of nursing standards.

Module II.2

V. PROFESSIONAL ORGANIZATION ACTIVITY

A. Policy Statements and Action by Professional Nursing Organizations

1. The American Nurses' Association and specialty nursing organizations, such as the National Nurses' Society on Addictions, have developed policy statements and established educational initiatives on impaired nursing practice and/or the impaired nurse.

2. These statements include the rights of the nurse to fair treatment, confidentiality, and the right to work.

3. Statements define the appropriate use of urinalysis in relation to substance use.

4. Outreach by recovering nurses is advocated by professional organizations and consists of nurse-organized efforts.

5. The National Council of State Boards for Nursing outlines approaches to interventions in impaired nursing practice and provisions for State Board of Nursing action.

B. Models of Peer Assistance Programs

1. State nurses' associations have developed models of peer assistance, including committees on impaired nursing practice, peer assistance programs, and programs of education, consultation, and referral, to assist nurses experiencing addictive and psychiatric problems.

    a. Peer assistance programs provide referral and consultation services; some may monitor recovering nurses.

    b. Some peer assistance programs provide outreach, including visiting individuals in need of treatment and supporting their entry to treatment, and participation in interventions by employers and family members.

    c. Peer assistance programs are financed by contributions to a foundation, by portions of dues payments identified for peer assistance, and by state nurses' association staff and services.

    d. Such programs provide alternatives to disciplinary action by offering nurses the option of seeking treatment prior to being reported.

    e. Program members may advocate for the nurse in various capacities.

2. Support groups of recovering nurses are often sponsored by state or district nurses' associations or are freestanding. They are a useful resource for education and peer support.

    a. Support groups serve as adjuncts to aftercare. Twelve Step programs exist in most regions. 12–Step programs include Alcoholics Anonymous (A.A.), Narcotics Anonymous (N.A.), Al-Anon, Adult Children of Alcoholics (A.C.O.A.).

    b. Support groups may be composed exclusively of nurses or mixed groups of health professionals.

    c. Support groups are self-help efforts dependent on the efforts of participants. They are not considered treatment as they are voluntary and conducted by the members.

VI. EMPLOYMENT-BASED RESOURCES TO ASSIST THE PRACTITIONER WITH DRUG, ALCOHOL, AND PSYCHIATRIC PROBLEMS

Resources within the agency or institution assist nurses, coworkers, and employers in addressing impaired practice and related job performance and health issues.

A. Employee Assistance Programs

1. Employee Assistance Programs (EAPs) are organized systems, with trained personnel and established protocols, directed toward the identification of, intervention for, and motivation of the employee who needs to seek professional help.

2. Employee Assistance Programs offer health screening, counseling of the employee and family members, and referral for all categories of health care workers.

3. The health care industry has lagged behind other industries in developing Employee Assistance Programs.

4. Hospitals and academic institutions without Employee Assistance Programs use health services and mental health programs to provide counseling, monitoring, and referrals of nurses and nurse educators experiencing or recovering from alcohol and/or drug dependencies and psychiatric problems.

B. Mechanisms for Consultation and Referral

1. When organized employer-based services are not available, employers can utilize consultation and referral to external agencies, independent care providers, or treatment facilities as a means of assisting the nurse.

2. Consultation and referral services are available through state nurses' associations and community agencies.

C. In-Service Education

1. Education and staff development programs assist nurses and other health care providers to:

    a. Identify risk factors and problems in themselves, family members, and coworkers.

    b. Learn about health and health promotion.

    c. Learn ways to utilize resources within their institutions, communities, and professional organizations.

    d. Understand and promote workplace efforts and modifications to prevent substance dependence in employees and support the nurse returning to work.

D. Return to Work Contracts

1. Employer/employee contracts structure the mutual expectations for nurse and employer.

Module II.2

2. Institutional policies on the management of impaired practice should be reflected in the return to work contract:

   a. Restrictions on work functions and hours should be identified.

   b. Position statements on body fluid analysis methods and agreements should be described.

   c. Conditions of continuing employment, e.g., one relapse, no relapses, should be described.

   d. Individuals and mechanisms for coordinating information and monitoring compliance with treatment for the recovering individual should be identified.

   e. Motivating a person to seek treatment can emerge from prevention, outreach, and education programs. Peers and employers should be alert to signs in the workplace that individuals are experiencing problems.

MODULE II.2
IMPAIRED PRACTICE
BY HEALTH PROFESSIONALS

INSTRUCTOR'S GUIDE

Madeline A. Naegle, PhD, RN, FAAN

Madeline A. Naegle, PhD, RN, FAAN
Project Director
Janet S. D'Arcangelo, MA, RN, C
Project Coordinator

Project SAEN
SUBSTANCE ABUSE
EDUCATION IN NURSING

CONTENTS

Component	Page
Module Description	130
Time Frame	130
Placement	130
Learner Objectives	131
Recommended Readings	132
Faculty Readings	132
Student Readings	132
Recommended Audiovisual and Other Resources	133
Overhead Masters	134
Handout Masters	141
Recommended Teaching Strategies and Sample Assignments	211
Test Questions and Answers	213
Bibliography	217

Module II.2

MODULE DESCRIPTION

This module provides an overview of impaired professional practice among health professionals. Relevance of the problem in nursing, medicine, and other health professions, identification and intervention techniques, and legal and ethical implications are presented.

TIME FRAME

3 hours

PLACEMENT

Co-Requisite with Professional Role Courses

Instructor's Guide

LEARNER OBJECTIVES

Upon successful completion of this module, the learner will:

1. List signs that indicate that work performance may be impaired due to the use of alcohol and/or drugs or psychiatric illness.
2. Describe patterns of drug/alcohol dependence common among health professionals.
3. Identify factors specific to the work setting which relate to health and contribute to substance abuse among health professionals.
4. List the key components of intervention with practitioners whose practice is impaired.
5. Describe legal regulatory methods to address impaired practice.
6. Describe ethical aspects of intervention with impaired practitioners.
7. List resources for practitioners, administrators, employers, and family members addressing drug/alcohol dependence in others.
8. List voluntary professional organization activities in relation to impaired practice.
9. Describe implications for the recovering professional on returning to the workplace.

Module II.2

RECOMMENDED READINGS

FACULTY READINGS

Cannon, B. L., & Brown, J. S. (1988, Summer). Nurses' attitudes toward impaired colleagues. *Image: Journal of Nursing Scholarship, 20,* 96–101.

Haack, M., & Hughes, T. (Eds.). (1987). *Addiction in the nursing profession: Approaches to intervention and recovery.* New York: Springer Publishing Co.

Stafen, R. R., & Farley, B. P. (1989). The use of group therapy for assisting the recovery and reentry of impaired nurses. In M. Haack & T. Hughes (Eds.), *Addiction in the nursing profession: Approaches to intervention and recovery* (pp. 113–128). New York: Springer Publishing Co.

Sullivan, E. J., Bissell, L., & Williams, E. (1987). *Chemical dependency in nursing: The deadly diversion.* Redwood City, CA: Addison-Wesley Publishing, Inc.

Veatch, D. (1987). When is the recovering impaired nurse ready to work? *Journal of Nursing Administration, 17*(2), 14–16.

STUDENT READINGS

Connell, C. C., & Murphy, J. F. (1987). New dimensions of regulating the practice of professional nursing. *Nursing Management, 18*(8), 62–64.

Cross, L. (1985). Chemical dependency in our ranks: Managing a nurse in crisis. *Nursing Management, 16*(11), 15–16.

Floyd, J. (1991). Nursing students' stress levels, attitudes toward drugs, and drug use. *Archives of Psychiatric Nursing, V*(1), 46–53.

Hutchinson, S. A. (1987, November/December). Toward self-integration: The recovery process of chemically dependent nurses. *Nursing Research, 36*(6), 339–343.

Moore, G., & Hogan, R. L. (1987). Substance abuse and the nurse: A legal and ethical dilemma. *Journal of Professional Nursing, 3*(1), 5–9.

Naegle, M. A. (1989). Patterns and implications of drug use by students of nursing. *Imprint, 36*(2), 85, 87–88.

RECOMMENDED AUDIOVISUAL AND OTHER RESOURCES

AUDIOVISUAL RESOURCES

1. **Impaired Nursing Practice: Assessment and Intervention**

   Describes the phenomenon and steps taken to address it by professional nursing organizations. 28 minutes. **Available from American Journal of Nursing Company, Educational Services Division/E49, 555 West 57th Street, New York, New York 10019-2961.** Videocassette #7089V rental ($60) or #7809S sale ($275).

2. **Managing Job-Related Stress**

   Emphasizes ways to prevent stress and to provide support for employees. 30 minutes. **Available from American Journal of Nursing Company, Educational Services Division/E49, 555 West 57th Street, New York, New York 10019-2961.** Film rental ($60) or sale ($350). Videocassette rental ($60) or sale ($250).

Module II.2

OVERHEAD MASTERS

MODULE II.2 IMPAIRED PRACTICE BY HEALTH PROFESSIONALS

1. Reentry Issues for the Nurse
2. Professional Factors Related to Reentry
3. Nurses' Rights in Relation to Impaired Practice

Instructor's Guide

Module II.2—Overhead #1

REENTRY ISSUES FOR THE NURSE

A. Successful Negotiation of Treatment and Progress Toward Recovery.

B. Continuing Treatment.

C. Action for Licensure Reinstatement, if Necessary.

D. Negotiation of an Employment Contract with Employing Institution:

    1. Agreement with contract stipulations.

    2. Plans for the monitoring of compliance with employment provisions:

        a. Physical exams.

        b. Random body fluid analysis.

    3. Periodic job performance evaluations.

E. Involvement with Peer Assistance Program or Peer Support Network or Group.

F. Option to Utilize Employee Benefits for Treatment/Hospitalization as Necessary.

G. Documentation and Communication with Regulatory Agencies as Required.

Instructor's Guide

Module II.2—Overhead #2

PROFESSIONAL FACTORS RELATED TO REENTRY

A. Ability to Function According to the Provisions of the Nurse Practice Act.

B. Recognition of Need for Employment Contract.

C. Ability to Meet Role-Specific Standards of Practice.

D. Utilization of the Supervisory Relationship.

E. Identification of Work-Related Stress Factors.

F. Willingness to Modify Career Goals to Facilitate Job Placement.

G. Knowledge and Acceptance of Ethical Constraints.

Module II.2—Overhead #3

NURSES' RIGHTS IN RELATION TO IMPAIRED PRACTICE

A. Recognition as an Individual with a Disease: Importance of Assigning and Assuming the Sick Role.

B. Referral to Comprehensive Treatment Programs.

C. Confidentiality and Protection from Slander and Stigmatic Behavior.

D. Appraisal of Legal Rights Regarding Self-Incriminating Testimony.

E. Benefits and Health Provisions, Including Disability, Accorded Other Diseases.

Instructor's Guide

HANDOUT MASTERS

MODULE II.2 IMPAIRED PRACTICE BY HEALTH PROFESSIONALS

1. A Technique for Intervention and Confrontation of Substance Abusers
2. Relationship Between Alcohol Abuse and Employee Behaviors
3. Assessment Tools
4. Return to Work Contracts
5. Resources/Groups for the Impaired Health Professional
6. New York State Nurses Association, Council on Nursing Practice: *Position Statement on Drug Testing of Professional Nurses*
7. New York State Nurses Association, Task Force on Alcohol and Substance Abuse in the Profession of Nursing: *Concepts of Peer Assistance* (7A), Interventions in the Work Place (7B), Peer Intervention Assistance (7C)
8. American Nurses' Association: *Supplement to Addictions and Psychological Dysfunctions in Nursing: The Profession's Response to the Problem*

Contents	160
Program Activities of State Nurses' Associations, Constituents of the American Nurses' Association	161
State Boards of Nursing	189
Specialty Nursing Groups	194
Agencies and Professional Groups	195

9. State Nurses' Associations—Peer Assistance Activities Overview
10. Guidelines for Developing a Hospital-Based Employee Assistance Program (10 A–R)

Module II.2

Module II.2—Handout #1

A TECHNIQUE FOR INTERVENTION AND CONFRONTATION OF SUBSTANCE ABUSERS

The concept behind the intervention technique is that the substance habituation is usually a progressive illness and very rarely goes into remission without outside help. The following technique is only one of several approaches.

1. **Three Key Attitudes for Intervention**

    a. Express genuine concern.

    b. Maintain a non-judgmental approach.

    c. Be honest.

2. **Goals of an Intervention**

    The goal of the intervention is to bring the substance-abusing person into treatment by using a dramatic confrontation to help penetrate his or her denial mechanism.

3. **The Team Approach**

    In most cases, the family and/or friends have previously tried unsuccessfully to get the chemically dependent person to cut down or to stop chemical use; usually these attempts have failed because:

    a. The approach was made in an inflammatory and accusatory fashion that placed the chemically dependent person on the defensive and only increased the denial mechanism.

    b. These concerned persons were uninformed about the diagnosis and proper treatment of chemical dependency.

    c. Each attempt was made at a different time. Consequently, the chemically dependent person was able to use his denial mechanism in an effective manner and, at times, an available "enabler" may have helped him to further resist help; e.g., after his wife threw him out of the house, his mother took him in. This type of person is called an "enabler" because such relatives or friends "enable" the chemically dependent person to continue the pattern of abuse; without the "enabler" the substance abuser may be forced to stop.

4. **Techniques**

    a. A concerned person seeks help for a problem related to the chemical dependency of the person he or she cares about. (The concerned person is usually a spouse but may be a child, employer, or friend.) Keep the process in the open and have the spouse inform the substance abuser about the meetings. Be sure the substance abuser is

Instructor's Guide

Module II.2—Handout #1 *(continued)*

       informed that the therapist (not the concerned person) has invited the participants. This procedure describes the reality of the situation and directs the anger away from the concerned person.

  b. This person is enlisted to gather other significant persons into a meeting about the intervention process. This group will be organized into an intervention team.

  c. Team members are educated about the chemical dependency, the treatment, and the intervention process (discussion of the denial or sincere self-deception of the substance abuser, symptoms of the illness, prognosis, and so on).

  d. Each team member is asked to make a list of three to five significant events in the relationship in which he or she was hurt in some way by the chemically dependent person. The lists should be specific as to time, place, and circumstances and non-judgmental, without using labels, just detailed descriptions and reactions to the behavior.

  e. Each event should be presented in a non-judgmental way, emphasizing the connection between the use of chemicals and the event; e.g., "You came late to my school play. You were drinking and made a scene in the audience. The principal finally asked you to leave. I was *so* embarrassed, Dad." Note that the statements should include the team member's feelings: "I felt helpless, scared, frustrated, angry," etc.

  f. All team members are cautioned to temporarily suspend past quarrels among themselves for the benefit of the team effort. It is important to present a united front with a consistent message: "We are concerned about your drinking (or drug-taking) and its effect on your behavior. We can no longer stand helplessly in the wings while you destroy yourself and us. You need treatment."

  g. A chairperson is selected to serve as coordinator, keeping the team together and on target. This person may be a professional in the field of alcoholism, a physician, or one of the interveners; i.e., spouse, brother, employer, or neighbor.

  h. If some members of the team feel unable to carry out their roles, they are encouraged to share that feeling and exclude themselves from the intervention. They may plan with the team how they will be involved in the future.

  i. Treatment options are discussed, selected, and arranged prior to the intervention.

5. **Commitment of the Team**

  a. If the chemically dependent person rejects the intervention team (this is rare), the team must be ready to assert itself by honestly stating what is at stake if there is no treatment.

  b. Each team member must have thought out what he or she is prepared to do if the person refuses to see the therapist. The power of this strategy is consolidating all of the consequences into a single time frame and making it very clear that the only remedy is treatment as defined by the team (e.g., "If you refuse to see Dr. _____, you can't come home.").

Module II.2—Handout #1 *(continued)*

  c. Each team member must be ready to present the ultimatum in a clear and unyielding fashion. If a team member falters on the commitment, the team must rally to hold that member to the commitment. Because of this possibility, it is very important that "b" is carefully thought out and understood by all team members. Rash but empty threats will be of no use in the intervention process. These threats only increase the denial mechanism.

6. Rehearsal

Having reviewed the above material and prepared their lists of "significant events," the team stages a practice session of the intervention. This is helpful in:

a. Identifying unexpected problems.

b. Enhancing the ability to be concise and work together.

c. Exploring resistance.

d. Increasing the confidence of the treatment team.

In summary, the intervention technique attempts to telescope or compress the events associated with substance abuse into an early therapeutic confrontation in order to precipitate a crisis in the present rather than waiting for years of suffering to take place and risking the future loss of family, job, or other important life factors.

Modified by Dr. Donald Gallant of the Tulane University School of Medicine from a handout by Dr. Michael Liepman of the University of Michigan Medical School. Copyright 1981 by Michael Liepman.

Instructor's Guide

Module II.2—Handout #2

RELATIONSHIP BETWEEN ALCOHOL ABUSE AND EMPLOYEE BEHAVIORS

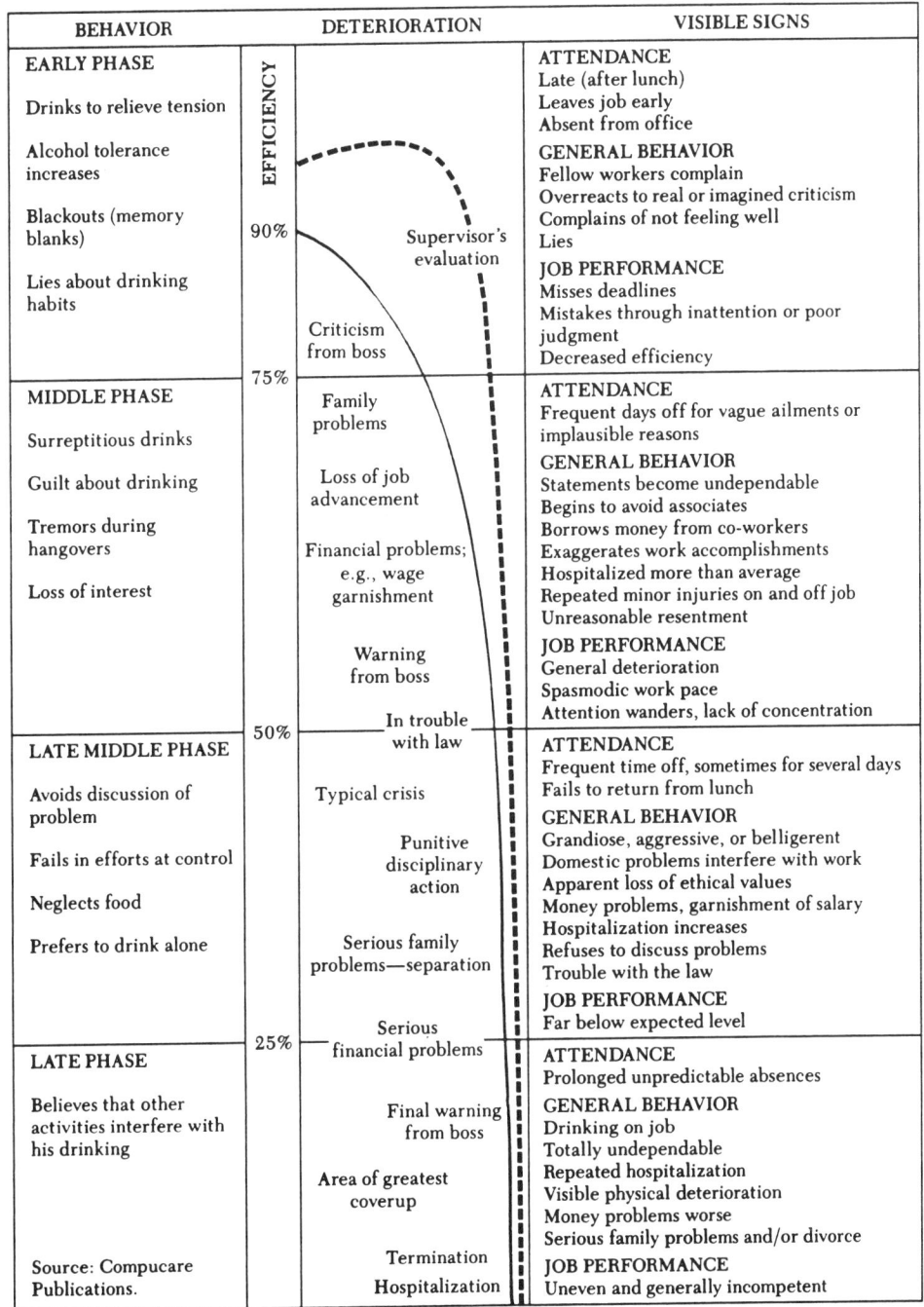

BEHAVIOR	DETERIORATION		VISIBLE SIGNS
EARLY PHASE Drinks to relieve tension Alcohol tolerance increases Blackouts (memory blanks) Lies about drinking habits	EFFICIENCY 90% 75%	Supervisor's evaluation Criticism from boss	**ATTENDANCE** Late (after lunch) Leaves job early Absent from office **GENERAL BEHAVIOR** Fellow workers complain Overreacts to real or imagined criticism Complains of not feeling well Lies **JOB PERFORMANCE** Misses deadlines Mistakes through inattention or poor judgment Decreased efficiency
MIDDLE PHASE Surreptitious drinks Guilt about drinking Tremors during hangovers Loss of interest	50%	Family problems Loss of job advancement Financial problems; e.g., wage garnishment Warning from boss In trouble with law	**ATTENDANCE** Frequent days off for vague ailments or implausible reasons **GENERAL BEHAVIOR** Statements become undependable Begins to avoid associates Borrows money from co-workers Exaggerates work accomplishments Hospitalized more than average Repeated minor injuries on and off job Unreasonable resentment **JOB PERFORMANCE** General deterioration Spasmodic work pace Attention wanders, lack of concentration
LATE MIDDLE PHASE Avoids discussion of problem Fails in efforts at control Neglects food Prefers to drink alone	25%	Typical crisis Punitive disciplinary action Serious family problems—separation Serious financial problems	**ATTENDANCE** Frequent time off, sometimes for several days Fails to return from lunch **GENERAL BEHAVIOR** Grandiose, aggressive, or belligerent Domestic problems interfere with work Apparent loss of ethical values Money problems, garnishment of salary Hospitalization increases Refuses to discuss problems Trouble with the law **JOB PERFORMANCE** Far below expected level
LATE PHASE Believes that other activities interfere with his drinking Source: Compucare Publications.		Final warning from boss Area of greatest coverup Termination Hospitalization	**ATTENDANCE** Prolonged unpredictable absences **GENERAL BEHAVIOR** Drinking on job Totally undependable Repeated hospitalization Visible physical deterioration Money problems worse Serious family problems and/or divorce **JOB PERFORMANCE** Uneven and generally incompetent

From: Lawrence, C., Jr. (1983, October 24). As workers get high, so do prices. *The Miami Herald*, C-1.

Module II.2—Handout #3

ASSESSMENT TOOLS

A. **Assessment Tools**

   Have you ever:

   - Avoided initiating discussion about drinking or drug-abusing behavior when a particular coworker was around?
   - Not followed up on a report that a coworker was drinking too much or abusing drugs?
   - Tolerated or covered up for a coworker's behavior when you thought it was alcohol- or drug-related?
   - Been uncomfortable when coworkers discussed drinking or drug use at work?

   If you answer "yes" to any of the above questions, you may wish to use the resources in this guide for assisting a coworker to get help.

B. **Self-Assessment Tool**

   - Did you drink any alcoholic beverage during the past 24 hours?
   - Have you ever wondered if you drink too much?
   - Do you ever drink more than you intend?
   - Do you crave a drink at a definite time?
   - Do you like to or often drink alone?
   - Does your drinking bother your family or friends?
   - Have you ever decided to quit drinking for a while or cut down on your drinking?
   - Have you ever used sleeping pills, tranquilizers, or other drugs?
   - Have you used medication(s) for such problems as back pain, anxiety, depression, fatigue, or weight loss?
   - Are you taking or do you have more than one medication for these problems?
   - Have drinking or medications ever made you careless about your clients'/patients' welfare or your nursing responsibilities?
   - Are you harder to get along with since drinking or taking medications?

   If you answer "yes" to three or more of these questions, there is a good possibility that alcoholism or addiction may be present.

Instructor's Guide

Module II.2—Handout #4

RETURN TO WORK CONTRACTS

The use of Return to Work Contracts is designed to establish a set of conditions for an employee returning to work following treatment for alcoholism or other substance abuse. Generally, such agreements are negotiated among the employer, the treatment provider, the employee, and when applicable, the collective bargaining agent. These agreements have been useful in defining the employee's responsibilities, especially during early recovery, for maintaining those activities, relationships, and therapeutic follow-up deemed necessary for sustained abstinence.

Return to Work Contracts may include restrictions about areas of practice or hours of practice in order to avoid situations that increase the risk of relapse. In determining the elements that should be included in such a contract, individual circumstances must be considered. Consultation with the treatment provider should also be sought. On the following page is a sample of a Return to Work Contract that includes the elements most often included in such agreements. This is offered merely as a sample and should be modified to meet specific institutional and individual needs.

Module II.2—Handout #4 *(continued)*

A SAMPLE OF A RETURN TO WORK CONTRACT

Case No. _____ Date: _____

This agreement is executed in connection with the undersigned licensed nurse's participation in the _____ (*Employer*) Program for Impaired Nurses and the _____ (*Treatment Program*). It is the purpose of this Agreement to prevent any misunderstanding as to the terms and time specified. This agreement is specifically designed to meet the needs of the facility and the individual and is uniquely adapted to the recovering individual.

I, _____ (*Nurse*), enter into this agreement on the above date with _____ (*Employer*) and the _____ (*Treatment Program*).

In consideration of my being permitted to continue in or return to the employ of _____ (*Employer*), I agree to the Terms and Conditions set out in this Agreement. I understand that the Employer agrees to employ me only on these terms and conditions and that failure to comply with the terms of this Agreement shall be grounds for either additional disciplinary action or possible termination.

I understand that my failure to meet the Terms and Conditions set out in the Agreement violates the terms of my participation in the Program for Impaired Nurses.

The Terms and Conditions of this Agreement shall remain in force for a period of two (2) years from the above date but are subject to modification if the Employer, in its sole discretion, decides such modification is in the best interest of the Nurse's rehabilitation or necessary to protect the health and safety of clients/patients. I understand and agree that this Agreement does not obligate the Employer to employ me for a two (2) year period and that, except as provided in the Agreement, I am employed on the same terms and conditions as the Employer's other employees.

This Agreement consists of this page plus the attached Terms and Conditions for Return to Work, each page of which is initialed by the undersigned parties.

Any modification of the printed terms of the Agreement must be approved by _____ (*Employer*) and the undersigned nurse.

Executed on the date shown above.

Employee's Name	Employee's License Number
Supervisor's Name	Supervisor's Title
Counselor's Name (*Treatment Prog.*)	Counselor's Title
Nurse's Advocate	

Module II.2—Handout #4 *(continued)*

TERMS AND CONDITIONS OF
RETURN TO WORK AGREEMENT

Section 1: General Provisions

1.1 I agree to abstain completely from mood-changing chemicals except as prescribed by my primary physician, to notify my Employer of such prescriptions, and to provide Employer with such documentation as may be required to verify a prescription.

1.2 I agree to use as my primary physician the physician identified below, who I believe is thoroughly knowledgeable about chemical dependency, and to inform him/her of all aspects of my chemical dependency. I further agree to his/her receiving a copy of this agreement and to his/her consulting with my Employer about my chemical dependency and rehabilitation.

Name: _____

Street: _____

City: _____ Zip: _____

Phone—Work: _____ Home: _____

1.3 I agree to provide random urine/blood samples for drug screens obtained in the presence of a qualified witness at the discretion of the Employer. Such screens shall occur a minimum of once every _____ for the first ninety (90) days, and once every _____ for the second ninety (90) days of this Agreement, and as required by Employer and Treatment Center after that. Employer agrees to be responsible for the production of the specimen and maintaining chain of custody. The costs of the laboratory tests shall be the responsibility of _____ (Nurse/Employer). Positive urine will be cause for immediate assessment by supervisor, Director of Nursing, and myself. Relapse, a hallmark of chemical dependency, may or may not necessarily result in termination.

1.4 I agree to execute any consent forms and/or medication authorization forms required for Employer and Treatment Center to obtain information and records needed to monitor my compliance with this Agreement.

Case No.: _____ Nurse: _____

Date: _____ Employer: _____

Modification Approved: _____

1.5 I understand and agree that all expenses associated with my treatment and rehabilitation, except as otherwise provided by this Agreement, are my sole responsibility, and the Employer assumes no responsibility for such expenses.

Module II.2—Handout #4 *(continued)*

1.6 I understand that my continued employment depends not only on meeting the terms of this Agreement but also on satisfactory performance of my job. Employer will monitor my job performance and an unsatisfactory performance evaluation may be grounds for my termination consistent with the general employment criteria for all employees.

1.7 I understand the responsibilities of my job and am capable of meeting those responsibilities. I agree to notify Employer if at any time I believe I am not capable of performing any of my required job functions.

1.8 Employer agrees to maintain this Agreement and other information relating to my chemical dependency in a confidential file separate from my personnel records. If I successfully complete this Agreement, Employer agrees to expunge this Agreement and all other reference to my chemical dependency from its employment records. This paragraph does not preclude Employer from making an appropriate entry in my personnel file, if I am terminated or disciplined because of relapse of a drug-related incident.

Case No.: _____   Nurse: _____

Date: _____   Employer: _____

Modification Approved: _____

Nurse Advocate: _____

Instructor's Guide

Module II.2—Handout #4 *(continued)*

Section 2: Restrictions on Practice

2.1 Experience of recovering nurses indicates that the successful recovering nurse's return to practice needs to be in a work environment supportive to recovery. The restrictions set out below are ones that have proven to be the most successful in providing this support.

2.2 The parties agree to the following restrictions. Each restriction should be initialed by the parties to indicate acceptance.

Restrictions	Initials		
	Emplr.	Nurse	Conslt.
1. Day shift is preferred, but 3–11 shift is acceptable based on careful evaluation of the circumstances; i.e., staffing patterns, familiarity of coworkers on the shift with the nurse's dependency, availability of daytime support/group/therapy/aftercare meetings. Nurse will not work 11–7 shift for minimum of one year.			
2. Shift rotation will not be permitted; i.e., must work the same shift, either days or evenings, continually for one year.			
3. Nurse will work only on regularly assigned, identified, and predetermined units and will not be used for coverage on other units (e.g., "PRN" or "floating") for one year. It is preferred that staff on unit be knowledgeable and willing to work with a recovering nurse.			
4. Nurse will not work any overtime or on-call assignments for first six months. After six months, overtime and on-call assignments must be mutually agreed upon by employer, consultant, and nurse.			
5. Nurse agrees not to work for multiple employers for one year.			
6. Nurse will not do private duty nursing nor engage in any type of self-employed practice for one year.			
7. Nurse will not accept employment with temporary or supplementary agencies/registries/services, home health care, or other isolated areas of practice for one year.			
8. Nurse will not have access to mood-altering medications during first six months. Access to mood-altering medications after the first six months will occur only as mutually agreed upon by nurse, employer, and consultant. In certain cases where handling of narcotics cannot be avoided, the nurse must be on Trexan and monitored for compliance in use.			

Case No.: _____

Date: _____

Modification Approved: _____

Nurse: _____

Employer: _____

Nurse Advocate: _____

Module II.2—Handout #5

RESOURCES/GROUPS FOR
THE IMPAIRED HEALTH PROFESSIONAL

Do It Now Foundation
P.O. Box #21126
Phoenix, Arizona 85036

Drug and Alcohol Nursing Association
113 West Franklin Street
Baltimore, Maryland 21201

Drug-Anon Focus
P.O. Box #9108
Long Island City, New York 11103

Drugs Anonymous
P.O. Box #473, Ansonia Station
New York, New York 10023

Hazelden Foundation
Box #11
Center City, Minnesota 55012

Impaired Physician Program
(*Alcohol abuse*)
938 Peachtree Street, N.E.
Atlanta, Georgia 30309

International Advisory Council
for Homosexual Men and Women in Alcoholics Anonymous
P.O. Box #90
Washington, D.C. 20044

Narcotics Anonymous
P.O. Box #9999
Van Nuys, California 91409

Narcotics Education, Inc.
6830 Laurel Street, NW
Washington, D.C. 20012

National Association for Children of Alcoholics
31706 Coast Highway
Suite #201
South Laguna, California 92677

National Black Alcoholism Council
417 South Dearborn Street
Suite #700
Chicago, Illinois 60605

Instructor's Guide

Module II.2—Handout #6

THE NEW YORK STATE NURSES ASSOCIATION
COUNCIL ON NURSING PRACTICE

POSITION STATEMENT ON
DRUG TESTING OF PROFESSIONAL NURSES

OVERVIEW: In response to numerous requests from the professional nursing community in New York State, the Council on Nursing Practice, in collaboration with the Council on Ethical Practice and the Task Force on Alcohol and Substance Abuse in the Profession of Nursing, offers the following opinion and these recommendations regarding drug testing of professional nurses in the workplace.

PREMISE: The Council bases this opinion on the New York State Nurse Practice Act, the ANA Code for Nurses, ANA's "Statement on Drug Testing for Health Care Workers," the 1985 NYS Impaired Professionals Law, and existing NYS regulations which address the health screening of employees (NYCRR, Chapter 5, 405.21).

RATIONALE: The abuse of alcohol and other substances among health care workers is an unfortunate but real health problem. Professional nurses who abuse alcohol and/or other drugs endanger their own well-being as well as the health and safety of the consumer. Measures taken to address this problem must provide protection and assistance for professional nurses as well as promote the safe delivery of health care.

The ANA Code for Nurses requires the professional nurse to safeguard the client from harm, to assume responsibility and accountability for all of her/his actions, to maintain competency, and to participate in the profession's efforts to establish and maintain conditions of employment conducive to the delivery of high-quality nursing care.

In New York State, the Regent's Rules on Unprofessional Conduct (Section 29.1), the General Provisions for the Health Professions (Section 29.2), and Title VIII of the Education Law (Article 130, Subsections 3 and 4) address the state's concern with the unprofessional conduct of a licensee. The NYS Impaired Professionals Law (1985) provides a system which encourages a licensed health care professional to voluntarily surrender her/his license while undergoing rehabilitation for alcohol or other substance abuse.

NYSNA's Task Force on Alcohol and Substance Abuse in the Profession of Nursing has identified a three-fold responsibility for the professional association regarding the issue of drug testing:

1. To safeguard quality of patient care.

2. To provide and promote education, consultation, guidance, and assistance so that professional nurses can obtain appropriate treatment and regain health.

3. To promote self-regulation by the members of the profession.

Module II.2

Module II.2—Handout #6 *(continued)*

In addition, the Task Force believes that the workplace provides an ideal setting for early intervention with employees who are affected by health problems, including the diseases of alcohol and drug abuse. This belief is expanded in NYSNA's document, "Guidelines for Developing a Hospital-Based Employee Assistance Program."

OPINION: The Council on Nursing Practice endorses the American Nurses' Association's "Statement on Drug Testing for Health Care Workers." The Council supports such a practice when it is based on objective evidence that job performance is or has been impaired by alcohol or other drug usage. However, the Council opposes random screening of body fluids of health care workers for alcohol or other drugs.

RECOMMENDATIONS: The Council strongly suggests that any drug-testing program of professional nurses by employing facilities include the following recommendations. These recommendations suggest actions which acknowledge the rights and responsibilities of employees and employers.

An employer or employing agency should:

1. Prior to any testing, advise employees or potential employees, in writing, if they are classified in "sensitive positions" which are subject to drug testing.

2. Provide a policy statement regarding the employer's position when job performance is affected by alcohol or other drug usage. This information should be included in the employee policy manual, prominently displayed for employee information, and clearly stated on the employment application.

Instructor's Guide

Module II.2—Handout #7A

NEW YORK STATE NURSES ASSOCIATION
TASK FORCE ON ALCOHOL AND SUBSTANCE ABUSE IN THE PROFESSION OF NURSING

CONCEPTS OF PEER ASSISTANCE

Introduction

Peer assistance describes those activities of professional colleagues which are directed toward providing help to chemically dependent colleagues through personal relationships or within formal structures. Formal structures include organized programs, peer support groups, and professional networks. Both informal and professional contacts or networking channels within institutions also provide avenues for peer assistance.

Peer assistance activities demonstrate accountability within the nursing profession for the maintenance of high levels of standards of professional practice. Activities with Constituent District Associations and the state nurses association serve to uphold the responsibilities of the profession to ensure quality care to the consumer. Professional self-regulation includes accountability for the well-being and practice of one's colleagues. The ANA Code for Nurses with Interpretive Statements in Tenet 3 states, "The nurse acts to safeguard the client and the public when health care and safety are affected by incompetent, unethical, or illegal practice of any person,"° The origins of such practice include substance abuse as well as many other problems.

Elements of Peer Assistance

In providing peer assistance two elements must be considered; either or both may provide the basis for action:

1. Voluntary response of the practitioner to efforts of assistance by a peer.

2. Alternative efforts wherein disciplinary action is initiated in compliance with legal regulations.

While the term "peer assistance" is frequently associated with Constituent District Associations or the New York State Nurses Association action which may parallel or precede action by regulatory agencies, peer assistance does not necessarily eliminate the possibility of action by a colleague to report a nursing practitioner to appropriate legal authorities. When colleagues have implemented outreach efforts which have brought no response, the stated intention to take action which threatens licensure may be a necessary step toward motivating the individual to seek treatment and may be the only means to protect clients. Because the nursing practitioner's license represents a primary source of income as well as legal permission to practice as a professional nurse, its importance may represent a reality of greater weight than the other losses associated with alcohol and substance abuse. Nurses who are recovering have identified intentions stated by nursing care coordinators or colleagues to act on licensure as the final event which motivated them to seek treatment.

Module II.2

Module II.2—Handout #7A *(continued)*

Peer assistance may mean that a coworker or colleague acts as an advocate for the nursing practitioner in a variety of ways. The nursing practitioner may intercede in situations involving impaired practice by nurses as an advocate for the practitioner, for the patient/consumer, or for professional standards. In each situation the nurse assumes a position in support of another or of professional standards. The willingness to assume that position is an essential aspect of peer assistance.

Guidelines

Peer assistance takes a variety of forms.

Education as peer assistance ranges in scope from informal teaching to formally organized educational efforts. By identifying alcohol and substance abuse as "cause for concern," the nurse raises the level of awareness about these illnesses, their recognition, and what constitutes appropriate treatment. This type of information sharing may take place in small groups and informal work relationships or may be incorporated as formal educational offerings. Peers are responsible for disseminating knowledge and sharing expertise in this area.

Consultation is also a form of peer assistance. In the area of alcohol and substance abuse, consultation provides information and support directly to the individual who must deal with the addicted nurse or coworkers, families, or friends who assist the nurse. The consultant, who is knowledgeable about these illnesses, forms of intervention, and methods of treatment, confers directly with the concerned individual. In two-tiered intervention, the consultant confers with coworkers, family, or friends, who then intervene with the impaired nurse. This has the advantage of providing consultation on direct intervention techniques, as well as assistance in identifying actions of colleagues and/or family which support the continuing use/abuse of alcohol or drugs. This behavior is known as "enabling." These activities are generally not perceived by those demonstrating them as related to the ongoing problem. Because of knowledge and perspective, the consultant is able to work with others in the system in order to identify actions which impede constructive change.

Intervention is frequently utilized as a basic form of peer assistance. It may consist of outreach to individuals in early stages of illness or efforts by peers in collaboration with supervisors or other concerned persons to move the individual toward treatment. The concerned persons may be changing their behavior in response to the addicted individual. Such behavior is called "cobehavior." A primary advantage of peer assistance interventions is the capability of quick mobilization in response to a request for help from the nursing practitioner or whenever there is cause for concern by others. This concern may originate when the individual demonstrates signs of illness or when there is evidence that the nurse is practicing while judgment is impaired.

Components of Intervention

When peer assistance is implemented as intervention, the following components must be present:

Instructor's Guide

Module II.2—Handout #7A *(continued)*

- *Goals and interventions* to act on behalf of the nurse toward restoration of health, to protect the consumer, and maintain professional standards.

- *Accessibility* of individuals who can assess the origins and ramifications of the practice problems. Individuals who are part of the system in which the nurse works may be best able to communicate a combination of caring concern and a firm imperative for action. If peer assistance activities are available, these should be widely publicized.

- *Visibility and recognition* of the intervener as a resource person. The knowledgeable and experienced peer who initiates steps toward assistance must be committed and capable of beginning and completing, or helping others to complete the intervention process.

- *Knowledge.* The peer participating in intervention must be able to recognize and assess a colleague with this illness, be knowledgeable about nurses' and consumers' rights, and be able to use techniques to motivate individuals toward treatment resources which are timely and appropriate to the problem.

- *Established guidelines for intervention.* Who intervenes and how interventions take place must be established early. Experiences of others suggest that two concerned individuals intervening with the nurse in difficulty are most effective in confronting the denial and illuminating enabling attitudes and behaviors which impede action to correct the situation. The complexities of interacting with the ill nurse require skill and objectivity which may be compromised in highly emotional and upsetting circumstances. Interventions by two individuals and/or including concerned colleagues often clarify the problem and its implications.

- *Referral and follow-up mechanisms.* Efforts to assist the nurse will not always result in action to correct the problem. Mechanisms need to be developed to feed back outcomes to concerned individuals who have sought assistance or expressed worry about the nurse. Continued outreach activities may be necessary to help the nurse acknowledge the illness. The peer participating in intervention must be knowledgeable about nurses' and consumers' rights, be able to recognize and assess a colleague with this illness, and be able to use techniques to motivate individuals toward treatment resources which are timely and appropriate to the problem.

- *Confidentiality.* A method must be devised to ensure confidentiality and to protect the rights of the nursing practitioner in regard to health care and licensure. Confidentiality should be a central component of the development of employee assistance and peer assistance protocols.

The title "nursing practitioner" refers to the NYSNA Position Descriptions approved by the NYSNA Board, June 1972.

°*From:* American Nurses' Association, *Code for Nurses With Interpretive Statements*, Tenet 3, p. 8, 1977, April.

Module II.2

Module II.2—Handout #7B

INTERVENTIONS IN THE WORK PLACE

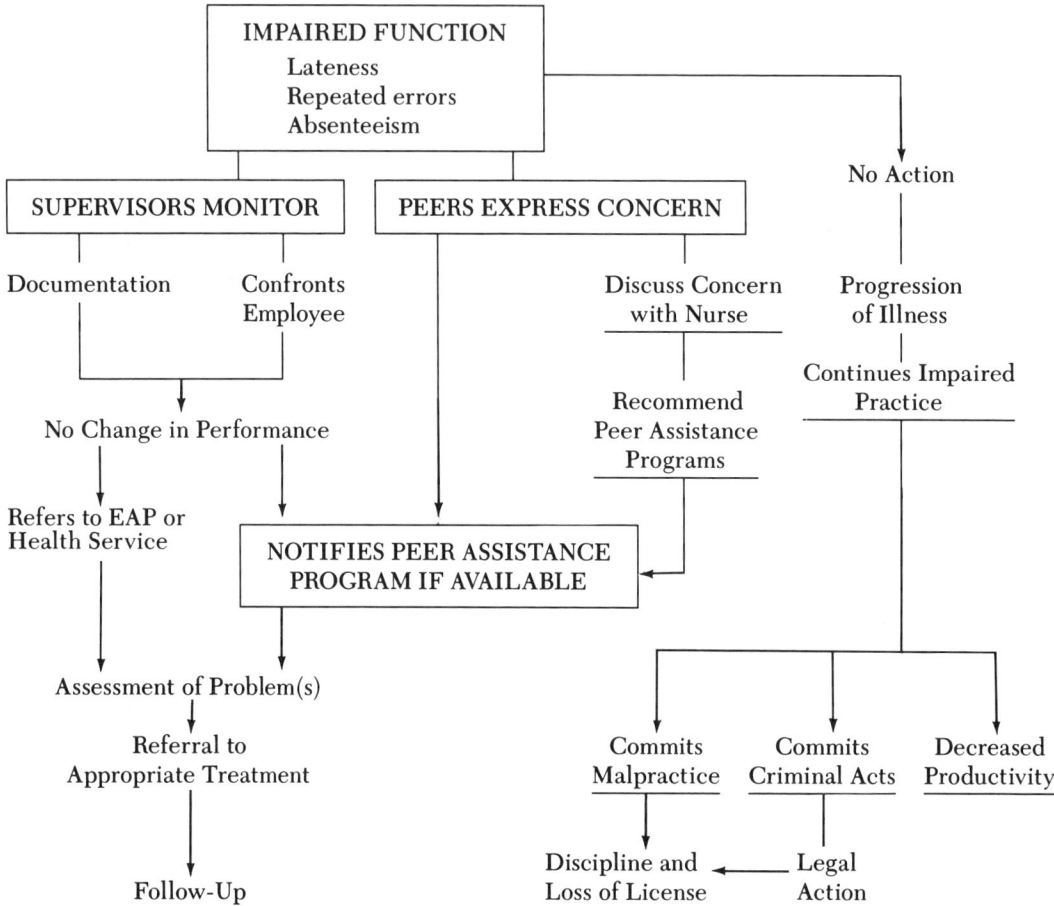

From: New York State Nurses Association. (1985, April). *NYSNA Task Force Report on Alcohol and Substance Abuse in the Profession of Nursing.* Albany, NY: NYSNA.

Instructor's Guide

Module II.2—Handout #7C

PEER INTERVENTION ASSISTANCE

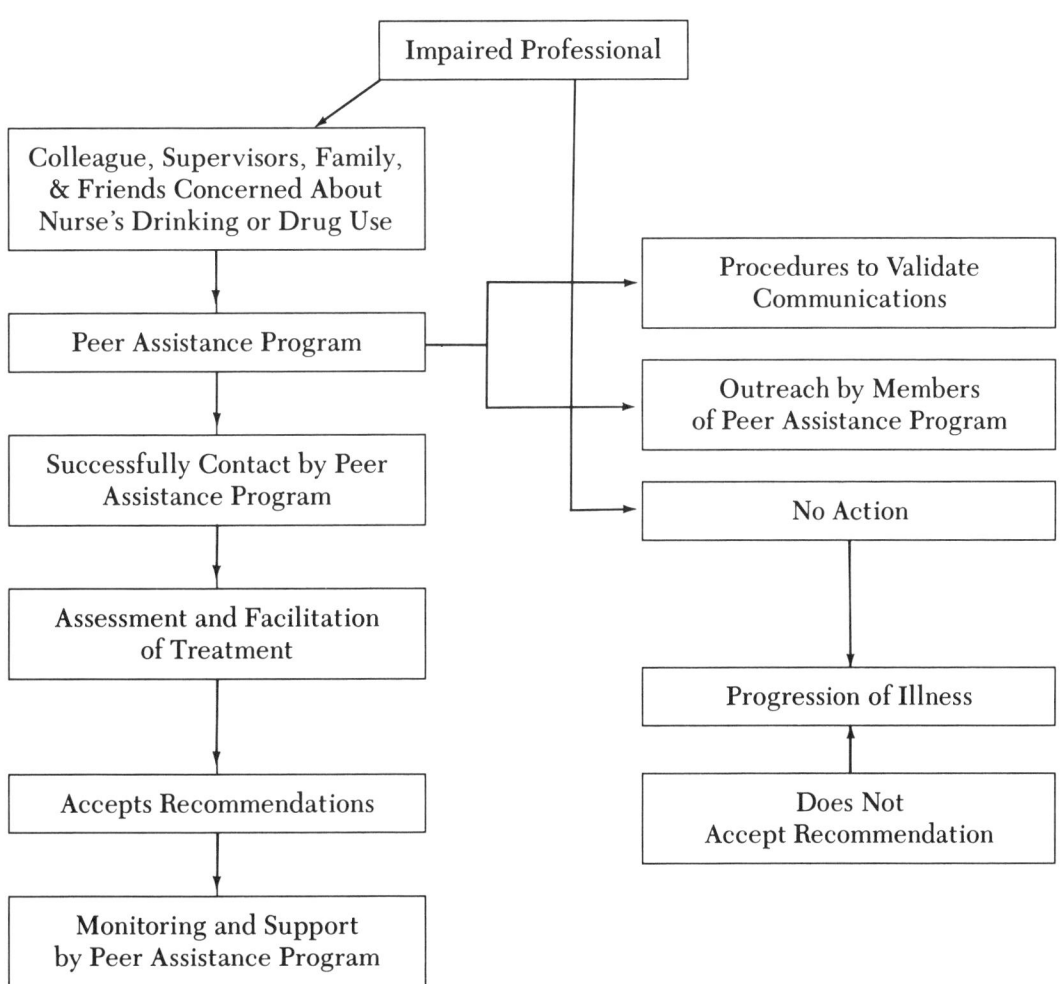

From: New York State Nurses Association. (1985, April). *NYSNA Task Force Report on Alcohol and Substance Abuse in the Profession of Nursing.* Albany, NY: NYSNA.

Module II.2

Module II.2—Handout #8

AMERICAN NURSES' ASSOCIATION
SUPPLEMENT TO
ADDICTIONS AND PSYCHOLOGICAL DYSFUNCTIONS IN NURSING
THE PROFESSION'S RESPONSE TO THE PROBLEM*
Revised 1989

Contents

Program Activities of State Nurses' Associations, Constituents of the American Nurses' Association	161
State Nurses' Associations, Executive Directors	184
State Boards of Nursing	189
Specialty Nursing Groups	194
Agencies and Professional Groups	195

This supplement will be updated annually. The American Nurses' Association requests your help to identify agencies and organizations that provide educational materials, program development assistance, and prototypes of assistance programs. If you know of any organization or agency not listed in this supplement, please send pertinent information to:

Marin Goodier, Coordinator
Office of Constituent Relations
American Nurses' Association
1102 14th Street N.W.
Washington, D.C. 20005

---

*Published by the American Nurses' Association, Kansas City, Missouri, 1984.

Instructor's Guide

Module II.2—Handout #8 *(continued)*

PROGRAM ACTIVITIES OF STATE NURSES' ASSOCIATIONS, CONSTITUENTS OF THE AMERICAN NURSES' ASSOCIATION

During May 1984, and again in December 1984, January 1986, March 1987, April 1988, and June 1989, the state nurses' associations, constituents of the American Nurses' Association, had an opportunity to describe program activities in their states related to the problem of nurses whose practice is impaired by addiction or psychological dysfunction. Following are program descriptions submitted by state nurses' associations.

ALABAMA STATE NURSES' ASSOCIATION

The Alabama State Nurses' Association has appointed a Task Force on the Impaired Nurse with the following goals: (1) to develop and provide ongoing educational programs related to the problems of the impaired nurse, (2) to work collaboratively with other existing groups in the encouragement of treatment, the recovering process, and reentry into nursing practice, and (3) to work collaboratively in establishing and implementing a peer assistance program for the impaired nurse. Education programs are currently available and the task force is working on a model program and necesary legislation. The program will include intervention, referral, peer support groups, and reentry monitoring.

Name of contact person: Charlene Roberson, MSN, RN

Address: Alabama State Nurses' Association
360 North Hull Street
Montgomery, Alabama 36197
(205) 262-8321 (daytime)

Daytime hrs./days contact person is available by phone: 9:00 a.m.–5:00 p.m., Monday–Friday

ALASKA NURSES ASSOCIATION

The Alaska Nurses Association has developed guidelines for a peer assistance program entitled "New Directions." Currently, educational activities are under way. For the actual implementation of its program, AaNA is looking into combining efforts with other health care providers (physicians, pharmacists, dentists) to help overcome the difficulties of reaching impaired professionals in outlying bush communities. The Alaska Board of Nursing uses agreements as alternatives to discipline and has the only monitored aftercare for nurses. In addition, a local chapter of Nurses House has been established in Anchorage.

Name of contact person: Gail McGuill, RN

Address: Alaska Nurses Association
237 East Third Avenue
Anchorage, Alaska 99501
(907) 274-0827 (daytime)

Module II.2

Module II.2—Handout #8 *(continued)*

ARIZONA NURSES' ASSOCIATION

The Arizona Nurses' Association Impaired Nurse Committee is involved in the following activities to assist impaired nurses: (1) conducts needs assessment; (2) works with the Arizona State Board of Nursing and agencies with assistance programs and with nurses who work in chemical dependency to develop criteria for identifying the impaired nurse; (3) developed a model for confrontation and intervention; (4) presents workshops to educate other nurses; and (5) compiles educational information on ethical/legal issues.

Name of contact person: Sarah Withgott, MS, RN, Chairperson,
Impaired Nurse Committee

Address: Arizona Nurses' Association
1850 East Southern Avenue, Suite 1
Tempe, Arizona 85282
(602) 831-0404 (daytime)

Daytime hrs./days contact person is available by phone: 8:30 a.m.–4:30 p.m., Monday–Friday

ARKANSAS STATE NURSES' ASSOCIATION

District 10, ASNA has established the Nurses for Recovery Task Force. The following are objectives that have been met or are in progress: A support group for recovering nurses is available; philosophy, policies, and job descriptions are written; collaboration is ongoing with the state board of nursing; and educational programs for nurses are taught by members of the task force. Emphasis of education for administrators is upon health care facilities setting policies with which every employee is familiar.

Name of contact person: Charlene Bradham, MNSc, RN, or Nancy Burris

Address: Charlene Bradham
5016 Western Hills Avenue
Little Rock, Arkansas 72204
(501) 569-8084 (daytime)
(501) 562-2444 (evening)

Nancy Burris
(501) 663-2363 (daytime)
(501) 686-6090 (evening)

Daytime hrs./days contact person is available by phone: Ms. Bradham (7:00 a.m.–3:00 p.m., Monday–Friday); Ms. Burris (10:00 a.m.–3:00 p.m., every day)

Evening hrs./days contact person is available by phone: Ms. Bradham (3:00 p.m.–7:00 a.m., every day); Ms. Burris (3:00 p.m.–11:00 p.m., Monday–Friday)

Module II.2—Handout #8 *(continued)*

CALIFORNIA NURSES ASSOCIATION

The California Nurses Association established a Well-Being Committee to assist nurses with chemical dependency and stress as it relates to their work. The committee members are knowledgeable in the area of drug and alcohol addiction, mental health, and legal issues. The purpose is to educate nurses, nursing service directors, and hospital administration regarding these problems.

Name of contact person: David Fabun, RN, Labor Representative, Oakland Office

Address: California Nurses Association
            1855 Folsom Street, Suite 670
            San Francisco, California 94103
            (415) 562-2883 (daytime)

Daytime hrs./days contact person is available by phone: 9:00 a.m.–5:00 p.m., Monday–Friday

Hotline telephone number: none established. Currently developing the person power and assessing the cost.

COLORADO NURSES' ASSOCIATION

The Colorado Nurses' Association houses NURSES of Colorado Corporation which is a separate corporate entity. NURSES (Nurses United for Recovery, Support, and Education Successfully) of Colorado Corporation is a peer employee assistance program providing assessment, referral, peer intervention, monitoring/follow-up, support groups, training/consultation, and a confidential information phone line 24 hours a day. CNA-sponsored legislation to establish a Nursing Peer Health Assistance Diversion Program has been passed; the new law took effect July 1, 1989.

Name of contact person: Elizabeth M. Pace, BS, RN, CEAP, Executive Director

Address: N.U.R.S.E.S. of Colorado Corporation
            P.O. Box 61294
            Denver, Colorado 80206
            (303) 758-0596 (daytime/evening)

Daytime hrs./days contact person is available by phone: 8:00 a.m.–4:00 p.m., Monday–Friday

Hotline telephone number: (303) 758-0596   (This is an answering service, available 24 hours every day.)

CONNECTICUT NURSES' ASSOCIATION

The Connecticut Nurses' Association offers educational programs and refers nurses with addiction problems to treatment programs, such as Nurses for Nurses.

Module II.2

Module II.2—Handout #8 *(continued)*

Name of contact person: Karen Stonkas Ponton, MA, RN, Executive Director

Address: Connecticut Nurses' Association
Meritech Business Park
377 Research Parkway, Suite 2D
Meriden, Connecticut 06450
(203) 238-1207 (daytime)

Daytime hrs./days contact person is available by phone: 9:00 a.m.–5:00 p.m., Monday–Friday

Hotline telephone number: none established.

DELAWARE NURSES' ASSOCIATION

The Impaired Nurse Hotline has been in existence since December 1986. Volunteers are prepared to conduct crisis intervention, refer nurses whose lives are affected by substance abuse or mental health problems to treatment/rehabilitation programs, and offer appropriate support.

Name of contact person: L. Alberta Regan, MSN, RN, Chairperson,
Impaired Nurse Peer Assistance Committee

Address: 2109 Milltown Road
Wilmington, Delaware 19808
(302) 454-3942 (daytime)
(302) 994-5638 (evening)

Hotline telephone number: (302) 366-1775   (This is an answering service, available 24 hours every day.)

DISTRICT OF COLUMBIA NURSES' ASSOCIATION, INC.

The District of Columbia Nurses' Association offers educational programs, makes available resource materials and refers nurses with addiction problems to treatment programs. Peer review legislation that will make possible intervention through the professional association is pending. DCNA's intervention activities will begin following successful passage of that legislation.

Name of contact person: Evelyn Sommers, MBA, Executive Director

Address: District of Columbia Nurses' Association, Inc.
Suite 306
5100 Wisconsin Avenue, N.W.
Washington, D.C. 20016
(202) 244-2705 (daytime)

Daytime hrs./days contact person is available: 9:00 a.m.–5:00 p.m., Monday–Friday

Hotline telephone number: none established.

Instructor's Guide

Module II.2—Handout #8 (continued)

FLORIDA NURSES ASSOCIATION

The Florida Nurses Association Council on Chemical Dependency provides nurses interested in or working in the field of addiction with a statewide organization to address current issues, continuing education, and networking. The activity of council members is focused on educating nurses and nursing students about the Board of Nursing's Intervention Project for Nurses (in lieu of disciplinary proceedings) and treatment resources, as well as identification and education of the "at risk" nurse or student and appropriate management, including standardized curriculum in nursing programs.

Name of contact person: Mary Martin, RN, Chairperson, Council on Chemical Dependency

Address: Florida Nurses Association
           P.O. Box 536985
           Orlando, Florida 32853-6985
           (407) 896-3261 (daytime)

Daytime hrs./days contact person is available by phone: 8:30 a.m.–4:30 p.m., Monday–Friday

Hotline telephone number: none established.

GEORGIA NURSES ASSOCIATION, INC.

The overall goal of the Georgia Nurses Association Impaired Nurse Committee is to identify and assist impaired nurses to seek treatment for addictive diseases so they can remain useful members of our profession. The committee provides information, referral, intervention, support groups, education, consultation, and advocacy when the need is identified.

Name of contact person: Rose Robertson, MSN, RN, Chairperson,
                        Impaired Nurse Committee

Address: 277 Ashtonwood Drive   or   Georgia Nurses Association
           Martinez, Georgia 30907   1362 West Peachtree Street, N.W.
           (404) 828-2079 (daytime)   Atlanta, Georgia 30309
           (404) 863-7383 (evening)   (404) 876-4624

Daytime hrs./days contact person is available by phone: 8:30 a.m.–4:30 p.m.

Hotline telephone number: (404) 876-8416   (This is an answering service, available 24 hours every day. Rose Robertson responds to these calls personally or refers them to district advocates.)

HAWAII NURSES' ASSOCIATION

The Hawaii Nurses' Association is assisting the Board of Nursing in its development of a program.

Module II.2—Handout #8 *(continued)*

IDAHO NURSES ASSOCIATION

The Idaho Nurse Peer Assistance Program (INPAP) provides education, awareness, and practices which promote prevention, early intervention, and support strategies for nurses and their patients at high risk for chemical dependency. INA has joined the Idaho Health Professionals Recovery Organization, IHPRO, a multi-discipline educational and early intervention program to assist impaired health professionals. IHPRO is seeking grant funding to support a shared recovery coordinator.

Name of contact person: Diane Johnson, President of INPAP

Address: 1763 East Boise Avenue or Idaho Nurses Association
Boise, Idaho 83706 200 North 4th Street, Suite 20
(208) 336-5100, ext. 7225 (daytime) Boise, Idaho 83702-6001
(208) 345-5547 (evening) (208) 345-0500 (daytime)

Daytime hrs./days contact person is available by phone: 8:00 a.m.–5:00 p.m., Monday–Friday

Hotline telephone number: none established.

ILLINOIS NURSES ASSOCIATION

The Illinois Nurses Association developed a support network for nurses whose professional performance is hampered by abuse of chemicals or any mental or resulting physical illness. This support network is the Peer Assistance Network for Nurses (P.A.N.N.). P.A.N.N. was incorporated as a foundation on November 13, 1987.

Name of contact person: Monica M. Russell, BSN, RN, Associate Administrator

Address: Illinois Nurses Association
20 North Wacker Drive, Suite 2520
Chicago, Illinois 60606
(312) 236-9708 (daytime)

Daytime hrs./days contact person is available by phone: 9:00 a.m.–5:00 p.m., Monday–Friday

Hotline telephone number: none established.

INDIANA STATE NURSES' ASSOCIATION

The Peer Review and Assistance Program for Registered Nurses is a network of support, monitoring, and referral for treatment to nurses whose professional performance is hampered by alcohol and/or other drug abuse.

Instructor's Guide

Module II.2—Handout #8 *(continued)*

Name of contact person: Ernest C. Klein, Jr., Assistant Director

Address: Indiana State Nurses' Association
2915 North High School Road
Indianapolis, Indiana 46224
(317) 299-4575 (daytime)

Daytime hrs./days contact person is available by phone: 9:00 a.m.–4:00 p.m., Monday–Friday

Hotline telephone number: (317) 299-4575 (24 hours every day, on answering machine).

IOWA NURSES' ASSOCIATION

The Iowa Nurses' Association has established a Peer Assistance Program Planning Committee. A three-component design is in process: prevention, education, and intervention. Whether the program will be implemented depends on funding. The INA met with other Iowa professional organizations in March 1989, to discuss voluntary programs of assistance. All the professional associations are cooperating in arranging a statewide conference on impaired professionals.

Name of contact person: Marcene Moran, RN, Chairperson,
Peer Assistance Program Planning Committee

Address: 2525 Apache Drive
Sioux City, Iowa 51104
(712) 279-2446 (daytime)

Hotline telephone number: none established.

KANSAS STATE NURSES ASSOCIATION

The Kansas State Nurses Association's Peer Assistance Program works to find and refer all Kansas State Board of Nursing licensees (RNs, LPNs, LMHTs) with physical, emotional, or mental disabilities, including deterioration through the aging process, disease, loss of motor skill, or abuse of drugs or alcohol, into treatment and provide intervention, monitoring, education, lab testing where appropriate, and collegial support through the recovery process.

Name of contact person: Diana M. Glynn, JD, RN, Program Administrator or
Pat Green, LMSW, RN, Program Director

Address: Kansas State Nurses Association
820 Quincy Street
Topeka, Kansas 66612
(800) 666-4571 (daytime)
(913) 233-8638 (24 hours per day)

Daytime hrs./days contact person is available by phone: 9:00 a.m.–5:00 p.m., Monday–Friday

Module II.2

Module II.2—Handout #8 *(continued)*

Hotline telephone number: none established, but members of the committee can be called at any time:

Pat Green, MSW, RN
Lawrence, Kansas
(816) 254-3652 (work)
(913) 842-3893 (home)

John Aker, MS, CRNA
3417 S.W. Birchwood
Topeka, Kansas 66614
(913) 588-6612 (work)

Sr. Mary Theresa Morris, RN
801 South 8th
Atchison, Kansas 66002
(913) 367-6110 (work/home)

Evelyn Westhoff Maxwell, MN, RN
414 Wayne
Salina, Kansas 67401
(913) 827-3304 (work/home)

KENTUCKY NURSES ASSOCIATION

Nurses Assisting Nurses (NAN) is sponsored by the University of Kentucky College of Nursing in cooperation with the Kentucky Nurses Association and the Kentucky Board of Nursing. The project consists of clinical counseling services, advocacy, public and professional education, and a longitudinal research study. Services are provided by doctoral and master's-prepared psychiatric/mental health nurses.

Name of contact person: Melva Jo Hendrix, DNSc, RN, Professor and Project Director, NAN

Address: University of Kentucky College of Nursing
800 Rose Street
Lexington, Kentucky, 40536
(606) 257-1587 (daytime/evening)

Hotline telephone number: (606) 257-1587   (Answering service available 24 hours every day.)

LOUISIANA STATE NURSES ASSOCIATION

The Louisiana State Nurses Association statewide program (LaNNIP—Louisiana Nurses' Network for the Impaired Professional) provides for (1) early detection and identification of impaired nurses or potentially impaired nurses; (2) confrontation of and intervention with such nurses; (3) evaluation of the conditions underlying their impairment; (4) assistance in identifying, securing, and pursuing effective treatment; (5) license protection, two years monitoring in practice and the recovery process; and (6) educational programs focused on developing the awareness and understanding of addiction and peer assistance among nurses, nursing administration, related health professionals, and the public.

Name of contact person: Bobby G. Huskey, MA, BSN, RN, LSNA Coordinator

Address: Louisiana State Nurses Association
712 Transcontinental Drive
Metairie, Louisiana 70001
(504) 889-1030 (daytime)
(504) 738-0281 (evening)

Instructor's Guide

Module II.2—Handout #8 *(continued)*

Daytime hrs./days contact person is available by phone: 8:00 a.m.–4:00 p.m., Monday–Friday

Evening hrs./days contact person is available by phone: 4:00 p.m.–8:00 a.m., Monday–Saturday

Hotline telephone number: (800) 456-6378 (available 8:00 a.m.–4:00 p.m.)

MAINE STATE NURSES' ASSOCIATION

The Maine State Nurses' Association has been involved with (1) testifying before the Maine legislature on bills relating to substance abuse (i.e., random drug testing and establishment of employee assistance programs); (2) negotiating contract language for the establishment of employee assistance programs; (3) pursuing a grant to study the needs of Maine nurses regarding the extent of the problem; (4) license protection; and (5) client protection.

Name of contract person: Anne Sassong, RN, Executive Director

Address: Maine State Nurses' Association
P.O. Box 2240
Augusta, Maine 04330
(207) 622-1057 (daytime)

MARYLAND NURSES ASSOCIATION, INC.

The Maryland Nurses Association Impaired Nurses Committee recognizes that impaired nursing practice impacts on the individual, the patient, and the nursing profession. It is committed to addressing the problem through education, information sharing, and networking with other groups and professions. It supports referral of a nurse into treatment and rehabilitation. The committee has supported and encouraged the development of a peer support group, "Nurses Recovering Together"; has developed a statewide directory of information and referral resources; provides committee-sponsored speakers to assist with in-service presentations, staff development, and conference planning; participates in interdisciplinary networks through the Professional Rehabilitation Council and national networks; has a pamphlet which is designed to provide information of referral, identification, and education as well as describe the committee's services and activities; and has active involvement with the Maryland Board of Nursing.

Name of contact person: Maureen Sheppard-Smith, RN, Chairperson,
MNA Impaired Nurses Committee

Address: 1513 Carriage Hill Drive
Westminster, Maryland 21157
(800) 233-7770 (daytime/evening)
(301) 461-9922 (daytime/evening)

Daytime hrs./days contact person is available by phone: 8:30 a.m.–5:00 p.m., Monday–Friday or 24 hours every day by beeper

Hotline telephone number: none established.

Module II.2

Module II.2—Handout #8 *(continued)*

MASSACHUSETTS NURSES ASSOCIATION

The Massachusetts Nurses Association Voluntary Peer Assistance Committee is designed to provide support, assessment, referral, and follow-up support through a network of peer assistants-volunteers throughout the state who know about chemical dependency and recovery. The program also offers education and management consultation regarding chemical dependency.

Name of contact person: Margaret M. Shea, MS, RN

Address: Massachusetts Nurses Association
340 Turnpike Street
Canton, Massachusetts 02021
(617) 821-4625 (daytime)

Daytime hrs./days contact person is available by phone: 8:30 a.m.–4:30 p.m., Monday–Friday

Hotline telephone number: (800) 882-2056 (8:30 a.m.–4:30 p.m., Monday–Friday)

MICHIGAN NURSES ASSOCIATION

The Michigan Nurses Association has established the Nurse Peer Assistance Referral Line (NPAL) to provide a referral service for requests for information about chemical dependency and impaired professional functioning by nurses in Michigan. Individuals who phone NPAL are put in touch with chemical dependency resources who can provide information, assistance, or additional referrals. This line serves all nurses in Michigan. The Michigan Nurses Association's Impaired Professional Functioning Committee has adopted the following goals: (1) educate the profession on the extent and nature of chemical dependency; (2) disseminate research on the problem; (3) ensure the availability of peer assistance programs; (4) support and promote the passage of recently introduced legislation (HB 4712, the Health Professional Treatment Act) to allow the Board of Nursing to establish a voluntary program which would accept diversion into treatment and voluntary suspension of license during the treatment program as an alternative to disciplinary action.

Name of contact person: Carol E. Franck, MSN, RN, Executive Director

Address: Michigan Nurses Association
120 Spartan Avenue
East Lansing, Michigan 48823
(517) 337-1653 (daytime)

Daytime hrs./days contact person is available by phone: 8:00 a.m.–5:00 p.m., Monday–Friday

Hotline telephone number: (517) 337-3050 (8:00 a.m.–5:00 p.m., Monday–Friday)

Instructor's Guide

Module II.2—Handout #8   (continued)

MINNESOTA NURSES ASSOCIATION

The Minnesota Nurses Association's Peer Assistance Program for Nurses (PAPN) has the following components: (1) *referral:* chemically dependent nurses are followed by the Regional Liaison Person (RLP) from time of referral through 2–3 years into recovery; (2) *education:* in-services, workshops, printed information, and consultation are tools used to educate others about chemical dependency in nurses; (3) *consultation:* assistance is provided to anyone with questions and concerns about chemical dependency in nurses; (4) *back to work issues:* assistance with the development of return to work contracts and assistance to receiving staffs are provided.

Name of contact person: Lou Erickson, MPH, RN, Coordinator, PAPN

Address: Minnesota Nurses Association
          1295 Bandana Boulevard North, Suite 140
          St. Paul, Minnesota 55108-5115
          (612) 646-4807 (daytime)

Daytime hrs./days contact person is available by phone: 8:15 a.m.–4:30 p.m., Monday–Friday

Hotline telephone number: none established.

MISSISSIPPI NURSES' ASSOCIATION

The Mississippi Nurses' Association's Educational Resource Committee is offering educational and referral services throughout the state. Nurses seeking assistance are encouraged to call for more information at (601) 982-9182. As a healing and preventative profession, nursing has a commitment to educate the public, peers, and colleagues on the disease concept, rehabilitation, and reentry of those who are chemically dependent. The state of Mississippi, recognizing the importance of such a program, gave additional funding to the Board of Nursing for a staff person for the board's Recovering Nurse Program.

Name of contact person: Betty Dickson, Executive Director

Address: Mississippi Nurses' Association
          135 Bounds Street, Suite 100
          Jackson, Mississippi 39206
          (601) 982-9182 (daytime)

Daytime hrs./days contact person is available by phone: 8:00 a.m.–4:30 p.m., Monday–Friday

Hotline telephone number: none established.

Module II.2

Module II.2—Handout #8 *(continued)*

MISSOURI NURSES ASSOCIATION

The Missouri Nurses Association Peer Assistance Program was formally incorporated into the association bylaws in 1983. MONA's newly refocused program will develop educational programs for nurses and others in chemical impairment, conduct nursing research on chemical impairment, and provide information on chemical impairment and/or treatment centers within the state.

Name of contact person: Belinda Heimericks, MSN, RN

Address: Missouri Nurses Association
P.O. Box 325
206 East Dunklin Street
Jefferson City, Missouri 65102
(314) 636-4623 (daytime)

Daytime hrs./days contact person is available by phone: 8:00 a.m.–4:30 p.m., Monday–Friday

Hotline telephone number: none established.

MONTANA NURSES' ASSOCIATION

The Montana Nurses' Association's affiliated Program for Recovering Nurses (PRN) serves four purposes: (1) to assist nurses (RNs and LPNs) who have been identified as needing rehabilitation into treatment programs; (2) to educate health care workers and the public about the Montana Program for Recovering Nurses; (3) to provide aftercare through a recovery contract for monitoring recovery; and (4) to provide a support group for nurses in recovery. A task force has been developed to support the introduction of bills into the upcoming legislative session to allocate funds for a diversion program for nurses and to establish limited licensure guidelines for nurses in recovery. The Program for Recovering Nurses (PRN) is a special interest group of Montana Nurses' Association, but is in no other way a direct program. MNA successfully promoted legislation empowering the Board of Nursing to develop a diversion program, enabling PRN to function as a peer assistance group.

Name of contact person: Marge Vanderhoof, RN, Liaison to PRN, or Carol Sem, BSN, RN

Address: Marge Vanderhoof, RN
4732 North Montana Avenue
Helena, Montana 59601
(406) 442-2480 (daytime)
(406) 422-1306 (evening)

Carol Sem, BSN, RN
127 North Higgins, Suite H
Missoula, Montana 59802
(406) 721-4610 (daytime)
(406) 721-6971 (evening)

Daytime hrs./days contact person is available by phone: Ms. Vanderhoof (4:00 p.m.–7:00 a.m., any day); Ms. Sem (anytime, Monday–Friday)

Instructor's Guide

Module II.2—Handout #8 *(continued)*

NEBRASKA NURSES' ASSOCIATION

Nebraska Nurses' Association has an Impaired Nurse Committee and support group in place. The committee holds educational sessions for nurses. Volunteers work with nurses reported to the group and also work with nurses' employers and monitoring during recovery. The committee continues to work with other health care disciplines for diversion legislation.

Name of contact person: Kathy Wright, RN, Chairperson, NNA Impaired Nurse Program

Address: University of Nebraska Medical Center
NICU
42nd and Dewey
Omaha, Nebraska 68105
(402) 559-5815 (daytime)
(402) 551-4023 (evening)

Daytime hrs./days contact person is available by phone: 7:00 a.m.–4:00 p.m.

Evening hrs./days contact person is available by phone: 4:00 p.m.–7:00 p.m.

Hotline telephone number: none established.

NEVADA NURSES' ASSOCIATION

The Peer Assistance Committee is composed of volunteer members who hold support group meetings and are available for one-on-one private counseling. Educational seminars may also be held for impaired and unimpaired nurses. Committee goals are: (1) to educate health care professionals in the state of Nevada on practice issues with impaired professionals; and (2) to act as an advisory or information service on impairment issues.

Name of contact person: Pat Erdmann, RN, Peer Assistance Committee

Address: Carson Tahoe Hospital
1715 Fleishmann Way
Carson City, Nevada 89702
(702) 885-8866 (daytime)
(702) 825-3555 (daytime)
(702) 827-1245 (evening)

Daytime hrs./days contact person is available by phone: 8:00 a.m.–5:00 p.m., Monday–Friday or call NNA office: (702) 825-3555

Hotline telephone number: (702) 825-3555 (9:00 a.m.–3:00 p.m., Monday–Friday)

NEW HAMPSHIRE NURSES' ASSOCIATION

In 1989, New Hampshire passed a new Nurse Practice Act. Within this document was a mandatory reporting clause. There is not, as yet, diversion legislation in New Hampshire, thus creating a greater need for the state association and state board to work cooperatively

Module II.2—Handout #8 *(continued)*

in program planning. A work group has been established in conjunction with the Medical Society's PAD's project. At present, the education and information component of NHNA's Peer Assistance group is unchanged. Consultation and referral are in limbo pending further work with the Board of Nursing and the legislative process. The volunteer group continues to be small and informal, and desires increased participation of other interested professional members. Legislative, economic, and referral issues need to be addressed, and more volunteers are needed.

Name of contact person: Lonnie Larrow, MS, RN, Nurses' Peer Assistance Group, or Marsha Day-Donahue, RN

Address: New Hampshire Nurses' Association
48 West Street
Concord, New Hampshire 03301
(603) 225-3783 (daytime)

Daytime hrs./days contact person is available by phone: 8:00 a.m.–4:30 p.m., Monday–Friday

NEW JERSEY STATE NURSES ASSOCIATION

Funding has been received from the New Jersey Department of Health, Division of Alcoholism, for an 800 number peer assistance line which is voice answered 24 hours a day, seven days a week. Volunteers from the Impaired Nurse Committee have developed an on-call schedule to cover calls when the New Jersey State Nurses Association's office is closed. Presently there are six Nurse Recovery Groups (NRG) with the anticipation of adding more this year. The *Resource Directory* is under revision and will be reissued in the Fall of 1989, financed in part through committee donations and the "Self Development of People," Presbytery of New Brunswick, New Jersey. The committee continues to provide continuing education throughout the state as well as a program at the annual convention. The Impaired Nurse Committee has expanded and has representatives from all backgrounds and areas of the state. Assisting the main committee is an advisory group composed of recovering nurses, LPNs, and others who work with recovering nurses.

Name of contact person: Dorothy Flemming, MSN, RN, Executive Director

Address: New Jersey State Nurses Association
320 West State Street
Trenton, New Jersey 08618
(609) 392-4884 (daytime/evening)

Daytime hrs./days contact person is available by phone: 8:30 a.m.–4:30 p.m., Monday–Friday

Hotline telephone number: (800) 662-0108 (24 hours every day).

Instructor's Guide

Module II.2—Handout #8 *(continued)*

NEW MEXICO NURSES ASSOCIATION

CAN Recover (Committee to Assist Nurses Recover) provides intervention, education, and referral for nurses with chemical addiction on a confidential and anonymous basis. CAN Recover also conducts educational seminars about chemical dependency among nurses. Diversion legislation has been passed in New Mexico, and the New Mexico Regulation and Licensing Department/Nursing has a monitoring program in place.

Name of contact person: Courtney Cook, RN, CAN Recover

Address: P.O. Box 1273
  Santa Fe, New Mexico 87501
  (505) 989-5277 (daytime)

Hotline telephone number: (505) 293-5146 (9:00 a.m.–5:00 p.m., Monday–Friday. NMNA does not provide crisis service.)

NEW YORK STATE NURSES ASSOCIATION

The Committee on Impaired Nursing Practice focuses on education and encouraging peer assistance activities. DNA 1 (Buffalo) has "Nurses Helping Nurses"; DNA 4 (Syracuse) has "Lamplighters" Support Group; DNA 9 (Albany) has "Support Group for Chemically Dependent Nurses"; DNA 13 has "Impaired Nurse Task Force"; DNA 14 (Long Island) has "The Impaired Nursing Practice Assistance Committee." Materials are available on peer assistance, the state of New York's Impaired Professionals Program, hospital-based employee assistance programs, New York's Professional Assistance Program, and reentering the work force.

Name of contact person: Gail DeMarco, MS, RN, Associate Director,
  Nursing Practice and Services Program

Address: New York State Nurses Association
  2113 Western Avenue
  Guilderland, New York 12084
  (518) 456-5371 (daytime)

Daytime hrs./days contact person is available by phone: 9:00 a.m.–5:00 p.m., Monday–Friday

Hotline telephone number: none established.

NORTH CAROLINA NURSES ASSOCIATION

The North Carolina Nurses Association Peer Assistance Program (PAP) focuses on education regarding the hazards of substance abuse and services to impaired nurses. Four continuing education programs have been developed, and a resource referral file listing services available at facilities in the state has been compiled. Guidelines and an orientation for volunteers have been developed and implemented. NCNA has implemented the self-referral component of its peer assistance program. Nurses whose practice is impaired who call NCNA are put in contact with NCNA Area Liaison Team volunteers for follow-up.

Module II.2—Handout #8 *(continued)*

Name of contact person: Janice Millns, MSN, RN, Assistant Executive Director

Address: North Carolina Nurses Association
P.O. Box 12025
Raleigh, North Carolina 27605
(919) 821-4250 (daytime)

Daytime hrs./days contact person is available by phone: 9:30 a.m.–1:30 p.m., Monday–Friday

Hotline telephone number: none established.

NORTH DAKOTA NURSES' ASSOCIATION

The North Dakota Nurses' Association is currently working with seven other groups of health-related licensed professionals in the North Dakota Coalition for Impaired Health Professionals. The primary goal of the coalition is to assist impaired professionals to receive appropriate treatment and support to enable their return to the safe and productive practice of their profession. Coalition activities dealing with impairment are based on an advocacy model. Program elements include: (1) education, (2) identification and verification, (3) intervention, (4) referral and treatment, (5) aftercare and monitoring, and (6) support and advocacy. Appropriate confidentiality measures are assured throughout, and health professionals voluntarily seeking help through the coalition will not be automatically reported to licensing authorities. Legislation has mandated that a $1.00 surcharge be assessed on every nursing licensure fee, and this money will be used to help support the coalition's impaired professionals program. (More information about the North Dakota Coalition for Impaired Health Professionals is available from Bob Freise, Executive Director, North Dakota Coalition for Impaired Health Professionals, P.O. Box 2701, Bismarck, North Dakota 58502, or by calling (701) 224-1708.) The North Dakota Nurses' Association Task Force on the Impaired Nurse has prepared a handbook entitled *Chemical Dependency and the Professional Nurse: A Resource Guide*, which was distributed to all health care facilities in the state. Copies are available at the NDNA office for a fee of $5.00.

Name of contact person: Christeen M. Curran, MS, RN, C, LAC, Chairperson,
Task Force on the Impaired Nurse, or Ms. Nola Helm, RN,
North Dakota Nurses' Association

Address: Christeen M. Curran   or   Nola Helm
1012 16th Street, North   North Dakota Nurses' Association
Fargo, North Dakota 58102   212 North Fourth Street
(701) 232-5579   Bismarck, North Dakota 58501
                                       (701) 223-1385

Daytime hrs./days contact person is available by phone: Ms. Curran (8:00 a.m.–5:00 p.m., Monday–Friday); Ms. Helm (1:00 p.m.–5:00 p.m.)

Instructor's Guide

Module II.2—Handout #8 *(continued)*

OHIO NURSES ASSOCIATION

The Ohio Nurses Association's Peer Assistance Program for Nurses is a volunteer program that provides intervention, referral, and support services to registered nurses who are chemically dependent or physically or mentally impaired. Nurses in the program are monitored for at least two years. Volunteers also assist nurses reentering the job market. ONA is in its tenth year of providing peer support services. ONA offers the only peer support program approved by the Ohio Board of Nursing.

Name of contact person: Carol A. Jenkins, MS, RN, Director, Nursing Practice

Address: Ohio Nurses Association
 4000 East Main Street
 Columbus, Ohio 43213-2950
 (614) 237-5414 (daytime, or leave message on answering machine
  after hours)

Daytime hrs./days contact person is available by phone: 8:30 a.m.–4:30 p.m., Monday–Friday

Hotline telephone number: none established.

OKLAHOMA NURSES ASSOCIATION

The Oklahoma Nurse Assistance Program, Inc., "was created to respond to nurses who are at risk or are actively engaged in substance abuse. ONAP facilitates treatment and expedites re-entry into the workforce. ONAP's cornerstone is peer assistance—Regional Liaison Nurses (RLNs) helping other nurses. . . . A statement of understanding between ONAP and the Oklahoma Board of Nurse Registration and Nursing Education (OBNR&NE) was finalized December 1987. The statement addressed the working relationships of the two groups in matters relating to chemical dependency among nurses. . . . ONAP functions independently of, but cooperatively with, the OBNR&NE." The program is focused on prevention (continuing education), intervention, and referral.

Name of contact person: Frances I. Waddle, MSN, RN, Program Director

Address: Oklahoma Nurse Assistance Program, Inc.
 6414 North Santa Fe, Suite A
 Oklahoma City, Oklahoma 73116
 (405) 840-3478 (daytime)

Daytime hrs./days contact person is available by phone: 8:00 a.m.–4:30 p.m.

Hotline telephone number: (405) 556-4152 (available 24 hours every day)

Module II.2

Module II.2—Handout #8 *(continued)*

OREGON NURSES ASSOCIATION, INC.

The Oregon Nurse Association, Inc. founded the Nurse Assistance Network (NAN) as a peer referral and advocacy service offered to: (1) Oregon nurses (RN, LPN, SN) experiencing problems with chemical addiction or emotional distress; (2) employers and colleagues concerned about the problems of nurses in the work setting; (3) family members who want to help a troubled nurse.

Name of contact person: Ginny Pecora, RN, Chairperson,
                                Nurse Assistance Network Committee

Address: 616 East 16th   2825 Greentree Way
            Eugene, Oregon 97401   Eugene, Oregon 97405
            (503) 687-1110 (daytime)   (503) 687-9429 (evening)

Daytime hrs./days contact person is available by phone: 8:00 a.m.–5:00 p.m., Monday–Friday

Evening hrs./days contact person is available by phone: 6:00 p.m.–9:00 p.m., Monday–Friday

Hotline telephone number: (503) 243-1244 (Portland); (503) 683-0120 (Eugene) (Answering service available 24 hours per day.)

PENNSYLVANIA NURSES ASSOCIATION

The Impaired Nurse Program has engaged in a series of educational programs, audiovisuals, brochures, and a manual to raise awareness of the problem. We are supporting development of recovering nurse support groups, information bureaus, assistance with interventions, referrals, and reentry. We have worked legislatively to promote a more effective approach to impaired nurses by the state board.

Name of contact person: Jessie F. Igou, DrPH, RN, Director, Programs and Services

Address: Pennsylvania Nurses Association
            2578 Interstate Drive
            P.O. Box 8525
            Harrisburg, Pennsylvania 17105-8525
            (717) 657-1222 (daytime)

Daytime hrs./days contact person is available by phone: 9:00 a.m.–5:00 p.m., Monday–Friday

Hotline telephone number: none established.

Instructor's Guide

Module II.2—Handout #8   *(continued)*

RHODE ISLAND STATE NURSES' ASSOCIATION

The Rhode Island State Nurses Association Peer Assistance Program is being professionally managed and staffed by the Rhode Island Employee Assistance Program. Services offered include assessment, referral to treatment, advocacy, aftercare planning, referral to peer support and self-help groups, and monitoring of reentry. The program also conducts educational programs. Problem areas include alcoholism, drug addiction, emotional problems, marital and family problems, and single parenting issues.

Name of contact person: Lorraine Hall, RN, CS

Address: c/o Rhode Island Employee Assistance Program
33 College Hill Road
Warwick, Rhode Island 02886
(401) 828-9560 (daytime/evening) (answering machine)

Daytime hrs./days contact person is available by phone: 8:30 a.m.–5:00 p.m., Monday–Friday

Hotline telephone number: (401) 828-9560   (This is an answering service only, available 24 hours a day.)

SOUTH CAROLINA NURSES' ASSOCIATION

The Peer Assistance Program for Chemically Dependent Nurses (PAPIN) is a volunteer advocacy program designed to assist nurses with alcohol and/or other drug problems. Major components of the program are education, intervention to facilitate entry into treatment, and peer support throughout treatment and recovery, with advocacy for reentry into nursing practice. Peer support groups have been established in regions throughout the state.

Name of contact person: Carol Beard, RN, Chairperson,
Peer Assistance Program for Chemically Dependent Nurses

Address: South Carolina Nurses' Association
1821 Gadsden Street
Columbia, South Carolina 29201
(803) 252-4781 (SCNA—daytime)
(803) 776-4000, ext. 315 (Ms. Beard—daytime)

Daytime hrs./days contact person is available by phone: SCNA (8:30 a.m.–4:00 p.m., Monday–Friday); Ms. Beard (9:00 a.m.–5:00 p.m., Monday–Friday)

Hotline telephone number: none established.

SOUTH DAKOTA NURSES' ASSOCIATION

The South Dakota Nurses' Association supports the efforts, including educational program activities, of the South Dakota Board of Nursing on behalf of nurses whose practice is impaired by substance abuse. SDNA refers callers to consultation and treatment programs.

Module II.2—Handout #8 *(continued)*

TENNESSEE NURSES' ASSOCIATION

The Tennessee Nurses' Foundation Peer Assistance Program for Chemically Dependent Nurses is an advocacy program to assist nurses in recognizing and seeking treatment for chemical dependency. Strict confidentiality is maintained. After completion of treatment, a two-year follow-up program is required of the recovering nurse. Caduceus support groups are utilized across the state, and each individual nurse is assigned an advocate for monitoring purposes.

Name of contact person: Douglas R. Arrington, MSN, RN

Address: Tennessee Nurses' Foundation
1720 West End Building, Suite 400
Nashville, Tennessee 37203
(615) 321-0455 (daytime/evening)

Daytime hrs./days contact person is available by phone: 24 hours per day.

Hotline telephone number: (615) 321-0455 (24 hours every day; on tape evenings and weekends.)

TEXAS NURSES ASSOCIATION

The Texas Peer Assistance Program for Impaired Nurses (TPAPIN) is an advocacy program implemented to assist licensed nurses whose practice is impaired by drug or alcohol abuse or by mental illness by allowing the opportunity for rehabilitation before their licenses are revoked. Confidentiality is strictly maintained. A two-year follow-up program is required of each recovering nurse.

Name of contact person: Andrea Brooks, MSHP, RN, CD, Program Director

Address: Texas Nurses Association
300 Highland Mall Boulevard, Suite 300
Austin, Texas 78752-3718
(512) 467-7027

Daytime hrs./days contact person is available by phone: 24 hours per day.

Hotline telephone number: (800) 288-5528 (inside Texas only); (512) 467-7027 (outside Texas, available 24 hours every day)

UTAH NURSES' ASSOCIATION

The Utah Nurses' Association sponsors Nurses Assisting Nurses with Substance Abuse (NANSA). The program assists nurses identified by the State Board of Nursing or referred directly to UNA with legal, professional, and treatment issues.

Module II.2—Handout #8 *(continued)*

Name of contact person: Executive Director

Address: Utah Nurses' Association
1058A East 900 South
Salt Lake City, Utah 84105
(801) 322-3439 (daytime)

Daytime hrs./days contact person is available by phone: 8:30 a.m.–4:30 p.m., Monday–Friday

Hotline telephone number: none established.

VERMONT STATE NURSES' ASSOCIATION, INC.

The Task Force on Impairment Among Nurses was directed by the members of VSNA at the 1986 convention to move ahead in the development of a peer support program. The task force assisted with the development of management principles and work with other state groups to develop a statewide impairment support program for physicians, dentists, veterinarians, pharmacists, and nurses. This interdisciplinary group, Vermont Recovering Professionals (VRP), has grown such that the VSNA task force has been disbanded, and VSNA sends official representatives to VRP. VRP continues to work on developing educational programs and developing a statewide impairment program for professionals.

Name of contact person: Lynne Dapice, MS, RN, Executive Director

Address: Vermont State Nurses' Association, Inc.
500 Dorset Street
South Burlington, Vermont 05403
(802) 864-9390 (daytime)

Daytime hrs./days contact person is available by phone: 8:30 a.m.–4:30 p.m., Monday–Friday

Hotline telephone number: none established.

VIRGINIA NURSES' ASSOCIATION

The Virginia Nurses' Association's Peer Assistance for Chemically Dependent Nurses Committee provides peer support/advocacy, education, consultation, and referral services. Information handouts for wide distribution have been developed which include a Fact Sheet, Selection Criteria for Treatment Programs, Bibliography, and Reentry Guidelines. Multiple training programs have been conducted for the Peer Assistance Volunteers who will form the cadre of peer interveners and monitors of proposed Regional Liaison Teams. The Peer Assistance Volunteer Program has been very well received around the state. A formal statement of understanding with the Virginia Board of Nursing is near completion. This understanding will provide for intervention in lieu of disciplinary action.

Module II.2—Handout #8 *(continued)*

Name of contact person: Lee Crigler, MSN, RN, CS, Chairperson,
Peer Assistance for Chemically Dependent Nurses Committee,
or Jay Douglas, MSN, RN

Address: Virginia Nurses' Association
1311 High Point Avenue
Richmond, Virginia 23230
(804) 353-7311 (daytime)

Daytime hrs./days contact person is available by phone: 8:00 a.m.–6:00 p.m., Monday–Friday

Evening hrs./days contact person is available by phone: Per arrangement.

Hotline telephone number: none established.

WASHINGTON STATE NURSES ASSOCIATION

The Washington State Nurses Association maintains a list of nurses willing to assist their chemically dependent peers. A position paper on the "Need for Employee Assistance Programs for Chemically Dependent Nurses" has been written. An audiotape, "Reaching Out: Nurses Share Recovery," a discussion with a group of recovering nurses, is available for $10.00, with discounts available on quantities.

Name of contact person: Executive Director

Address: Washington State Nurses Association
83 South King Street, Suite 500
Seattle, Washington 98104
(206) 622-3613 (daytime)

Daytime hrs./days contact person is available by phone: 8:00 a.m.–4:30 p.m., Monday–Friday

WEST VIRGINIA NURSES ASSOCIATION, INC.

The Nurse Care Network is a voluntary peer information and support network for nurses suffering from problems such as: addiction, stress, burnout, and others, with a strong emphasis on post-treatment individual and group support. Education and prevention information, seminars, and workshops are provided to nurses, supervisors, and students. The Nurse Care Network is endorsed by, but not sponsored by, the West Virginia Nurses Association, Inc.

Name of contact person: Barbara C. Banonis, BSN, RN, OPC, Chairperson,
Nurse Care Network

Address: Barbara C. Banonis Associates
P.O. Box 8491
South Charleston, West Virginia 25303
(304) 342-5110 (daytime/evening)

Module II.2—Handout #8 *(continued)*

Daytime/evening hrs./days contact person is available by phone: Variable hours; on answering machine when not available by phone.

Hotline telephone number: none established.

WISCONSIN NURSES ASSOCIATION, INC.

The Wisconsin Nurses Association Board of Directors, on July 21, 1988, took action to establish a task force to further explore a peer assistance program for nurses whose practice is impaired by substance abuse. The task force includes representatives of WNA, the WNA Economic and General Welfare Commission, and ten other nursing organizations in the state.

Name of contact person: Nancy Cervanansky, MSN, RN, Chair,
    Peer Assistance Task Force

Address: Wisconsin Nurses Association, Inc.
    6117 Monona Drive
    Madison, Wisconsin 53716
    (608) 221-0383 (daytime)

WYOMING NURSES ASSOCIATION

The Wyoming Nurses Association is currently investigating options related to peer assistance. Because of limited resources, WNA is currently able only to refer nurses whose practice is impaired by substance abuse to treatment programs in the state.

Name of contact person: Mary Lou Scavnicky-Mylant, PhD, RN

Address: Box 306S
    University Station
    Laramie, Wyoming 82071
    (307) 766-4291

Daytime hrs./days contact person is available by phone: 9:00 a.m.–3:00 p.m., Monday–Friday

Module II.2

Module II.2—Handout #8 *(continued)*

STATE NURSES' ASSOCIATIONS

Alabama
Elizabeth Barker Morris, MSEd, RN
Executive Director
Alabama State Nurses' Association
360 North Hull Street
Montgomery, Alabama 36197
(205) 262-8321

Alaska
Barbara Miller, BS, RN, CNA
Acting Executive Director
Alaska Nurses Association
237 East Third Avenue
Anchorage, Alaska 99501
(907) 274-0827

Arizona
Cathleen K. Wilson, PhD, RN
Executive Director
Arizona Nurses' Association
1850 East Southern Avenue, Suite 1
Tempe, Arizona 85282
(602) 831-0404

Arkansas
Billie Larch, MSE, MA, RN
Executive Director
Arkansas State Nurses' Association
117 South Cedar Street
Little Rock, Arkansas 72205
(501) 664-5853

California
Barbara L. Nichols, MS, RN, FAAN
Executive Director
California Nurses Association
1855 Folsom Street, Suite 670
San Francisco, California 94103
(415) 864-4141

Colorado
Alison Biggs, RN
Interim Executive Director
Colorado Nurses' Association
5453 East Evans Place
Denver, Colorado 80222
(303) 757-7484

Connecticut
Karen Stonkas Ponton, MA, RN
Executive Director
Connecticut Nurses' Association
Meritech Business Park
377 Research Parkway, Suite 2D
Meriden, Connecticut 06450
(203) 238-1207

Delaware
Ruth Bashford, MN, RN
Executive Director
Delaware Nurses' Association
2634 Capitol Trail, Suite C
Newark, Delaware 19711
(302) 368-2333

District of Columbia
Evelyn Sommers, MBA
Executive Director
District of Columbia Nurses'
Association, Inc., Suite 306
5100 Wisconsin Avenue, N.W.
Washington, D.C. 20016
(202) 244-2705

Florida
Paula Massey, MN, RN
Executive Director
Florida Nurses Association
P.O. Box 536985
Orlando, Florida 32853-6985
(407) 896-3261

Module II.2—Handout #8 *(continued)*

Georgia
Susan Williamson, MPH, RN
Executive Director
Georgia Nurses Association, Inc.
1362 West Peachtree Street, N.W.
Atlanta, Georgia 30309
(404) 876-4624

Guam
Rosita Yamashita, RN
Secretary
Guam Nurses' Association
P.O. Box 3134
Agana, Guam 96910
(671) 646-5801

Hawaii
Rosalind F. Wagner, RN
Executive Director
Hawaii Nurses' Association
677 Ala Moana Boulevard, Suite 301
Honolulu, Hawaii 96813
(808) 531-1628

Idaho
Maria Eschen, PhD, RN
Executive Director
Idaho Nurses Association
200 North 4th Street, Suite 20
Boise, Idaho 83702-6001
(208) 345-0500

Illinois
Louise Shores, EdD, RN
Executive Administrator
Illinois Nurses Association
20 North Wacker Drive, Suite 2520
Chicago, Illinois 60606
(312) 236-9708

Indiana
Naomi R. Patchin
Executive Director
Indiana State Nurses' Association
2915 North High School Road
Indianapolis, Indiana 46224
(317) 299-4575/4576

Iowa
JoAnne H. Kennebeck, JD, RN
Executive Director
Iowa Nurses' Association
100 Court Avenue, 9LL
Des Moines, Iowa 50309
(515) 282-9169

Kansas
Terri R. Roberts, JD, RN
Executive Director
Kansas State Nurses Association
820 Quincy Street
Topeka, Kansas 66612
(913) 233-8638

Kentucky
Barbara Dermody, MSN, RN, C
Executive Director
Kentucky Nurses Association
1400 South First Street
P.O. Box 2616
Louisville, Kentucky 40201
(502) 637-2546/2547

Louisiana
Mical DeBrow, MSN, RN, CCRN
Executive Director
Louisiana State Nurses Association
712 Transcontinental Drive
Metairie, Louisiana 70001
(504) 889-1030

Maine
Anne Sassong, RN
Executive Director
Maine State Nurses' Association
P.O. Box 2240
Augusta, Maine 04330
(207) 622-1057

Maryland
Robin Platts
Executive Director
Maryland Nurses Association, Inc.
5820 Southwestern Boulevard
Baltimore, Maryland 21227
(301) 242-7300

Module II.2—Handout #8 *(continued)*

Massachusetts
Barbara Roderick, MS, RN
Acting Executive Director
Massachusetts Nurses Association
340 Turnpike Street
Canton, Massachusetts 02021
(617) 821-4625

Michigan
Carol E. Franck, MSN, RN
Executive Director
Michigan Nurses Association
120 Spartan Avenue
East Lansing, Michigan 48823
(517) 337-1653

Minnesota
Sonja Meyerholz, MSN, RN
Executive Director
Minnesota Nurses Association
1295 Bandana Boulevard North, Suite 140
St. Paul, Minnesota 55108-5115
(612) 646-4807

Mississippi
Betty Dickson
Executive Director
Mississippi Nurses' Association
135 Bounds Street, Suite 100
Jackson, Mississippi 39206
(601) 982-9182/9183

Missouri
Mary E. Riner, MN, RN, CNA
Executive Director
Missouri Nurses Association
P.O. Box 325
206 East Dunklin Street
Jefferson City, Missouri 65102
(314) 636-4623

Montana
Barbara E. Booher
Executive Director
Montana Nurses' Association
715 Getchell
P.O. Box 5718
Helena, Montana 59604
(406) 442-6710

Nebraska
Donna R. Baker, MS, RN
Executive Director
Nebraska Nurses' Association
941 "O" Street, Suite 707–711
Lincoln, Nebraska 68508
(402) 475-3589

Nevada
Linda Roide
Office Manager
Nevada Nurses' Association
3660 Baker Lane, Suite 104
Reno, Nevada 89509
(702) 825-3555

New Hampshire
Theresa Bonanno, MSN, RN, C
Executive Director
New Hampshire Nurses' Association
48 West Street
Concord, New Hampshire 03301
(603) 225-3783

New Jersey
Dorothy Flemming, MSN, RN
Executive Director
New Jersey State Nurses Association
320 West State Street
Trenton, New Jersey 08618
(609) 392-4884/2031
FAX (609) 396-2330

New Mexico
Florence Hendrickson, RN
Executive Director
New Mexico Nurses Association
525 San Pedro, N.E., Suite 100
Albuquerque, New Mexico 87108
(505) 268-7744

New York
Martha L. Orr, MN, RN
Executive Director
New York State Nurses Association
2113 Western Avenue
Guilderland, New York 12084
(518) 456-5371
FAX (518) 456-0697

Instructor's Guide

Module II.2—Handout #8 *(continued)*

North Carolina
Executive Director
North Carolina Nurses Association
103 Enterprise Street
Box 12025
Raleigh, North Carolina 27605
(919) 821-4250

North Dakota
Ida Rigley, MSN, RN, C
Executive Director
North Dakota Nurses' Association
212 North Fourth Street
Bismarck, North Dakota 58501
(701) 223-1385

Ohio
Joanne F. Easterling, MSN, RN
Executive Director
Ohio Nurses Association
4000 East Main Street
Columbus, Ohio 43213-2950
(614) 237-5414

Oklahoma
Frances I. Waddle, MSN, RN
Executive Director
Oklahoma Nurses Association
6414 North Santa Fe, Suite A
Oklahoma City, Oklahoma 73116
(405) 840-3476

Oregon
Paula A. McNeil, BSN, RN
Executive Director
Oregon Nurses Association, Inc.
9700 S.W. Capitol Highway, Suite 200
Portland, Oregon 97219
(503) 293-0011

Pennsylvania
David R. Ranch, MSEd, RN
Executive Administrator
Pennsylvania Nurses Association
2578 Interstate Drive
P.O. Box 8525
Harrisburg, Pennsylvania 17105-8525
(717) 657-1222
FAX (717) 657-3796

Rhode Island
Judy L. Sheehan-Beliveau, MSN, RN
Rhode Island State Nurses' Association
Hall Building South
345 Blackstone Boulevard
Providence, Rhode Island 02906
(401) 421-9703

South Carolina
Judith C. Thompson
Executive Director
South Carolina Nurses' Association
1821 Gadsden Street
Columbia, South Carolina 29201
(803) 252-4781

South Dakota
Kate Heligas, RN
Executive Director
South Dakota Nurses' Association, Inc.
1505 South Minnesota, Suite 6
Sioux Falls, South Dakota 57105
(605) 338-1401

Tennessee
Louise Browning, CAE
Executive Director
Tennessee Nurses' Association
1720 West End Building, Suite 400
Nashville, Tennessee 37203
(615) 329-2511

Texas
Clair B. Jordan, MSN, RN
Executive Director
Texas Nurses Association
Community Bank Building, Suite 300
300 Highland Mall Boulevard
Austin, Texas 78752-3718
(512) 452-0645
FAX (512) 452-0648

Utah
Nancy Lundgren
Business Manager
Utah Nurses' Association
1058A East 900 South
Salt Lake City, Utah 84105
(801) 322-3439/3430

Module II.2—Handout #8 *(continued)*

Vermont
Lynne Dapice, MS, RN
Executive Director
Vermont State Nurses' Association, Inc.
500 Dorset Street
South Burlington, Vermont 05403
(802) 864-9390

Virgin Islands
Verna C. Garcia, BSN, RN
Executive Secretary
Virgin Islands Nurses' Association
P.O. Box 583
Christiansted
St. Croix, U.S. Virgin Islands 00820
(809) 773-2323, Ext. 116/118

Virginia
Jan Marshall Johnson, MS, RN
Executive Director
Virginia Nurses' Association
1311 High Point Avenue
Richmond, Virginia 23230
(804) 353-1775

Washington
Patty Jones, MN, RN
Acting Executive Director
Washington State Nurses Association
83 South King Street, Suite 500
Seattle, Washington 98104
(206) 622-3613

West Virginia
Carol S. Fulks
Executive Director
West Virginia Nurses Association, Inc.
2 Players Club Drive, Building 3
P.O. Box 1946
Charleston, West Virginia 25327
(304) 342-1169

Wisconsin
JoAnn G. Hanaway, MSN, RN, C
Executive Administrator
Wisconsin Nurses Association, Inc.
6117 Monona Drive
Madison, Wisconsin 53716
(608) 221-0383

Wyoming
Margaret L. Pouppirt, MBA
Executive Director
Wyoming Nurses Association
Majestic Building, Room 305
1603 Capitol Avenue
Cheyenne, Wyoming 82001
(307) 635-3955

Instructor's Guide

Module II.2—Handout #8   *(continued)*

STATE BOARDS OF NURSING

Alabama
Shirley Dykes
Executive Officer
Alabama Board of Nursing
500 Eastern Boulevard, Suite 203
Montgomery, Alabama 36117
(205) 261-4060

Alaska
Gail M. McGuill
Executive Officer
Alaska Board of Nursing Licensing
Department of Commerce and Economic
  Development
Division of Occupational Licensing
P.O. Box D-LIC
Juneau, Alaska 99811-0800
(907) 465-2544

Arizona
Fran Roberts
Executive Director
Arizona Board of Nursing
2001 W. Camelback Road, Suite 350
Phoenix, Arizona 85015
(602) 255-5092

Arkansas
June Garner
Executive Director
Arkansas State Board of Nursing
University Tower Building
1123 South University Avenue, Suite 800
Little Rock, Arkansas 72204
(501) 371-2751

California
Catherine Puri
Executive Director
California Board of Registered Nursing
P.O. Box 944210
1030 13th Street, Suite 200
Sacramento, California 94244-2100
(916) 322-3350

Colorado
Karen Brumley
Program Administrator
Colorado Board of Nursing
1650 Broadway, Suite 670
Denver, Colorado 80202
(303) 894-2430

Connecticut
Bette Jane Murphy
Chairperson
Connecticut Board of Examiners
  for Nursing
Department of Health Services
150 Washington Street
Hartford, Connecticut 06106
(203) 566-1041

Delaware
Rosalee Seymour
Executive Director
Delaware Board of Nursing
Margaret O'Neill Building
Federal and Court Streets
P.O. Box 1401
Dover, Delaware 19903
(302) 736-4522

District of Columbia
Barbara J. Hatcher
Chairperson
District of Columbia Board of Nursing
614 H Street, N.W., Room 112
P.O. Box 37200
Washington, D.C. 20013-7200
(202) 727-7468

Florida
Judie Ritter
Executive Director
Florida State Board of Nursing
111 Coastline Drive, East, Suite 540
Jacksonville, Florida 32202
(904) 359-6331

Module II.2—Handout #8 *(continued)*

Georgia
Carolyn Hutcherson
Executive Director
Georgia Board of Nursing,
  Registered Nurses
166 Pryor Street, S.W., Suite 400
Atlanta, Georgia 30303
(404) 656-3943

Guam
Teofila P. Cruz
Nurse Examiner Administrator
Guam Board of Nurse Examiners
P.O. Box 2816
Agana, Guam 96910
(617) 477-8766/8517

Hawaii
Jerold Sakoda
Executive Secretary
Board of Nursing, State of Hawaii
P.O. Box 3469
Honolulu, Hawaii 96801
(808) 548-3086

Idaho
Phyllis T. Sheridan
Executive Director
Idaho Board of Nursing
500 South 10th Street, Suite 102
Boise, Idaho 83720
(208) 334-3110

Illinois
Gary Clayton
Director
Illinois Department of Professional
  Regulation
320 West Washington Street, 3rd Fl.
Springfield, Illinois 62786
(212) 785-0800

Indiana
Linda D. McClain
Board Administrator
Indiana State Board of Nursing
Health Professions Service Bureau
One American Square, Suite 1020
P.O. Box 82067
Indianapolis, Indiana 46282-0004
(317) 232-2960

Iowa
Ann E. Mowery
Executive Director
Iowa Board of Nursing
1223 East Court
Des Moines, Iowa 50319
(515) 281-3255

Kansas
Dr. Lois Rich Scibetta
Executive Administrator
Kansas Board of Nursing
Landon State Office Building
900 S.W. Jackson, Room 551 S
Topeka, Kansas 66612-1256
(913) 296-4929

Kentucky
Sharon Weisenbeck
Executive Director
Kentucky State Board of Nursing
4010 Dupont Circle, Suite 430
Louisville, Kentucky 40207
(502) 897-5143

Louisiana
Merlyn M. Maillian
Executive Director
Louisiana State Board of Nursing
907 Pere Marquette Building
150 Baronne Street
New Orleans, Louisiana 70112
(504) 568-5464

Maine
Jean C. Caron
Executive Director
Maine State Board of Nursing
295 Water Street
Augusta, Maine 04330
(207) 289-5324

Maryland
Donna M. Dorsey
Executive Director
Maryland Board of Nursing
201 West Preston Street
Baltimore, Maryland 21201
(301) 225-5880

Module II.2—Handout #8 *(continued)*

Massachusetts
Mary H. Snodgrass
Executive Secretary
Massachusetts Board of Registration
  in Nursing
100 Cambridge Street, Room 1519
Boston, Massachusetts 02202
(617) 727-7393

Michigan
Administrative Assistant
Michigan Board of Nursing
P.O. Box 30018
Lansing, Michigan 48909
(517) 373-1600

Minnesota
Joyce M. Schowalter
Executive Director
Minnesota Board of Nursing
2700 University Avenue W., Suite 108
St. Paul, Minnesota 55114
(612) 642-0567

Mississippi
Marcella McKay
Executive Director
Mississippi Board of Nursing
239 North Lamar, Suite 401
Jackson, Mississippi 39206
(601) 359-6170

Missouri
Florence McGuire
Executive Director
Missouri State Board of Nursing
3523 North Ten Mile Drive
P.O. Box 656
Jefferson City, Missouri 65102
(314) 751-2334

Montana
Phyllis McDonald
Executive Secretary
Montana State Board of Nursing
Department of Commerce
1424 Ninth Avenue
Helena, Montana 59620-0407
(406) 444-4279

Nebraska
Vicky Burbach
Nursing Practice Consultant
Nebraska Board of Nursing
State House Station, Box 95007
Lincoln, Nebraska 68509
(402) 471-2115

Nevada
Lonna Burress
Executive Director
Nevada State Board of Nursing
1281 Terminal Way, Suite 116
Reno, Nevada 89502
(702) 786-2778

New Hampshire
Doris E. Nay
Executive Director
New Hampshire Board of Nursing
Division of Public Health Services
Health and Welfare Building
6 Hazen Drive
Concord, New Hampshire 03301-6527
(603) 271-2323

New Jersey
Sister Teresa Louise Harris
Executive Director
New Jersey Board of Nursing
1100 Raymond Boulevard, Room 319
Newark, New Jersey 07102
(201) 648-2490

New Mexico
Nancy Twigg, Executive Director
New Mexico Regulation and Licensing
  Department/Nursing
4125 Carlisle, N.E.
Albuquerque, New Mexico 87107
(505) 841-6524

New York
Milene A. Megel, Executive Secretary
New York State Board for Nursing
State Education Department
Cultural Education Center, Room 3013
Albany, New York 12230
(518) 474-3843

Module II.2

Module II.2—Handout #8 *(continued)*

North Carolina
Carol A. Osman
Executive Director
North Carolina Board of Nursing
P.O. Box 2129
Raleigh, North Carolina 27602
(919) 782-3211

North Dakota
Karen MacDonald
Executive Director
North Dakota Board of Nursing
919 S. 7th Street, Suite 504
Bismarck, North Dakota 58504
(701) 224-2974

Ohio
Rosa Lee Weinert
Executive Secretary
Ohio Board of Nursing Education and
 Nurse Registration
65 South Front Street, Suite 509
Columbus, Ohio 43266-0316
(614) 466-3947

Oklahoma
Sulinda Moffett
Executive Director
Oklahoma Board of Nurse Registration and
 Nursing Education
2915 No. Classen Boulevard, Suite 524
Oklahoma City, Oklahoma 73106
(405) 525-2076

Oregon
Dorothy J. Davy
Executive Director
Oregon State Board of Nursing
1400 S.W. Fifth Avenue, Room 904
Portland, Oregon 97201
(503) 229-5623

Pennsylvania
Miriam H. Limo
Executive Secretary
Pennsylvania State Board of Nursing
P.O. Box 2649
Harrisburg, Pennsylvania 17105-2649
(717) 783-7146

Rhode Island
Bertha Mugurdichian
Executive Secretary
Rhode Island Board of Nurse Registration
 and Nursing Education
Cannon Health Building, Room 104
75 Davis Street
Providence, Rhode Island 02908
(401) 277-2827

South Carolina
Renatta Loquist
Executive Director
State Board of Nursing
 for South Carolina
1777 St. Julian Place, Suite 102
Columbia, South Columbia 29204
(803) 737-6594

South Dakota
Carol Stuart
Executive Secretary
South Dakota Board of Nursing
304 South Phillips Avenue, Suite 205
Sioux Falls, South Dakota 57102
(605) 335-4973

Tennessee
Elizabeth Lund
Executive Director
Tennessee State Board of Nursing
Bureau of Manpower and Facilities
283 Plus Park Boulevard
Nashville, Tennessee 37219-5401
(615) 367-6232

Texas
Louise Waddill
Executive Secretary
Board of Nurse Examiners
 for the State of Texas
P.O. Box 140406
Austin, Texas 78714
(512) 835-4880

Module II.2—Handout #8 *(continued)*

Utah
Executive Secretary
Utah State Board of Nursing
Division of Occupational and Professional Licensing
Heber M. Wells Building, 4th Floor
160 E. 300 Street, P.O. Box 45802
Salt Lake City, Utah 84145-0801
(801) 530-6733

Vermont
Dennis Ross
Chairperson
Vermont State Board of Nursing
Redstone Building
26 Terrace Street
Montpelier, Vermont 05602
(802) 828-2396

Virgin Islands
Juanita Molloy
Executive Secretary
Virgin Islands Board of Nurse Licensure
Knud-Hansen Complex
P.O. Box 7309
Charlotte Amalie
St. Thomas, Virgin Islands 00801
(809) 774-9000

Virginia
Executive Director
Virginia State Board of Nursing
1601 Rolling Hills Drive
Richmond, Virginia 23229
(804) 662-9909

Washington
Constance Roth
Executive Secretary
Washington State Board of Nursing
Division of Professional Licensing
Healthcare RN Department
P.O. Box 9649
Olympia, Washington 98504
(206) 753-2206

West Virginia
Garnette Thorne
Executive Secretary
West Virginia Board of Examiners for Registered Nurses
Embleton Building, Suite 309
922 Quarrier Street
Charleston, West Virginia 25301
(304) 348-3596

Wisconsin
Ramona W. Warden
Director
Wisconsin Board of Nursing
P.O. Box 8935
Madison, Wisconsin 53708-8935
(608) 266-3735

Wyoming
Joan Bouchard
Executive Director
Wyoming State Board of Nursing
Barrett Building, 4th Floor
2301 Central Avenue
Cheyenne, Wyoming 82002
(307) 777-7601

Module II.2

Module II.2—Handout #8 *(continued)*

SPECIALTY NURSING GROUPS

Drug and Alcohol Nursing Association
720 Light Street
Baltimore, Maryland 21230-2186

International Nurses Anonymous
c/o Patricia Green, MSW, RN
1020 Sunset Drive
Lawrence, Kansas 66044

National Consortium of Chemical
   Dependency Nurses
99 West 10th, Suite 319
Eugene, Oregon 97401

National Nurses Society on Addictions
5700 Old Orchard Road
Skokie, Illinois 60877

Instructor's Guide

Module II.2—Handout #8 *(continued)*

AGENCIES AND OTHER PROFESSIONAL GROUPS

Alcohol and Drug Problems Association
 of North America
444 North Capitol Street, N.W., Suite 706
Washington, D.C. 20001

American Bar Association
750 North Lake Shore Drive
Chicago, Illinois 60611

American Council for Drug Education
204 Monroe Street
Rockville, Maryland 20850

American Council on Alcoholism
White Marsh Business Center
5024 Campbell Blvd., Suite H
Baltimore, Maryland 21236

American Dental Association
211 East Chicago Avenue
Chicago, Illinois 60611

American Medical Association
535 North Dearborn Street
Chicago, Illinois 60610

American Medical Society on Alcoholism
 and Other Drug Dependencies
12 West 21st Street, 8th Floor
New York, New York 10010

American Pharmaceutical Association
2215 Constitution Avenue, N.W.
Washington, D.C. 20037

Association of Medical Education and
 Research in Substance Abuse Center for
 Alcohol and Addiction Studies
Brown University, Box G
Providence, Rhode Island 02912

Center for Alcohol Studies
Chapel Hill, North Carolina 27514

Center for Alcohol Studies
Smithers Hall, Busch Campus
Rutgers, State University of New Jersey
Piscataway, New Jersey 08854

Drug Enforcement Administration
Lincoln Place-East
600 Army and Navy Drive
Arlington, Virginia 22202

Employee Assistance Professionals
 Association
4601 North Fairfax Drive, Suite 1001
Arlington, Virginia 22203

International Commission for the
 Prevention of Alcoholism and Drug
 Dependency
12501 Old Columbia Pike
Silver Spring, Maryland 20904

National Association of Addiction
 Treatment Providers
2082 Michelson Drive, Suite 101
Irvine, California 92715

National Association of Social Workers
7981 Eastern Avenue
Silver Spring, Maryland 20910

National Association of State Alcohol and
 Drug Abuse Directors
Suite 520
444 North Capitol Street, N.W.
Washington, D.C. 20001

National Association on Drug Abuse
 Problems
355 Lexington Avenue
New York, New York 10017

Module II.2

Module II.2—Handout #8 *(continued)*

National Clearinghouse for Alcohol
  Information
16C-10 Parklawn Building
5600 Fishers Lane
Rockville, Maryland 20857

National Council on Alcoholism
12 West 21st Street
New York, New York 10010

National Institute on Alcohol Abuse and
  Alcoholism
16-105 Parklawn Building
5600 Fishers Lane
Rockville, Maryland 20857

National Institute on Drug Abuse
10-05 Parklawn Building
5600 Fishers Lane
Rockville, Maryland 20857

Oregon Institute of Alcoholism Studies
Willamette University
900 State Street
Salem, Oregon 97301

Pharmacists Against Drug Abuse
Welsh and McKean Roads
Spring House, Pennsylvania 19477

Society for Professional Well-Being
5102 Chapel Hill Boulevard
Durham, North Carolina 27707

University of California at San Diego
  Summer School of Alcohol and Other
  Drug Studies
UCSD Extension X-001
LaJolla, California 92093

University of Utah School on Alcoholism
  and Other Drug Dependencies
P.O. Box 2604
Salt Lake City, Utah 84110

Women for Sobriety
P.O. Box 618
Quakertown, Pennsylvania 18951

Instructor's Guide

Module II.2—Handout #9

STATE NURSES' ASSOCIATIONS—PEER ASSISTANCE ACTIVITIES OVERVIEW

	Services Offered							Assistance Limited To		Program Run By			Diversion Legislation			
	Intervention	Referral	Education	Peer Support Group	Regionalized Contracts Statewide	Reentry Monitoring	Hotline	RNs Only	Nurses Who Are State Residents	Volunteers	Volunteers Reimbursed for Expenses	Paid Staff	Passed	Introduced	Considered	Rejected
Alabama			x													
Alaska			x													
Arizona		x	x	x	x			yes		x		x		x		
Arkansas°		x	x	x				no	no	x						
California		x	x	x	x			yes	no		x	x	x			
Colorado	x	x	x	x	x	x	x	no	yes		x	x	x		x	
Connecticut		x	x							x					x	
Delaware	x	x	x				x	no		x						
Dist. of Columbia		x	x					yes		x		x		x		
Florida		x	x										x			
Georgia	x	x	x	x	x	x	x	no	no	x						
Guam																
Hawaii																
Idaho	x	x	x												x	
Illinois		x	x		x			no	no	x		x	x			
Indiana	x	x	x		x	x	x	yes	yes	x	x	x				
Iowa																
Kansas	x	x	x		x	x		no	no		x	x			x	
Kentucky		x	x	x			x	yes	no	x						
Louisiana	x	x	x	x	x	x	x	yes	no	x	x	x			x	
Maine																
Maryland		x	x	x	x			yes	no	x		x	x			
Massachusetts		x	x	x	x			yes	yes	x			x			
Michigan		x	x		x			no	no	x		x		x		
Minnesota	x	x	x		x	x		yes	no		x	x			x	
Mississippi		x	x													
Missouri		x	x					no	yes	x						
Montana			x	x	x	x		no	no	x			x			
Nebraska	x		x	x		x		no	yes	x				x	x	
Nevada			x	x						x					x	

197

Module II.2

Module II.2—Handout #9 (continued)

	Services Offered							Assistance Limited To		Program Run By			Diversion Legislation			
	Intervention	Referral	Education	Peer Support Group	Regionalized Contracts Statewide	Reentry Monitoring	Hotline	RNs Only	Nurses Who Are State Residents	Volunteers	Volunteers Reimbursed for Expenses	Paid Staff	Passed	Introduced	Considered	Rejected
New Hampshire			x					no	no	x						
New Jersey		x	x	x	x			no	no	x		x				
New Mexico		x	x	x									x			
New York			x		x			no	no		x	x	x			
N. Carolina		x	x		x			yes	yes	x		x			x	
N. Dakota°°°		x	x							x		x				
Ohio	x	x	x	x	x	x		no	no		x	x				
Oklahoma	x	x	x	x	x	x	x	no	yes	x	x	x			x	
Oregon	x	x	x	x	x		x	no	no	x					x	
Pennsylvania	x	x	x	x	x						x	x			x	
Rhode Island	x	x	x	x	x	x	x		yes							
S. Carolina	x	x	x	x	x	x			yes	x						
S. Dakota°°			x			x										
Tennessee	x	x	x	x	x	x	x	no	no	x	x	x			x	
Texas	x	x	x	x	x	x	x	no	yes		x	x	x			
Utah		x														
Vermont°°°			x						yes	x					x	
Virgin Islands																
Virginia		x	x	x	x			yes	yes	x					x	
Washington		x	x					yes	no			x	x			
W. Virginia°°	x	x	x	x	x	x	x		yes	x						
Wisconsin																
Wyoming		x														

°Program is sponsored by ASNA District 10.
°°Program is endorsed by, but not sponsored by the SNA.
°°°Program is sponsored by a coalition, of which the SNA is a part.

Instructor's Guide

Module II.2—Handout #10

GUIDELINES FOR DEVELOPING A HOSPITAL-BASED EMPLOYEE ASSISTANCE PROGRAM

These Guidelines were developed by the Task Force on Alcoholism and Substance Abuse in the Profession of Nursing and were based on a document which was originally developed with the assistance of the New York State Division of Alcoholism and Alcohol Abuse.

Approved by the NYSNA Board of Directors
June 6, 1986

INTRODUCTION

An Employee Assistance Program (EAP) is a confidential, work-based system for the identification, motivation for treatment, referral, and follow-up of employees with problems that may interfere with the ability to function at work. Access to the system may be by self-referral or a mandatory recommendation when job performance has been affected. Behavioral/health problems directly associated with one's ability to function in the work setting include, but are not limited to alcoholism, drug use and abuse, financial, family, or psychosocial difficulties.

NEED FOR PROGRAM

Employees with behavioral/health problems are often unable to devote needed time and attention to their position performance and as a result represent a severe human and economic burden. This is reflected in increased absenteeism, decreased productivity, excessive waste, accidents, poor decision making, and higher insurance premiums. In a hospital setting these problems interfere with the quality of patient care and are often reflected in illegal activities, such as drug diversion, theft, or sale. Licensed professionals who practice while under the influence of drugs or alcohol are in violation of their license.

 The workplace provides an ideal setting for early intervention with employees who are affected by behavioral/health problems. Such employees often use employment as a factor in their denial that the problem exists. However, when these employees are confronted with a choice of losing their position or accepting a referral for help, they will choose assistance. Therefore, work-based programs are recognized as a means for effective early intervention with employees with health problems. Within these programs, activities must be provided to intervene appropriately with employees who have specific problems. The legal implications associated with alcohol and/or other mood-altering substances require these activities in order to assure the accurate identification of alcoholism and drug abuse.

 Employee Assistance Programs provide a system within the work setting whereby employees with problems are referred for needed assistance, treatment or rehabilitation, and follow-up, thus minimizing disruption at the workplace. While the programs generally do not provide direct treatment services, they are invaluable for motivating, referral, and monitoring. The follow-up provided to employees makes it possible to identify needed

Module II.2—Handout #10 (continued)

additional services and assures that recommended treatment and rehabilitation services are utilized by program participants.

Program services can be obtained by employees who either voluntarily seek assistance or are referred through established procedures. Some programs are available to the family members of employees. All information concerning program participation is confidential, and participation in the program does not jeopardize an employee's standing in the workplace or promotional opportunities. These programs do not replace existing disciplinary procedures. They provide an additional system for preserving valuable staff resources and for reducing the economic and human toll that results from health problems.

SPECIAL NEEDS FOR NURSES

Every year a significant number of nurses are referred for license review because of unprofessional conduct related to alcohol abuse and/or other chemical dependencies. While Employee Assistance Programs are highly effective in the identification, motivation, and referral of most employees in need of assistance, there are existing barriers to program participation for nurses. These barriers include (1) the limited employment of nurse counselors in EAPs, (2) limited personal control of work time, and (3) shift rotations.

The attitudes of health care providers, the gender-oriented nature of treatment approaches, and the absence of strategies designed for professional health care workers pose additional barriers. Additional assistance is necessary to coordinate with institutions that employ nurses. Such assistance should provide mechanisms to promote early intervention, motivate nurses to accept treatment, and, at the same time, safeguard the quality of patient care. Such a system does not replace the Employee Assistance Program but enhances it. Frequently, it is a peer assistance program which is developed as the component to providing this capability.

PROGRAM MODELS

The decision as to the type of program best suited to a specific setting must be based on several factors:

— Number of nursing personnel to be served by the program;

— Services available to employees; and

— Budgetary constraints.

Experience in program development and operation demonstrates that a qualified full-time staff best promotes optimal effectiveness. In hospital settings where the number of employees does not justify the designation of full-time EAP staff, the Employee Health Service or Personnel Department may be able to include EAP services with other functions. The staff must be properly trained. Program services can also be provided by external consultants through a contractual arrangement with the hospital.

Regardless of the type of services selected, an EAP must be tailored to meet the needs that exist within the institution where it will operate. Typical staff functions within an EAP include:

Instructor's Guide

Module II.2—Handout #10 *(continued)*

— Educating administrative personnel and labor representatives about the program;

— Orienting and educating personnel;

— Establishing and maintaining contact with referral resources;

— Liaison with a system of peer assistance for nurses;

— Assessing, referring, and follow-up of employees who voluntarily seek program services and those who are referred through established procedures; and

— Developing and maintaining a system of data collection and program evaluation.

PROGRAM ELEMENTS

A program must be integrated into the structure of a hospital and have the cooperation and participation of the administration, staff and representative labor groups. The following elements should be included in the program:

A. Committee of Concern (optional).

B. Program Coordinator (staff and position descriptions).

C. Program Definition.

D. Policy Statement.

E. Stated Procedures.

F. Insurance Coverage.

G. Educational Programs for Administrative Staff and Labor Personnel.

H. Employee Education and Information.

I. Designation of Referral Resources.

J. Data Collection—Privileged Information.

RECOMMENDED STEPS FOR PROGRAM IMPLEMENTATION

A. Committee of Concern

A Committee of Concern may be the initial step in the development of a program and can be utilized in the selection of a program coordinator. This Committee should include representatives from staff and administration. The Committee acts in an advisory capacity in determining the program's structure, its scope, and its functions. The Committee's role includes involvement in the development of a policy statement, procedures, and staff recruitment. The Committee may cease to exist when the program becomes functional, or it may continue to serve in an advisory role.

Steps:

— Identify committee members from administration, staff, and representative labor organizations.

Module II.2

Module II.2—Handout #10 *(continued)*

- Obtain assurance from administration and labor representatives that committee members will have work-release time to attend meetings.
- Define role and function of committee.

B. Program Coordinator

A program coordinator may be employed part-time or on a full-time basis. Size of program, number of employees, and budgetary considerations are some determining factors. Experiences has shown that a full-time staff person is recommended for 1,000 employees or more. Regardless of hours of function, a coordinator must fully understand EAPs and be able to assess employee problems, make appropriate referrals, and follow employees' progress. Responsibility includes training, education, and program promotion. Program coordination with an external EAP can be established through a liaison position within the hospital.

Identification and Designation of a Coordinator:

Steps:

- Determine position specification and competencies needed.
- Develop a position description and requirements for professional and educational background.
- Review with the administrator who has overall responsibility.
- Revise and obtain approval.
- Recruit, interview, and designate.
- Determine when additional education is needed.
- Inform employees about appointment of coordinator.

C. Program Definition

Steps:

- Review programs in other health care settings. Visit one or more established and active programs.
- Review existing needs in the health facility.
- Designate an office for overall program responsibility, or recommend a new office.
- Define nature and scope of program.
- Submit to appropriate administration and labor representatives for review and comment.
- Revise.
- Include definition in Policy Statement.

Instructor's Guide

Module II.2—Handout #10 *(continued)*

D. Policy Statement

Steps:

— Review existing policies on problem employees and disciplinary process.

— Recommend revision of existing policies.

— Meet with regional or local consultant to obtain assistance with policy development.

— Develop Policy Statement.

— Submit to appropriate administration and labor representatives for review and comment.

— Review and submit to appropriate governing body.

— Issue and circulate Policy Statement.

E. Stated Procedures

Steps:

— Review existing procedures with regard to:
  1. Employee performance evaluation.
  2. Documentation of absences.
  3. Disciplinary action.
  4. Management of employee health and safety.

— Recommend revision in existing procedures.

— Review guidelines.

— Develop procedures suitable for your facility.

— Submit to appropriate administrative and labor representatives for review and comment.

— Revise.

F. Insurance Coverage

Steps:

— Review existing insurance coverage for each employee group.

— Identify coverage, if any, to reimburse employees referred to outside services.

— Determine changes necessary for appropriate coverage.

— Meet with individuals responsible for employee/union benefits to determine feasibility of additional coverage through riders, increased insurance, or a fund to cover special treatment/rehabilitation services.

— Periodically review insurance coverage for adequacy. Make recommendations for change.

Module II.2

Module II.2—Handout #10 *(continued)*

G. Educational Programs for Administrative Staff and Labor Personnel

It is the responsibility of the program coordinator to ensure that appropriate educational programs are provided at all levels of the work setting. The coordinator is responsible for curriculum content.

Steps:

— Review education and staff development programs; e.g., in-service education, and program activity for management, supervisory, and union personnel.

— Determine whether educational and staff development programs can be incorporated into EAP training.

— Identify appropriate person(s) who will furnish training.

— Work with instructor(s) to develop educational outlines and content.

— Determine date(s), time, and location.

— Arrange for participation of appropriate persons with personnel, department heads, and union representatives.

H. Employee Education and Information

Employee education and information is an ongoing process. Posters, direct mailing to homes, newsletter articles, distribution of brochures, and audiovisual and verbal presentations are some ways to accomplish this. The coordinator, with the assistance of the Committee of Concern, can generate activities to meet the needs of a facility.

Steps:

— Develop materials with information specific to the setting.

— Establish and maintain contact with administrative and labor publications.

— Plan a campaign for information dissemination.

I. Designation of Referral Resources

Several factors must be considered in identifying resources to be used for referral. These include available services, fees, types of acceptable insurance, hours of operation, geographic location, and admission criteria. It is essential that treatment strategies recognize factors related to professional roles and responsibilities; e.g., attitudes and drug accessibility. Another important factor is the ease of coordination between program treatment staff. It is essential to maintain communication regarding employees referred for services. This is the responsibility of the program coordinator.

Steps:

— Identify services within your community.

— Visit facilities to determine:

Instructor's Guide

Module II.2—Handout #10 *(continued)*

      1. Type and quality of service.

      2. Fee structure.

      3. Insurance reimbursement policy.

      4. Admission procedures and limitations.

      5. Contact staff.

— Develop a referral list.

— Review and update list at regular intervals.

J. Data Collection Evaluation—Privileged Information

All information collected as part of program evaluation must be confidential. Program participants cannot be reported or identified.

Steps:

— Determine information to be recorded.

— Submit list to appropriate staff in the administration, personnel department, and labor groups.

— Develop a reporting form.

— Establish a reporting schedule.

— Review program utilization to determine if any program modifications are needed.

— Distribute aggregate data to designated staff.

POLICY STATEMENT

The policy statement defines the program, its scope, and activities. A policy statement about an Employee Assistance Program reflects the style and language of other policies issued by the employer. The following are recommended items for inclusion in statements about an Employee Assistance Program.

Policy:

A. It is recognized that behavioral health programs are legitimate concerns within the work setting. Their presence interferes with the ability to function on the job.

B. It is further recognized that behavioral/health problems are treatable:

— The majority of persons with such problems can be helped through assessment, referral, and follow-up.

— The decision to seek assistance through the Employee Assistance Program rests with the employee.

— The employer and union(s) will offer encouragement and assistance to employees.

Module II.2—Handout #10 (continued)

C. Any employee with a behavioral/health problem will receive the same access to services that is offered to employees with other illnesses.

D. Participation in the Employee Assistance Program will not jeopardize future promotions, pay increases, or any other employee benefits.

E. The Employee Assistance Program may supplement existing procedures for dealing with substandard job performance or illegal activities. If an employee does not cooperate or if rehabilitation efforts are unsuccessful, disciplinary action should be undertaken according to existing procedures.

F. All records related to program participation will be confidential and in a manner consistent with Federal guidelines.

APPENDIX: OUTLINE OF PROCEDURES FOR NURSING SUPERVISORY REFERRAL TO THE EMPLOYEE ASSISTANCE PROGRAM

Aim: To identify, motivate, refer and follow-up employees with behavioral/health problems.

It is not a function of supervisors/nursing care coordinators to diagnose underlying problems which may be the cause of position performance difficulties (such as alcoholism or abuse of mood-altering substances) even if the supervisor/nursing care coordinator is a clinical specialist certified to make such assessments. All supervisory referrals are based on position performance.

Procedure Format

I. *Identification:*

Nursing Supervisor/Coordinator

— Monitors position performance and job-related behavior and attendance.
— Documents job-related behaviors.
— Designates a time period in which performance must improve.

If Problem Persists:

II. *Confrontation and Referral:*

Nursing Supervisor/Coordinator

— Meets with employee to discuss failure to correct problem(s).
— Presents employee with documentation of problems.
— Informs employee that a referral to Employee Assistance Program (EAP) is indicated.
— Schedules an appointment with EAP staff.

Instructor's Guide

Module II.2—Handout #10 *(continued)*

If Employee Is a Licensed Professional and Problem Does Not Involve Professional Misconduct:

— Refer to EAP as recommended.

If Problem Involves Professional Misconduct:

— Inform employee that act will be reported. Current status may permit either a voluntary surrender or temporary suspension of license with reevaluation at a subsequent time.

III. *Motivation:*

EAP Staff

— Conduct an assessment to determine cause(s) of work difficulties.

— Determine course of treatment/peer assistance needed for the employee.

— Discuss recommendations with employee.

— Make arrangements for treatment/peer assistance.

— If required treatment necessitates a leave of absence, inform nursing supervisor/coordinator. No diagnosis is to be supplied. Information supplied allows nursing supervisor/coordinator to provide coverage.

IV. *Follow-up* (This process may require more than one session.):

EAP Staff

— Establish contact with treatment/peer assistance resource.

— Inform nursing supervisor/coordinator when employee can be expected to return to work.

— Be available to nursing supervisor/coordinator to discuss employee's return to work.

— Meet with employee on regular basis to discuss progress.

— Provide ongoing assistance for other services.

— Maintain contact with nursing supervisor/coordinator regarding employee's position performance.

— Maintain confidentiality but report employee's cooperation with the program if disciplinary action is undertaken.

Module II.2

Module II.2—Handout #10 *(continued)*

BIBLIOGRAPHY

American Journal of Nursing. (1974, September). Helping the nurse who misuses drugs. *American Journal of Nursing, 74*(9), 1665–1671.

American Journal of Nursing. (1982, April). Help for the helper (series of eight short articles). *American Journal of Nursing, 82*(4), 572–587.

American Medical Association. (1973). *The illness called alcoholism: An inquiry.* (Department of Mental Health Pamphlet, #OP–92). Chicago, IL: Author.

American Nurses' Association. (1984). *Addictions and psychological dysfunctions in nursing: The profession's response to the problem.* Kansas City, MO: Author.

American Nurses' Association. (1985). *Code for nurses with interpretive statements.* Kansas City, MO: Author

Bednarek, R. J., & Featherston, H. J. (1980, September/October). A program for hospital employees. *Labor-Management Alcoholism Journal.*

Bilski, A. (1985, April/May). The impaired nurse. *Imprint, 32,* 42–47.

Bissell, L., et al. (1973, November). The alcoholic hospital employee. *Nursing Outlook, 21*(11), 708–711.

Bissell, L., & Haberman, P. W. (1984). *Alcoholism in the professions.* New York: Oxford University Press.

Bissell, L., & Jones, W. (1981, February). The alcoholic nurse. *Nursing Outlook, 29*(2), 96–101.

Blair, B., & AHA Center for Health Promotion. (1985). *Hospital employee assistance programs.* Chicago, IL: American Hospital Publishing, Inc.

Blue Cross/Blue Shield. Problem-drinking employees. (1978, Winter). *Perspective, 13*(4), 30–36.

Brown, M. L. (1981). *Occupational Health Nursing.* New York: Springer Publishing Co.

Chinn, P. L. (Ed.) (1979, April). Ethics and values. *Advances in Nursing Science, 1*(3).

Cole, E., et al. (1985, Spring). Mini on the scene: State nurses associations and the impaired nurse. *Nursing Administration Quarterly, 9*(3), 27–43.

Federal Register. (1975, July 1). *Confidentiality of alcohol and drug abuse patient records. Federal Register, 40*(127), 27802–27821.

Cronin-Stubbs, D., & Schaffner, J. (1985, Spring). Professional impairment: Strategies for managing the troubled nurse. *Nursing Administration Quarterly, 9*(3), 44–54.

Darity, M. (1979, November). Drugs: Facing up to a problem on your staff. *RN, 10*(11), 21–26.

Finley, B. (1982, November). Primary and secondary prevention of substance abuse in nurses. *Occupational Health Nurse, 30,* 14–21.

Instructor's Guide

Module II.2—Handout #10 *(Bibliography continued)*

Green, P. (1983, June). Chemical dependency in the nursing profession. *Occupational Health Nursing, 28,* 15, 19.

Griffin, J. (1985, May). Chemical dependency: Nursing faculty and students are not immune. *Dean's Notes, 6*(5), 1–3.

Guida-Aaron, M. (1978, September/October). OHN's are in the best position to help workers fight alcoholism. *Occupational Health and Safety,* 48–52.

Herrington, R. E. (1986). *Alcohol and drug abuse handbook.* St. Louis, MO: Warren H. Green, Inc.

Isler, C. (1978, July). The alcoholic nurse: What we try to deny. *RN, 41*(7), 48–55.

Kabb, G. M. (1984, November). Chemical dependency: Helping your staff. *Journal of Nursing Administration, 14,* 18–23.

Kelley, R. D. (1978, July). Leadership at work: When a colleague's drinking becomes your headache. *RN, 41*(7), 31–34.

(1985, July/August). The fate of recovered chemically-dependent Michigan Board of Nursing disciplined RNs: A descriptive study. *Michigan Nurse, 58,* 8–10.

Lawrence, C., Jr. (1983, October 24). As workers get high, so do prices. *The Miami Herald,* C-1.

Levine, D. G., et al. (1974, September). A special program for nurse addicts. *American Journal of Nursing, 74*(9), 172–173.

Mereness, D. (1981, July/August). Protect your patients from nurse addicts. *Nursing Life, 1*(1), 71–73.

Naegle, M. A. (1985, April/May). Impaired nursing practice: Ethical and legal issues. *Imprint, 32,* 48–50, 53–54, 56.

Naegle, M. A. (1985, Spring). Creative management of impaired nursing practice. *Nursing Administration Quarterly, 9*(3), 16–26.

National Clearinghouse for Alcohol Information. (1977). *Selected publications on occupational alcoholism programs* (DHHS Publication No. (ADM) 78-271). Rockville, MD: DHHS.

New York State Division of Alcoholism and Alcohol Abuse. *Alcoholism services for women (regional resources).* New York: Author.

New York State Nurses Association. (1981). *Resolution regarding peer assistance program for nurses impaired by chemical dependency* (mimeo). Guilderland, NY: Author.

New York State Nurses Association, Council on Nursing Practice. (1981). *Guidelines for pre-employment reference checking.* Guilderland, NY: Author.

New York State Nurses Association. (1984). *Resolution regarding diversion program for chemically dependent nurses* (mimeo). Guilderland, NY: Author.

Ohio Nurses Association, Peer Assistance Program for Nurses Committee. (1980, March). Nurses will help each other in special program. *Ohio Nurses Review, 53*(1), 3.

Module II.2—Handout #10 *(Bibliography continued)*

Ridgeview Institute, Smyrna, Georgia. (1982, November). Impaired health professional program. *Hospital and Community Psychiatry, 33*(11), 934–935.

Shain, M., & Groenveld, J. (1980). *Employee assistance programs: Philosophy, theory and practice.* Lexington, MA: Lexington Books.

Sisk, B. A. (1981, March). Nursing roles in alcoholism: The employee assistance program in a one-nurse setting. *Occupation Health Nursing, 29*(3), 9–13.

Steinberg, S. L. (1981, February). Employee assistance program conserves human resources. *Hospital Progress, 2*(2), 50–51.

Tammelleo, A. D. (1980, June). Drug abuse by RN's: Unprofessional conduct? *The Regan Report on Nursing Law, 21*(1).

Tammelleo, A. D. (1984, November). ER nurse intoxicated: License revoked. *The Regan Report on Nursing Law, 25*(6).

Telephone reference check (Form 11.103). (1976). In *Modern health care forms: Hospital and nursing home administrators.* Boston, MA: Warren, Gorham, & Lamont.

Wilsnack. S., & Beckman, L. (1984). *Alcohol problems in women—Antecedents, consequences and intervention.* New York: Guilford Press.

Wolf, K. (1982, September/October). Casefinding models to identify and refer the impaired professional. *EAP Digest,* 37–39.

Reprinted with permission from New York State Nurses Association Committee on Impaired Nursing Practice.

Instructor's Guide

RECOMMENDED TEACHINGS STRATEGIES AND SAMPLE ASSIGNMENTS

RECOMMENDED TEACHING STRATEGIES

- Lecture
- Materials from organized professional efforts
- Videotapes
- Attendance at 12-Step meetings
- Interviews/presentations by recovering health professionals
- Small groups
- Role playing
- Selected field experiences; e.g., visits to employee assistance programs

CASE VIGNETTE

Amy McGowan

Amy is a 29-year-old head nurse in a busy CCU. She has held this position for two years now and finds the pace exhilarating and the intellectual challenge welcomed after working part-time for the past five years while she cared for her two children. Amy would like to return to graduate school but finds it difficult to stay awake in the evenings to study after working all day. She began using an over-the-counter stimulant last month but now finds that she needs something stronger. Since she needs to vary her work schedule for special conferences with her evening and night staff, she also drinks a half bottle of wine when she needs to get some sleep at unusual times. Her husband has expressed concern that she seems constantly irritable, has dark circles under her eyes, and spends so little time with her family. She "forgot" a late night call from her supervisor when a staff member called in sick at the last minute and asked for suggestions for possible staff who might be available.

Module II.2

Role-Play—Nurse's Script

Your task in this role play is to:

1. Assess the pattern of drug and alcohol dependence which this health professional manifests.

2. Identify factors specific to her work setting which relate to her health and contribute to her substance abuse.

3. Intervene on behalf of this nurse by:

    a. Establishing a daytime, regular schedule of activities that allows for adequate rest periods appropriate to her early withdrawal stage.

    b. Encouraging measures to reduce her anxiety, including expressing her feelings appropriately.

    c. Referring the client to a peer assistance group.

Instructor's Guide

TEST QUESTIONS AND ANSWERS

TEST QUESTIONS

Instructions: Questions 1–10 relate to the following patient/client vignettes. Answer the questions related to each vignette with the letter indicating the correct choice:

Florence P. needs to leave her job at an urban orthopedic unit because supervisors have noted her poor job performance, absenteeism, and frequent appearances at work with alcohol on her breath. Consultation indicates that she is in need of treatment for alcoholism.

1. The nurse who is experiencing dependence on a substance generally denies problems with job performance, despite poor interpersonal relations with patients and staff and poor psychomotor skills. The best way to provide realistic data on such problems is to:
    a. document observed omissions in patient care and problems in staff relations.
    b. tell the head nurse what you have observed.
    c. ask the nurse's best friend to speak to her about her behavior.
    d. point out to the nurse that her performance is below standards.

2. As the head nurse on the unit, you are concerned about resources available to Ms. P. as she attempts to treat her alcohol dependence. What resources are appropriate treatment referrals for the nurse in the community?
    a. Health professional support groups.
    b. Community-based rehabilitation centers.
    c. Psychotherapy.
    d. Peer assistance groups.

3. Staff development and in-service education programs are helpful resources inasmuch as they:
    a. Sensitize staff to one another's problems.
    b. Assist nurses in identifying impairment and its management.
    c. Identify activities which should be undertaken by management.
    d. Create networks for reporting impaired colleagues.

4. The employer and Ms. P. share responsibility for her successful return to work through:

Module II.2

    a. Additional supervision beyond that provided for other nurses.

    b. Close communication with the State Board for Nursing.

    c. Joint development of a return to work contract.

    d. Close communication with the nurse's A.A. sponsor.

5. Ms. P. denies that her activities, including alcohol consumption during non-working hours, affect her job performance. How can supervisors and peers address her denial?

    a. Provide objective feedback on medication and other nursing care errors.

    b. Point out that no one is strictly honest about alcohol intake.

    c. Tell her directly that you think she has a drinking problem.

    d. Develop a logical argument based on your observations to convince her of her problem.

Mr. H., aged 54, is the assistant vice president for nursing in a large psychiatric hospital. Staff nurses under his supervision have noted that his mood changes suddenly, and at times his speech is incoherent. In addition, he is often not available for consultation and is inconsistent in his record keeping on patient status as well as employee performance.

6. When staff attempt to address job performance problems of supervisors, issues which often inhibit their action include:

    a. Inadequate accounts of job performance problems.

    b. Ignorance about how to proceed.

    c. Fears that their perceptions are incorrect.

    d. Acknowledgment that supervisors are not subject to discipline.

7. Peer assistance programs provide a means of addressing performance problems in nurses by:

    a. Providing consultation to nurses and their employers.

    b. Reporting nurses to disciplinary bodies.

    c. Providing legal consultation on licensure.

    d. Evaluating employee performance.

8. Should Mr. H. need treatment for an impairment problem, what factors will enhance positive outcomes?

    a. Mr. H.'s age.

    b. A punitive stance by the state regulatory body.

    c. A progressively successful work history.

    d. Health care benefits of limited coverage.

9. When Mr. H. takes a medical leave of absence for treatment of cocaine dependence, which legal option offers the best means of protecting his nursing license?

Instructor's Guide

      a. Investigation by the local drug enforcement agency.

      b. Discipline hearing by the State Board for Nursing.

      c. Diversion legislation to bypass discipline.

      d. Residential treatment for 28 days.

10. National organizations provide the following for their members with psychiatric or drug problems:

      a. Peer support groups.

      b. Work place advocacy.

      c. Legal consultation.

      d. Policy statements and program models.

Module II.2

ANSWER KEY

1. a
2. b
3. b
4. c
5. a
6. b
7. a
8. c
9. c
10. d

BIBLIOGRAPHY

MODULE II.2 IMPAIRED PRACTICE BY HEALTH PROFESSIONALS

American Nurses' Association. (1984). *Addictions and psychological dysfunctions in nursing: The profession's response to the problem.* Kansas City, MO: Author.

American Nurses' Association. (1987, March). Impaired nursing practice (media backgrounder). In *ANA News.* Kansas City, MO: Author.

Assareh, S. (1987). Substance abuse testing in the work place: A review. *American Association of Occupational Health Nursing Journal,* 204–209, 246–248.

Bissell, L., & Haberman, P. (1984). *Alcoholism in the professions.* New York: Oxford University Press.

Bissell, L., & Royce, J. (1987). *Ethics for addiction professionals.* Center City, MN: Hazelden Foundation.

Bok, Sissela. (1980). Whistle-blowing and professional responsibility. *New York University Education Quarterly, 11*(4), 2–10.

Cannon, B. L., & Brown, J. S. (1988, Summer). Nurses' attitudes toward impaired colleagues. *Image: Journal of Nursing Scholarship, 20,* 96–101.

Clark, M. D. (1988). The recovering nurse: The employment interview. *Nursing Management, 19,* 33–37.

Connell, C. C., & Murphy, J. F. (1987). New dimensions of regulating the practice of professional nursing. *Nursing Management, 18*(8), 62–64.

Cross, L. (1985). Chemical dependency in our ranks: Managing a nurse in crisis. *Nursing Management, 16*(11), 15–16.

Dogoloff, L., & Angarola, R. (1985). *Urine testing in the work place.* New York: American Council for Drug Education.

Finagaretta, H., et al. (1978). Drinking on the job. *Hastings Center Report, 8*(6), 16–18.

Floyd, J. (1991). Nursing students' stress levels, attitudes toward drugs, and drug use. *Archives of Psychiatric Nursing, V*(1), 46–53.

Gerace, L. (1988). Patterns of alcohol use among nurse educators. *Issues in Mental Health Nursing, 9*(2), 189–200.

Haack, M., & Hughes, T. (Eds.). (1987). *Addiction in the nursing profession: Approaches to intervention and recovery.* New York: Springer Publishing Co.

Harben, K. (1982). Three-step recovery model aids impaired nurses. *Hospital Employee Health, 1*(2), 24–27.

Hutchinson, S. A. (1986). Chemically dependent nurses: The trajectory of self-annihilation. *Nursing Research, 35*(4), 196–200.

Hutchinson, S. A. (1987, November/December). Toward self-integration: The recovery process of chemically dependent nurses. *Nursing Research, 36*(6), 339–343.

Kilty, K. (1975). Attitudes toward alcohol and alcoholism among professionals and non-professionals. *Journal of Studies on Alcohol, 36*(3), 327–347.

McAuliffe, W. E., Rohman, M., & Wechsler, A. (1985). Alcohol and substance use and other risk factors in a sample of physicians in training. *Advances in Alcohol and Substance Abuse, 4*(2), 67–87.

McAuliffe, W. E., Santangelo, S. L., Gergias, J., Rohman, M., Sobol, A., & Magnussen, E. (1987). Use and abuse of controlled substances by pharmacists and pharmacy students. *American Journal of Hospital Pharmacy, 44*(2), 311–317.

Moore, G., & Hogan, R. L. (1987). Substance abuse and the nurse: A legal and ethical dilemma. *Journal of Professional Nursing, 3*(1), 5–9.

Morse, R. M., Martin, M. A., Swenson, W. M., & Niven, R. G. (1984). Prognosis of physicians treated for alcoholism and drug dependence. *Journal of the American Medical Association, 251*(6), 743–746.

Naegle, M. A. (1985, April/May). Impaired nursing practice: Ethical and legal issues. *Imprint, 32*, 48–56.

Naegle, M. A. (1989). Patterns and implications of drug use by students of nursing. *Imprint, 36*(2), 85, 87–88.

Rothstein, H. (1985–1986). Screening workers for drugs: A legal and ethical framework. *Employee Relations Law Journal, 11*(3), 422–437.

Smith, D. E., & Seymour, R. (1985). A clinical approach to the impaired health professional. *International Journal of Addictions, 39*, 1327–1332.

Stafen, R. R., & Farley, B. P. (1989). The use of group therapy for assisting the recovery and reentry of impaired nurses. In M. Haack & T. Hughes (Eds.), *Addiction in the nursing profession: Approaches to intervention and recovery* (pp. 113–128). New York: Springer Publishing Co.

Strickland, S. (1986). Critical health issues in the work place . . . Alcohol and substance abuse. *Journal of the American Association of Occupational Health Nurses, 34*(9), 443–444.

Sullivan, E. (1987). Comparison of chemically dependent and non-dependent nurses on familial, personal and professional characteristics. *Journal of Studies on Alcohol, 48*(6), 563–568.

Sullivan, E. J., Bissell, L., & Williams, E. (1987). *Chemical dependency in nursing: The deadly diversion.* Redwood City, CA: Addison-Wesley Publishing, Inc.

Van Servellen, G. M., Soccorso, E. A., Palermo, K., & Faude, K. (1985). Depression in hospital nurses: Implications for nurse managers. *Nursing Administration Quarterly, 9*, 74–84.

Veatch, D. (1987). When is the recovering impaired nurse ready to work? *Journal of Nursing Administration, 17*(2), 14–16.

Vogtsberger, K. N. (1984). Treatment outcomes of substance-abusing physicians. *American Journal of Drug and Alcohol Abuse, 10*(1), 23–27.

Wessells, D. T., Kutscher, A. H., Seeland, I. B., Selder, F. E., Chrico, D. J., & Clark, E. J. (Eds.). (1989). *Professional burnout in medicine and the helping professions.* New York: Haworth Press.

MODULE II.3
ADDICTIONS: NURSING DIAGNOSIS AND TREATMENT

Janet S. D'Arcangelo, MA, RN, C
Thomas Adamski, MEd, MSN, RNC, CRNA

Madeline A. Naegle, PhD, RN, FAAN
Project Director
Janet S. D'Arcangelo, MA, RN, C
Project Coordinator

Project SAEN
SUBSTANCE ABUSE
EDUCATION IN NURSING

CONTENT OUTLINE

I. Addiction
   A. Definitions
   B. Theoretical Perspectives, Briefly Reviewed
      1. Psychologic/psychoanalytic origins
      2. Physiologic models
      3. Interpersonal models of dependence
      4. Disease concept
   C. Addictions Manifested as Compulsive Behavior
   D. Dual Diagnosis
   E. Mixed Addictions

II. Manifestations of Addiction
   A. Denial: The Critical Symptom
   B. Manifestations of Alcohol and Other Psychoactive Substances
      1. Behavioral effects—DSM-III-R
      2. Physiologic effects, medical sequelae, and acute illness
   C. Manifestations of Impulse Control Disorders: Gambling and Sexual Addiction
   D. Related Concepts in Sexual Addiction
   E. Related Concepts in Eating Disorders
   F. Relapse

III. Nursing Diagnoses Congruent with Nursing and Interprofessional Classification Systems
   A. Relationship of Nursing Diagnoses to Medical Diagnoses
   B. Diagnosis of Actual and Potential Health Problems Related to Addictions

IV. Nursing Intervention
   A. Treatment Modalities for the Addictions
   B. Nursing Process in Intervention
      1. Establish plan of care based on nursing diagnosis
      2. Set care goals specific to the individual
      3. Identify anticipated outcomes
      4. Implement care, independently, or in collaboration with peers or members of other disciplines
   C. Referral
V. Generalist Nursing Roles
   A. Education on Addiction in the Adult Population
   B. Roles Implemented by the Nurse in the Acute and Chronic Care of the Addicted Individual and His/Her Family
   C. The Role of the Nurse in the Long-Term Rehabilitative Care of the Addicted or Substance Abusing Client
   D. Relapse
   E. Prevention

Addictions: Nursing Diagnosis and Treatment

CONTENTS

I. ADDICTION: ABUSE AND DEPENDENCE

A. Definitions

The definition of addictions is difficult and, more frequently than not, not all encompassing. Many conceptual lenses can be looked through without giving a clear, causal, or basic effect. Geneticists talk of a predisposition to addictions passed on from parents, while family practitioners seek to incorporate family dysfunction as the culprit. The reality is that each and every conceptual model maintains different levels of accuracy and no single model defines the phenomenon completely. Reviewing the literature shows attempts to define addiction by its conduct and description, not by its dynamics.

1. By its conduct, addiction is described as the force which drives toward pleasure and relief. It seeks to alter and change the subjective experience. In a 1987 American Nurses Association publication, addiction is defined as "an illness characterized by compulsion, loss of control, and continued patterns of abuse despite perceived negative consequences; obsession with a dysfunctional habit" (ANA, DANA, 1987).
2. Addiction is a phenomenon which affects all biophysical, psychosocial, and spiritual systems and experiences; it is irreducible.

B. Theoretical Perspectives, Briefly Reviewed

1. Psychological manifestations of addiction: Psychoanalytic origins.
    a. The Freudian view is that addiction stems from one or more of three unconscious tendencies: self-destruction, oral dependency, or latent homosexuality.
    b. Close to this view is the analytic concept that addictions develop as a response to inner conflict between dependency drives and aggressive impulses.
    c. The Adlerian view is that addictions represent a striving for power to compensate for the pervasive feelings of inferiority and use the substance to enhance low self-esteem (McLelland, 1972).
    d. Kohut's psychology of self sees addictions as part of a self-destructive suicide and absolute form of self-absorption, his or her own sole love object, and part of a narcissistic personality disorder (Levin, 1987).
    e. Sullivan notes that personalities under the control of substances are less competent at protecting themselves from anxiety and that addictions stem from problems of sexual adjustment most dominant in early adolescence. Addicts are unable to separate the dynamisms of lust and intimacy (Levin, 1987).
    f. Bradshaw sees substances as mood altering; and they add congruence and reinforce existing self-experiences of shame and guilt (Bradshaw, 1988).
    g. The common threads through the analytic theories seem to be the coexisting morbidities of diminished self-esteem as well as sexual maladjustment.

Module II.3

    The question which we must ask at this point is how many people who experience low self-esteem and sexual maladjustment are not addicts? Other conceptual lenses could be utilized to explain the phenomenon.

2. Physiologic Models.
   a. Physiologic dependence occurs with certain classes of drugs and nicotine.
   b. Ingestion of any substance necessarily alters the chemical composition and therefore the pattern and functioning of the whole organism on all levels including the cellular and systemic.
   c. Tolerance for the substance develops and increasing doses are necessary to achieve the desired effects. This is what distinguishes habituation from addiction. Habituation requires no increase to achieve effects; addiction requires increasing doses.
   d. Withdrawal symptoms appear upon cessation of the substance. Withdrawal syndromes may last from days to weeks and may be life threatening.
   e. Alleviation of withdrawal symptoms and craving for the substance contribute to continued use.
      (1) Episodic use is characterized by binges, followed by intense "crashes," during which the individual experiences anxiety, irritability, feelings of fatigue, and depression.
      (2) Continued use appears to be more of a response to the craving for the substance than the prevention of or relief from withdrawal. (Townsend, 1991) The craving is under limited control by the individual; it is characterized by intense feelings of loss and uneasiness; it is a psychological withdrawal response (Mello, 1977).
3. Interpersonal Models of Dependence.
   a. Bill Wilson, co-founder of Alcoholics Anonymous, identified the disturbances in self as central flaws in the addict's personality. The accepting attitude in the 12-step program for alcoholism and addictive behaviors allows the individual to identify with the collective self and extend the narcissistic disturbance from the self to the group. The "work" of group process then provides experiences which are emotionally curative.
   b. Stanton Peele describes addiction as a phenomenon that accomplishes something for the addict. Addictions are ways of coping with feelings and situations with which addicts cannot otherwise cope. Addictions involve three components: the person, the situation, and the environment, all of which are couched in the overall culture and social factors of the individual. He suggests that as the personal environments of situations change, so does the pattern of addiction. Using Vietnam as an example, he cites the war situation as stressful and out of control, encouraging addiction. Upon return most of the addicted soldiers were able to shed their addictions. Clearly this belief challenges the existing paradigm suggesting that addictions are always out of control and degenerative (Peele, 1989).
4. The Disease Concept of Addiction.
   a. Stein (*The Addicted Brain*, video, 1990) has identified the conduct of addiction to the level of the individual brain cell.

(1) Under laboratory conditions he has demonstrated that the individual brain cell, when exposed to a pleasure generating stimulus, in this case cocaine, exhibits excessive electrical discharging which subsides upon being ballasted with more cocaine.

(2) McGuire, as demonstrated in the video *The Addicted Brain* (video, 1990), used the process of neurometrics (the measurement of specific neurotransmitters in specific regions of the brain) to identify that:

   (a) People easily bored tend to seek excitement through alteration of biochemistry via a high with neuropiates.

   (b) Various centers of the brain are rich in some neurotransmitters and others are poor, resulting in conduct such as obsessive compulsive behavior, premenstrual irritability, and even dominance and leadership.

   (c) All are responsive to levels of serotonin, or monoamine oxidase.

   (d) Alcoholics experience a paucity of neurotransmitters in a specific area of the brain which, with the use of alcohol, increases pleasure. Non-alcoholics do not experience the same paucity of neurotransmitters.

b. Blume and Nobel (1990) researched a possible genetic link, reported by Waldholz (1991).

   (1) Feelings of pleasure in humans are associated with brain chemicals, known as dopamine receptors, which genetically come in different forms.

   (2) The "A1" form of dopamine receptor may produce an inadequate amount of dopamine.

   (3) A person with this "A1" form of dopamine receptor might require unusual stimulation to give a person normal feelings of pleasure, thereby putting these people at risk for alcohol, drugs, or other behaviors.

c. One pivotal theorist in the area of addictions, especially alcohol, was E. M. Jellinek, who in 1960 defined alcoholism as any use of alcohol that causes damage to the individual or society. Jellinek reduced his definition into five subsets.

   (1) Alpha alcoholism—The undisciplined and out-of-control drinker who is unable to abstain.

   (2) Beta alcoholism—Includes the process of alpha however is complicated by the biophysical toxic responses.

   (3) Gamma—The drinker becomes physically dependent including cravings, tissue tolerance, and psychosocial/socioeconomic alterations.

   (4) Delta—The drinker develops withdrawal symptoms upon withdrawal of alcohol.

   (5) Epsilon—The periodic "binge" drinker.

C. Addictions Manifested as Compulsive Behavior

1. Other forms of addictions are not psychoactive; they are not based on substances, but on behaviors. These are frequently identified as process addictions.

Module II.3

2. Compulsive behaviors.
   a. Repetitious.
   b. Performed in secret.
   c. Under limited control by the person engaging in the behavior.
   d. Bringing negative consequences to the person engaging in the behavior.
   e. Representing a major preoccupation for the person.
   f. Causing restlessness and irritability as a result of inability to engage in the behavior.
3. Common forms of process addiction.
   a. Gambling.
   b. Compulsive sexual activity.
   c. Eating disorders.
4. Common features among all addictions.
   a. Etiology: For example, compulsive gambling is reported to run in families.
   b. Denial.
   c. Craving: Anxiety produced by cessation of the activity is relieved by repetition, thereby reinforcing the addiction; for example, the binging and purging cycle of bulimia.
   d. They are maladaptive coping mechanisms.
   e. Incidence and type of process addiction may be culturally and situationally influenced; for example, cultural values about promiscuity and "workaholism." (Pasquali, Arnold, & DeBasio, 1989).
   f. Alcohol and substance abuse commonly occur among people with the process addictions.

D. **Dual Diagnosis**

1. Typically, the nurse generalist will not be encountering the substance abuser on a prima facie basis. More often, it would be in an emergency department, ambulatory care, or community setting. The patient would probably present with such standard psychiatric disorders as:
   a. Generalized anxiety disorder.
   b. Panic disorder.
   c. Social anxiety.
   d. Mood disturbances.
   These may or may not be indicators of substance abuse.
2. Although these diagnostic categories may be symptom specific, the nurse generalist must consider the use of psychoactive substances and chronic substance abuse as an understated disease process. Certainly not all of the psychiatric DSM-III-R diagnoses have substance abuse as correlates. However, most substance abuse diagnoses have psychiatric disorders as correlates.
   a. Anxiety.
   b. Dysthymia, cyclothymia.

Addictions: Nursing Diagnosis and Treatment

    c. Social anxiety.
    d. Personality disorder.
    e. Isolation.
    f. Panic attacks.
   These are part of the profile of a substance abuser.

3. Frequently, a patient will present with both an addictive disorder and a psychiatric disorder. MICA (Mentally Ill Chemical Abuser) and Dual Diagnosis are the terms now used to describe these individuals.
4. Prevalence of Dual Diagnosis (Regier, Farmer, Rael, et al., 1990).
    a. Among people with psychiatric disorders (primary diagnosis other than psychoactive substance abuse/dependence).
        (1) 22% also have an alcohol problem.
        (2) 15% have another drug problem.
        (3) Risk of alcohol or drug problems among people with psychiatric disorder is 3 times that in normal population.
        (4) Lifetime rate of substance abuse among selected psychiatric diagnosed groups.
            (a) Antisocial personality—84%
            (b) Schizophrenics—47%
            (c) Bipolar disorder—61%
            (d) Panic disorder—25%
    b. Among substance abusers.
        (1) 39% of alcoholics have concurrent psychopathology.
        (2) 53% are users of other drugs.
    c. Dual diagnosis is highly prevalent on psychiatric emergency units. More than 1/3 to 1/2 of these patients have substance abuse related problems.
5. Factors contributing to the complexity of dual diagnosis.
    a. Commonalities among risk factors; e.g., genetic predisposition, sociocultural factors.
    b. Overlap of symptoms; e.g., denial, impulsivity.
    c. Feedback loops of effects of disorders; e.g., depression as an outcome of withdrawal, abstinence, psychopathology preceding addiction or developing as a result of addiction.
    d. The self-medicating and self-soothing drives associated with emotional instabilities.
6. Problems in treating dual diagnosis.
    a. Interventions for the identified addiction are sometimes contraindicated as psychotherapeutic strategies. For example, the active confrontation of addictive denial stimulates social withdrawal, low self-esteem, and suicidal ideation.
    b. The use of medication for a psychiatric disorder may conflict with the position of abstinence in addiction treatment.
    c. Behavioral problems associated with psychopathology may be interpreted as "treatment resistance."

7. Key concepts in treating dual diagnosis.
   a. Psychopathology and addiction must be treated discretely yet concurrently.
   b. Untreated psychopathology increases the risk of relapse.

E. **Mixed Addictions**

1. These may be polysubstance addictions or process/substance addictions.
2. The issues of dual diagnosis also are features of mixed addictions.
3. Correlations are observed to exist among identified addictions underlying causes or manifestations.
   a. Drinking, drug use, and gambling are correlated.
   b. A drug of the same class may be substituted to enhance effects or substitute for unavailability of the drug of choice (d.o.c.).
   c. Certain social situations may cause anxiety, leading to the compulsive behavior of binge eating, leading to bulimia and substance use which enhances this addiction for the individual. There are several drugs of choice among the appetitional disorders including amphetamines and barbiturates.

II. **MANIFESTATIONS OF ADDICTION**

A. **Denial: The Critical Symptom**

1. The symptom of denial is exhibited by numerous components of the abusing system.
   a. Drug substance abuser—directly or indirectly.
   b. Employers.
   c. Nurses and other caregivers/health professionals.
   d. Internal mechanisms—defense against stress.
   e. Advertising and other economic structures.
   f. Loved ones—family and friends of the abuser.

B. **Manifestations of Alcohol and Other Psychoactive Substances**

1. Behavioral effects—DSM-III-R.
   DSM-III-R Diagnostic Criteria for Psychoactive Substance Dependence and Psychoactive Substance Abuse are used for interdisciplinary consistency. The following information from the DSM-III-R summarizes behavioral effects.[*]
   a. Diagnostic criteria for psychoactive substance dependence. At least three of the following:
      (1) Substance often taken in larger amounts or over a longer period than the person intended.

---

[*] *From:* American Psychiatric Association. (1987). *Diagnostic and statistical manual of mental disorders* (3rd ed., revised) (p. 325). Washington, DC: Author.

Addictions: Nursing Diagnosis and Treatment

- (2) Persistent desire, or one or more unsuccessful efforts, to cut down or control substance use.
- (3) A great deal of time spent in activities necessary to get the substance (e.g., theft), taking the substance (e.g., chain smoking), or recovering from its effects.
- (4) Frequent intoxication or withdrawal symptoms when expected to fulfill major role obligations at work, school, or home (e.g., does not go to work because hung over, goes to school or work "high," intoxicated while taking care of children), or when substance use is physically hazardous (e.g., drives when intoxicated).
- (5) Important social, occupational, or recreational activities given up or reduced because of substance use.
- (6) Continued substance use despite knowledge of having a persistent or recurrent social, psychological, or physical problem that is caused or exacerbated by the use of the substance; e.g., keeps using heroin despite family arguments about it, cocaine-induced depression, or having an ulcer made worse by drinking.
- (7) Need for markedly increased amounts of the substance (at least a 50% increase) in order to achieve intoxication or desired effect, or markedly diminished effect with continued use of the same amount.
- (8) Characteristic withdrawal symptoms of psychoactive substance-induced organic mental disorders.
- (9) Substance often taken to relieve or avoid withdrawal symptoms.

b. Some symptoms of the disturbance have persisted for at least one month, or have occurred repeatedly over a longer period of time.

c. Criteria for severity of psychoactive substance dependence.
- (1) Mild—Few, if any, symptoms in excess of those required to make the diagnosis, and the symptoms result in no more than mild impairment of occupational functioning or of usual social activities or relationships with others.
- (2) Moderate—Symptoms or functional impairment between "mild" and "severe."
- (3) Severe—Many symptoms in excess of those required to make the diagnosis, and the symptoms markedly interfere with occupational functioning or with usual social activities or relationships with others. (Because of the availability of cigarettes and other nicotine-containing substances and the absence of a clinically significant nicotine intoxication syndrome, impairment in occupational or social functioning is not necessary for a rating of severe nicotine dependence.)
- (4) Partial remission—During the past six months, some use of the substance and some symptoms of dependence.
- (5) Full remission—During the past six months, either no use of the substance, or use of the substance and no symptoms of dependence.

d. Psychoactive substance abuse.
- (1) General description of this category of diagnosis.

Module II.3

Psychoactive substance abuse is a residual category for noting maladaptive patterns of psychoactive substance use that have never met the criteria for dependence for that particular class of substance.

This diagnosis is most likely to be applicable to people who have only recently started taking psychoactive substances and to involve substances, such as cannabis, cocaine, and hallucinogens, that are less likely to be associated with marked physiologic signs of withdrawal and the need to take the substance to relieve or avoid withdrawal symptoms.

(2) Examples of situations in which this category would be appropriate are as follows:

(a) A college student binges on cocaine every few weekends. These periods are followed by a day or two of missing school because of "crashing." There are no other symptoms.

(b) A middle-aged man repeatedly drives his car when intoxicated with alcohol. There are no other symptoms.

(c) A woman keeps drinking alcohol even though her physician has told her that it is responsible for exacerbating the symptoms of a duodenal ulcer. There are no other symptoms.

(3) Diagnostic criteria for psychoactive substance abuse.

(a) A maladaptive pattern of psychoactive substance use indicated by at least one of the following:

(i) continued use despite knowledge of having a persistent or recurrent social, occupational, psychological, or physical problem that is caused or exacerbated by use of the psychoactive substance.

(ii) recurrent use in situations in which use is physically hazardous; e.g., driving while intoxicated.

(b) Some symptoms of the disturbance have persisted for at least one month, or have occurred repeatedly over a longer period of time.

(c) Never met the criteria for psychoactive substance dependence for this substance.

e. Other general information relevant to diagnosis by DSM-III-R.

(1) Classes of psychoactive substances.

(a) Nine classes of psychoactive substances are associated with both abuse and dependence: alcohol; amphetamine or similarly acting sympathomimetic; cannabis; cocaine; hallucinogens; inhalants; opioids; phencyclidine (PCP) or similarly acting arylcyclohexylamines; and sedatives, hypnotics, or anxiolytics. Dependence (but not abuse) is seen with nicotine. (Although nicotine abuse is logically possible, according to the definition of abuse noted above, in practice virtually no one who has not previously been dependent on nicotine uses nicotine-containing substances in a maladaptive way; e.g., episodic use of cigarettes that exacerbates a physical disorder.)

(b) Although these psychoactive substances appear in alphabetical order, the following classes share similar features:

i) Alcohol and sedatives, anxiolytics or hypnotics.

ii) Cocaine and amphetamine or similarly acting sympathomimetics.

iii) Hallucinogens and phencyclidine (PCP) or similarly acting arylcyclohexylamines.

(2) Use of multiple substances.

Psychoactive substance abuse and dependence often involve several substances, either simultaneously or sequentially. For example, people with cocaine dependence frequently use alcohol, anxiolytics, or opioids to counteract lingering dysphoric anxiety symptoms. People with opioid or cannabis abuse or dependence usually have several other psychoactive substance use disorders, particularly of sedatives, hypnotics, or anxiolytics, amphetamines, or similarly acting sympathomimetic, and cocaine.

When a person's condition meets the criteria for more than one psychoactive substance use disorder, multiple diagnoses should be made. The polysubstance dependence diagnosis is reserved for noting a period of at least six months during which the person was repeatedly using at least three categories of psychoactive substances (not including nicotine and caffeine), but no single psychoactive substance predominated. Further, during this period the dependence criteria were met for psychoactive substances (as a group), but not for any specific substance.

(3) Recording specific diagnoses.

The clinician records the name of the specific psychoactive substance rather than the name of the class of substances, using the code number for the appropriate class. For example, the clinician should write 305.70 amphetamine abuse (rather than amphetamine or similarly acting sympathomimetic abuse), 304.10 diazepam dependence (rather than sedative, hypnotic, or anxiolytic dependence), and 305.90 cogentin abuse (rather than psychoactive substance abuse NOS).

f. Other features of psychoactive substance use disorders relevant to DSM-III-R diagnostic use.

(1) Route of administration.

The route of administration of a psychoactive substance is an important variable in determining the likelihood that its use will lead to dependence or abuse. It may also affect the particular pattern of psychoactive substance use; i.e., determine whether periodic binges or daily use is more likely. In general, routes of administration that produce more rapid and efficient absorption of the substance into the bloodstream tend to increase the likelihood of an escalating pattern of substance use that leads to dependence. In addition, for some substances there is an increased likelihood of a binge pattern of use; i.e., a form of episodic use consisting of compressed time periods of continuous high dose use followed by one or more days of nonuse. For example, a person is much more likely to develop dependence on cocaine and develop a binge pattern of use when the substance is smoked or taken intravenously than when it is "sniffed" or taken orally.

(2) Duration of psychoactive effects.

The duration of psychoactive effects associated with a particular psychoactive substance is also an important variable in determining the likelihood that use of the substance will lead to dependence or abuse and a pattern of binge use. In general, relatively short-acting psychoactive substances, such as amphetamine, cocaine, and certain anxiolytics, tend to be more commonly used than substances with similar psychoactive effects, but longer action. Consequently, the shorter-acting psychoactive substances have a particularly high potential for the development of dependence or abuse.

(3) Associated features.

   (a) Repeated episodes of psychoactive substance-induced intoxication are almost invariably present in psychoactive substance abuse dependence, although for some substances it is possible to develop dependence without ever exhibiting frank intoxication; e.g., alcohol.

   (b) Personality disturbance and disturbance of mood are often present, and may be intensified by the psychoactive substance use disorder. For example, antisocial personality traits may be accentuated by the need to obtain money to purchase illegal substances. Anxiety or depression associated with borderline personality disorder may be intensified as the person uses a psychoactive substance in an unsuccessful attempt to treat his or her mood disturbance.

   (c) In chronic abuse or dependence, mood lability and suspiciousness, both of which can contribute to violent behavior, are common.

(4) Age at onset.

Alcohol abuse and dependence usually appear in the 20s, 30s, and 40s. Dependence on amphetamine or similarly acting sympathomimetic, cannabis, cocaine, hallucinogens, nicotine, opioids, and phencyclidine (PCP) or similarly acting arylcyclohexylamines more commonly begin in the late teens and 20s. When a psychoactive substance use disorder begins in early adolescence, it is often associated with Conduct Disorder and failure to complete school.

(5) Complications.

   (a) The abuse or dependence associated with each class of psychoactive substances may cause an Organic Mental syndrome. For example, prolonged Alcohol Dependence may cause Alcohol Withdrawal Delirium, Alcohol Amnestic Disorder, or Alcohol Hallucinosis. Similarly, Hallucinogen Delusional Disorder may be a complication of chronic hallucinogen use. Complications of the specific intoxication states, such as traffic accidents and physical injury due to alcohol intoxication, have been noted in the organic mental disorders section.

   (b) Frequently there is a deterioration in the general level of physical health. Malnutrition and a variety of other physical disorders may result from failure to maintain physical health by proper diet and adequate personal hygiene.

Addictions: Nursing Diagnosis and Treatment

(c) Use of contaminated needles for intravenous administration of amphetamines, cocaine, and opioids can cause hepatitis, tetanus, vasculitis, septicemia, subacute bacterial endocarditis, embolic phenomena, malaria, and Human Immunodeficiency Virus (HIV)-related disorders; e.g., Acquired Immune Deficiency Syndrome (AIDS), AIDS-related Complex (ARC).

(d) Materials used to "cut" the substances can cause erosion of the nasal septum.

(e) Cocaine use can result in sudden death from cardiac arrhythmias, myocardial infarction, a cerebrovascular accident, or respiratory arrest.

(f) Physical complications of chronic alcohol dependence include hepatitis, cirrhosis, peripheral neuropathy, gastritis, and a variety of reproductive disorders. In addition, chronic alcohol dependence increases the risk and severity of heart disease, pneumonia, tuberculosis, and neurologic disorders. The long-term potential for respiratory disorder with chronic cannabis use is controversial. A review of physiologic manifestations of addictions appears later in the module.

(g) Depressive symptoms are a frequent complication of psychoactive substance use disorders and partly account for the high rate of suicide by people with these disorders. Suicide associated with alcohol and other psychoactive substances can occur in both intoxicated and sober states.

(h) Long-term dependence on certain psychoactive substances, particularly cannabis, hallucinogens, and PCP, is often associated with a generalized reduction in goal-directed behaviors (e.g., going to school, work, and the pursuit of hobbies), even when the person does not take the substance for long periods of time. This is often accompanied by depression, anxiety, irritability, and mild defects in cognitive functioning; e.g., difficulty concentrating. This has been called the "amotivational syndrome." It is unclear whether this syndrome is the direct consequence of the chronic effect of the psychoactive substances on the central nervous system or whether it is an expression of preexisting psychopathology.

(i) Impairment.

Impairment in social and occupational functioning is frequently marked, particularly with dependence.

(j) Course.

Brief, self-limited episodes of dependence or abuse may occur, particularly during periods of psychosocial stress. More commonly, the course is chronic, lasting several years, with periods of exacerbation and partial or full remission.

(k) Predisposing factors.

Conduct disorder in children, and personality disorders, particularly antisocial personality disorder, predispose to the development

Module II.3

of psychoactive substance use disorders. Children of people who themselves have psychoactive substance use disorders are at higher risk for developing these disorders.

(l) Sex ratio.

Psychoactive substance use disorders are diagnosed more commonly in males than in females.

(m) Differential diagnosis.
  i) Toxicologic analysis of body fluids is used in the differential diagnosis of psychoactive substance use disorders.
  ii) Psychoactive substance use disorders are diagnosed more commonly in males than in females.

(n) Nonpathologic psychoactive substance use for recreational or medical purposes is not associated with the dependence syndrome, or a maladaptive pattern of use (abuse).

(o) Repeated episodes of psychoactive substance-induced intoxication are almost invariably present in psychoactive substance abuse dependence, although for some substances (e.g., alcohol) it is possible to develop dependence without ever exhibiting frank intoxication. However, one or more episodes of psychoactive substance-induced intoxication alone are not sufficient for a diagnosis of either psychoactive substance dependence or abuse.

2. Physiologic effects, medical sequelae, and acute illness.
   a. Certain physiologic patterns are frequently seen as an outcome of substance dependence. The presentation of these patterns is a diagnostic indicator for nursing intervention for substance abuse.
   b. Physiologic alterations most frequently associated with alcohol dependence.
      (1) Hepatic.

      Hepatitis is characterized by enlarged liver, jaundice, right upper quadrant pain and fever; fatty liver; cirrhosis of the liver associated with alcoholism is also known as Laennec's cirrhosis, atrophic cirrhosis, or portal cirrhosis. The chronic accumulation of fatty acids in the liver causes fibrous and degenerative changes. The progression of symptoms includes:

      (a) Portal hypertension resulting from defective blood flow through the cirrhotic liver.

      (b) Ascites characterized by an accumulation of serous fluid in the peritoneal cavity.

      (c) Hepatic encephalopathy: The liver becomes unable to convert ammonia to urea. Rising serum ammonia levels result in confusion, restlessness, slurred speech, and fever; without intervention, coma or death can occur.

      (2) Gastrointestinal.
         (a) Gastritis.
         (b) Duodenal ulcers.

(c) Malabsorption syndromes.
(d) Cancer of the mouth.
(e) Esophageal varices: distended vein in the esophagus carry the risk of rupture and subsequent hemorrhage.
(f) Pancreatitis: early stages are characterized by pain, nausea, vomiting, and abdominal distention. As the pancreas deteriorates, symptoms of diabetes mellitus could occur.

(3) Neurologic.
(a) Peripheral neuropathy: the thiamine deficiency resulting from alcoholism causes numbness, tingling, and pain in the extremities.
(b) Wernicke-Korsakoff's syndrome: progressive thiamine deficiency results in mental confusion, agitation, and diplopia. Without thiamine replacement, rapid deterioration to coma and death can occur.
(c) Organic brain syndrome: cellular brain changes result in alteration in behavior and disposition, emotional stability, memory ideation, and orientation.

(4) Cardiovascular, hematologic.
(a) Hypertension, familial type IV hyperlipidemia, hypoglycemia, anemia, coronary artery disease, congestive heart failure. Cardiomyopathy is characterized by an enlargement of the heart due to accumulation of excess lipids in myocardial cells.

(5) Musculoskeletal.
(a) Skeletal myopathies.

(6) Immunologic.
(a) Immune suppression, and increased susceptibility to infection.

c. Physiologic alterations associated with ingestion of other substances are specific to the type of substance, and have effects from the cellular to the end organ levels.

d. Signs of tolerance or withdrawal symptoms known to be associated with substance ingestion are also indicators of physiologic dependence. For example, agitation, caffeine withdrawal headache, and hand tremors would be physiologic indicators of caffeine and alcohol dependence.

C. Manifestations of Impulse Control Disorders: Gambling

1. General features.
   a. Not related to obsessive compulsive personality disorder.
   b. Person is addicted to action.
   c. Two-thirds male.
   d. Begins in adolescence.
   e. Starts with "Big Win" (Quality of excitement, wants to recapture).
   f. Self-esteem becomes based on being a good gambler and a smart gambler.
   g. Diagnosis can be made during winning stage because of absorption in lifestyle.

h. Females use it as an escape.

i. Females hate less winning phases.

j. Addiction is a common form for women.

k. There is associated psychopathology of many types.

l. One-fifth of alcohol and drug patients have had a problem with gambling (Blume, 1988).

2. Phases (Custer, 1984).

   a. Winning phase.

   b. Losing phase.

   c. Desperation phase.

      (1) Wants bailout.

      (2) Thinks gambling is a bad idea.

      (3) Sometimes buoyed by an irrational belief that "the Big Win" is right around the corner.

      (4) Often ends with imprisonment, white collar crime, or suicide.

3. Assessment.

   a. South Oaks Gambling Screen.

      (1) This is a 20-item questionnaire based on DSM-IV criteria and cross validated to DSM-III-R. It can be given by generalist either as a paper and pencil test or in an interview format. There is an accompanying score sheet: A score of five or more indicates probable pathological gambling, less than five indicates some gambling problem (see handouts).

   b. DSM-III-R Criteria for Diagnosis.

      (1) Frequent preoccupation with gambling or with obtaining money to gamble.

      (2) Frequent gambling of larger amounts of money or over a longer period than intended.

      (3) A need to increase the size or frequency of bets to achieve the desired excitement.

      (4) Restlessness or irritability if unable to gamble.

      (5) Repeated loss of money by gambling and returning another day to win back losses ("chasing").

      (6) Repeated efforts to reduce or stop gambling.

      (7) Frequent gambling when expected to meet social or occupational obligations.

      (8) Sacrifice of some important social, occupational, or recreational activity in order to gamble.

      (9) Continuation of gambling despite inability to pay mounting debts or despite other significant social, occupational, or legal problems that the person knows to be exacerbated by gambling.

Addictions: Nursing Diagnosis and Treatment

4. Treatments.
   a. Self-help groups.
   b. Individual psychotherapy using psychodynamic, behavioral strategies, and group counseling.
   c. Group counseling.
   d. Psychodrama.
   e. Physical health care.
   f. Psychiatric management.
   g. Vocational rehabilitation.

D. Related Concepts in Sexual Addiction

1. This addiction is to be differentiated from the sexual disorders (exhibitionism, pedophilia) and sexual dysfunction (arousal disorder, organic disorder).
2. Sexual addiction is a pattern of compulsive sexual behavior resulting in negative consequences.
3. Carnes (1983) categorizes three levels of sexual addiction:
   (a) Level 1: Behaviors regarded as normal, acceptable, or tolerable.
      (1) Masturbation.
      (2) Use of pornography.
      (3) Homosexuality.
      (4) Prostitution.
   (b) Level 2: Behaviors that clearly victimize others and for which legal sanctions are enforced.
      (1) Exhibitionism.
      (2) Voyeurism.
   (c) Level 3: Behaviors that have grave consequences for the victims and legal consequences.
      (1) Incest.
      (2) Child molestation.
      (3) Rape.
4. Substance abuse is related to the addiction in that it increases risk by impairing judgment and sometimes enhancing sexual sensations.
5. Societal attitudes correlating drinking/drug use with enhanced sexuality increase vulnerability of individuals at risk; i.e., individuals with:
   (a) Low self-esteem.
   (b) Intimacy problems.
   (c) Weak sexual identity.
   (d) Inadequate sex education.

Module II.3

E. **Related Concepts in Eating Disorders**

1. Eating disorders as appetitional disorders.
   a. The etiology of normal appetite is biological, psychodynamic, and sociocultural, much like the multiple etiologies of addiction.
   b. Normal growth and functioning of the human body is dependent upon the concept of nutrition. This involves consistent episodic and continuous phenomena (ingestion, digestion).
   c. Under normal conditions, the consequences of the somewhat rigidly patterned behavior of eating results in positive consequences for the individual; dysfunctional eating patterns lead to negative consequences.
   d. Craving (dependence) and withdrawal (starvation) are associated with eating patterns.
2. Eating disorders, as addictions, have been described to include overeating, bulimia, anorexia, and pica (Haber, Hoskins, Leach, & Sideleau, 1987; Flood, 1989; Peele, 1989).
3. Psychiatric classification (DSM-III-R, 1987) describes three separate clinical entities:
   a. Anorexia Nervosa.
      (1) DSM-III-R diagnostic criteria:
         (a) Refusal to maintain body weight over a minimal normal weight for age and height (e.g., weight loss leading to maintenance of body weight 15% below that expected; or failure to make expected weight gain during period of growth, leading to body weight 15% below that expected).
         (b) Intense fear of gaining weight or becoming fat, even though underweight.
         (c) Disturbance in the way in which one's body weight, size, or shape is experienced; e.g., the person claims to "feel fat" even when emaciated, and believes that one area of the body is "too fat" even when obviously underweight.
         (d) In females, absence of at least three consecutive menstrual cycles when otherwise expected to occur (primary or secondary amenorrhea). A woman is considered to have amenorrhea if her periods occur only following hormone (e.g., estrogen) administration.
      (2) Ninety to ninety-five percent of cases are among females (Halmic, 1982).
      (3) Occurs predominantly among ages 12–18 (Townsend, 1991, p. 77) correlated with Caucasian ethnicity are affluent socioeconomic status.
      (4) However, people aged 10–60 from every ethnic background and socioeconomic level have been diagnosed as anoretic (Yoder, 1990, p. 169).
      (5) Starvation leads to hypothermia, dry skin, dependent edema, hypotension, lanugo, metabolic changes, deterioration of vital organs, and death due to heart failure (Kaplan & Sadock, 1988, p. 599).

Addictions: Nursing Diagnosis and Treatment

    b. Bulimia.
       (1) DSM-III-R diagnostic criteria:
          (a) The person has recurrent episodes of binge eating (rapid consumption of a large amount of food in a discrete period of time).
          (b) The person has a feeling of lack of control over eating behavior during the eating binges.
          (c) The person regularly engages in either self-induced vomiting, use of laxatives or diuretics, strict dieting or fasting, or vigorous exercise in order to prevent weight gain.
          (d) The person has had a minimum average of two binge eating episodes a week for at least 3 months.
          (e) The person is persistently overly concerned with body shape and weight.
       (2) Studies suggest a prevalence of 4% in women compared to less than .05% in men.
       (3) Although no familial incidence has been noted, obesity may be found in other family members.
    c. The course of the illness leads to dehydration and electrolyte imbalance requiring hospitalization. Eye hemorrhages and tooth decays result from forced vomiting. (Kaplan & Sadock, 1988; Yoder, 1990).
    d. Overeating.
       (1) This is no discrete classification for compulsive overeating. The medical field identifies obesity as a treatable symptom and DSM-III-R identifies obesity as a psychophysiological condition. Neither of these is adequate to put overeating in the perspective of a food addiction.
       (2) Diagnostic criteria for 316.00 psychological factors affecting physical condition:
          (a) Psychologically meaningful environmental stimuli are temporally related to the initiation or exacerbation of a specific physical condition or disorder (recorded on Axis III).
          (b) The physical condition involves either demonstrable organic pathology (e.g., rheumatoid arthritis), or a known pathophysiologic process (e.g., migraine headache).
          (c) The condition does not meet the criteria for a somatoform disorder.
4. Other perspectives on eating disorders.
    a. The uniqueness of food as an object of compulsivity has received little research attention.
    b. Even less is known about a deviance of appetite characterized by craving for non-nutritive substances such as clay or plaster. This appetite disorder is known as "pica."
    c. Dysynchromous eating patterns has been described as a maladaptive response to stress and includes anorexia, bulimia, pica, and obesity (Haber, Hoskins, Leach, & Sideleau, 1987).
    d. Out-of-control appetitive behavior, especially by the young is discussed by Peele (1989).

e. Not all obese people are food addicts and not all food addicts are obese (Yoder, 1990).

f. Stunkard (1980) notes when food is generally available, appetite is based on desire, rather than satisfaction of hunger which influences the choice and quantity of foods eaten.

g. Other dynamics such as the theme of control, and increased incidence of affective disorders in family members are discussed by Flood (1989).

5. Treatment.

Possible treatments include physical interventions to treat physiological sequelae, family therapy, individual and group psychotherapy, self-help groups, stress management techniques, and behavior modification.

6. Implications.

There are important implications of this range of perspectives on eating disorders. Appetite, craving, and drug of choice (d.o.c.) are factors which need further study, both individually and in correlation. Clearer insights into these factors, particularly from an etiologic perspective will lay groundwork for prevention and effective treatment strategies.

F. **Relapse.**

1. Relapse is an inherent factor in the treatment of addiction. However, that does not make it unpreventable.

2. The 12-step programs have two central principles to prevent relapse.

    a. The first is HALT, an acronym which stands for the avoiding of the experiences Hunger, Anger, Loneliness, and Tiredness.

    b. The second principle is a mandate to change persons, places, and things which facilitated the addictive process in its origins, and could inhibit recovery in the present.

3. Factors which are believed to affect relapse:

    a. Access to use.
    b. Failure to thrive.
        (1) Boredom.
        (2) Unemployment.
        (3) Poor self-concept.
    c. Protective social withdrawal.
    d. Alteration in mood.
    e. Untreated psychopathology.
    f. Nihilistic, self-destructive factors.
    g. Undiagnosed medical illness.
    h. Family/spousal dysfunction.
    i. Other drug or alcohol use.
    j. Non-compliance with aftercare plan.

Addictions: Nursing Diagnosis and Treatment

III. NURSING DIAGNOSES CONGRUENT WITH NURSING AND INTERPROFESSIONAL CLASSIFICATION SYSTEMS

A. Relationship of Nursing Diagnoses to Medical Diagnoses

It is important for the nurse generalist to become involved with the DSM-III-R. This system of codification was designed to allow all health providers to be able to reach consensus on a psychiatric/addictive diagnosis by virtue of assessing the patient's behaviors, which leads to the psychiatric diagnosis.

The goal of using DSM-III-R is to arrive at psychiatric diagnosis and treatment plan.

While formulating the nursing care plan, nurses must be familiar with medical diagnoses and treatment plans. The two diagnostic systems are meant to be complementary. A patient with one specific medical diagnosis may have a number of nursing diagnoses related to his or her various health responses. On the other hand, a patient may have a specific nursing diagnosis without any identified medical diagnosis (Stuart & Sundeen, 1991).

The critical point is that the diagnostic goals differ: one is toward identifying disease (medical diagnosis); the other is toward identifying an actual or potential response to a health problem (nursing diagnosis).

B. Diagnosis of Actual and Potential Health Problems Related to Addictions

1. Sensory-perceptual alteration.
   Defining characteristics.
   a. Confusion.
   b. Disorientation.
   c. Slow processing of information.
   d. Slow and slurred speech.
   e. Tremors and anxiety.
   f. Poor recent memory.
2. Sleep pattern disturbance.
   Defining characteristics.
   a. Verbal complaints of difficulty falling asleep.
   b. Verbal complaints of not feeling well rested.
   c. Reports of anxiety during the night.
   d. Sleep pattern reversal—sleeps during the day and is awake at night.
   e. Use of extra tranquilizers at night.
   f. Interrupted sleep.
   g. Restlessness during sleep.
3. Alteration in comfort—pain.
   Defining characteristics.
   a. Verbal reports of headache pain.
   b. Self-focusing withdrawal from social contact.

c. Distorted perception of pain.

d. Trips to emergency room for headache medication.

4. Dysfunctional family processes.

    Defining characteristics.

    a. Lack of open, effective communication within family.

5. Alteration in self-concept.

    Defining characteristics.

    a. Difficulty accepting or acknowledging bodily changes (hysterectomy).

    b. Negative statements about self.

    c. Feelings of inadequacy, guilt, and shame.

    d. Social withdrawal.

    e. Self-destructive behaviors.

    f. Limited problem-solving skills to use in raising level of self-esteem.

    g. Fluctuating feelings about self.

    h. Inability to relate to others on an intimate level.

    i. Feelings of emptiness.

6. Anxiety—moderate.

    Defining characteristics.

    a. Subjective feeling of discomfort.

    b. Interpersonal withdrawal.

    c. Tense, nervous, and fearful.

    d. Difficulty with concentration.

    e. Impaired attention span.

    f. Confusion.

    g. Fear of injury or death.

7. Self-care deficit.

    Defining characteristics.

    a. Intolerance of activity.

    b. Pain and discomfort.

    c. Depression.

    d. Decreased self-esteem.

    e. Compromised personal hygiene as evidenced by weight gain or poor grooming.

    f. Impaired nutritional status.

8. Sexual dysfunction.

    Defining characteristics.

    a. Actual or perceived limitation imposed by disease.

    b. Alterations in libido.

    c. Report of inability to achieve desired sexual satisfaction.

    d. Alteration in relationship with significant other.

Addictions: Nursing Diagnosis and Treatment

9. Impaired communication.
   Defining characteristics.
   a. Inability to express feelings.
   b. Lack of assertive behaviors.
   c. Slurring of speech and confusion.
   d. Inappropriate speech patterns.
10. Hopelessness.
    Defining characteristics.
    a. Passivity.
    b. Feelings of hopelessness related to addictions and outcomes of treatment.
    c. Lack of energy for normal activity.
    d. Social isolation.
    e. Increased need for attention, help, and reassurance.
    f. High risk of depression related to addiction.
    g. Lack of future plans.
    h. Flat, sad affect.

IV. **NURSING INTERVENTION**

A. **Treatment Modalities for the Addictions**

1. Primary.
   a. Detoxification.
      (1) Gradual withdrawal from drugs.
      (2) Medically supervised (defined).
      (3) Lasts two days to a week or longer.
      (4) May entail substitute drugs to wean patient off chemicals (such as methadone).
      (5) May entail drugs to ease the severity of withdrawal symptoms.
   b. Rehabilitation.
      (1) Residential.
         (a) Focus on breaking the cycle of addiction.
         (b) Recommended for people who need intensive support and education.
            i) Adolescents.
            ii) Drug addicts.
            iii) Chronic relapses.
            iv) Individuals at risk of harming self or others.
            v) Individuals from dysfunctional homes.
            vi) Dually diagnosed.
         (c) Majority of rehabilitation facilities are free-standing units, with chemical dependency as main focus.

Module II.3

   (d) Typical stay 4–6 weeks followed by 1–2 years of aftercare.
   (e) Usually incorporates family treatment, often in the form of weekend or short-term program.
  (2) Outpatient.
   (a) Recommended for individuals who are:
    i) Early stage addicts.
    ii) Securely employed.
    iii) From stable families.
    iv) In connection with adequate social supports.
   (b) Advantages.
    i) Evening programs allow continuation of functional patterns.
    ii) Practice of skills is reality-oriented, on a day-to-day basis.
    iii) Are an important resource for single parents; cost is 1/3 to 1/5 that of inpatient.
   (c) Typical programs consist of therapy, lectures, 12-step meetings, and family treatment.
   (d) Duration of programs is typically six weeks, four hours per night, five nights per week, or some variation of this format.
 c. Therapeutic community.
  (1) A residential setting in which the total social structure of the treatment unit is involved as part of the helping process.
  (2) Key concepts.
   (a) Participants are active in care planning.
   (b) Democratic, not hierarchic.
   (c) Rehabilitative, rather than custodial.
   (d) Permissive, instead of limited and controlled.
   (e) Communal, as opposed to emphasizing the therapeutic role of health professionals.
  (3) Typical components.
   (a) Daily community meeting followed by small groups.
   (b) Patient government.
   (c) Living-learning opportunities.
   (d) Feedback (Stuart & Sundeen, 1991).
  (4) General duration is one or more years.
 d. 12-step program.
  (1) Most popular recovery program.
  (2) Spiritual program based on fellowship and such universal spiritual values as honesty, humility, and forgiveness.
  (3) Goal of treatment: Abstinence.
  (4) Key concepts: The 12 steps of Alcoholics Anonymous.
   (a) We admitted we were powerless over alcohol—that our lives had become unmanageable.

Addictions: Nursing Diagnosis and Treatment

- (b) We came to believe that a Power greater than ourselves could restore us to sanity.
- (c) We made a decision to turn our will and our lives over to the care of God *as we understood Him.*
- (d) We made a searching and fearless moral inventory of ourselves.
- (e) We admitted to God, to ourselves, and to another human being the exact nature of our wrongs.
- (f) We were entirely ready to have God remove all these defects of character.
- (g) We humbly asked Him to remove our shortcomings.
- (h) We made a list of all persons we had harmed, and became willing to make amends to them all.
- (i) We made direct amends to such people wherever possible, except when to do so would injure them or others.
- (j) We continued to take personal inventory and when we were wrong promptly admitted it.
- (k) We sought through prayer and meditation to improve our conscious contact with God *as we understood Him,* praying only for knowledge of His will for us and the power to carry that out.
- (l) Having had a spiritual awakening as the result of these Steps, we tried to carry this message to others, and to practice these principles in all our affairs.

(5) Structure of the 12-step program: The 12 traditions of Alcoholics Anonymous.
- (a) Our common welfare should come first; personal recovery depends upon AA unity.
- (b) For our group purpose there is but one ultimate authority—a loving God as He may express Himself in our group conscience. Our leaders are but trusted servants; they do not govern.
- (c) The only requirement for AA membership is a desire to stop drinking.
- (d) Each group should be autonomous except in matters affecting other groups or AA as a whole.
- (e) Each group has but one primary purpose—to carry its message to the alcoholic who still suffers.
- (f) An AA group ought never endorse, finance, or lend the AA name to any related facility or outside enterprise, lest problems of money, property, and prestige divert us from our primary purpose.
- (g) Every AA group ought to be fully self-supporting, declining outside contributions.
- (h) AA should remain forever nonprofessional, but our service centers may employ special workers.
- (i) AA, as such, ought never be organized; but we may create service boards or committees directly responsible to those they serve.

(j) AA has no opinion on outside issues; hence the AA name ought never be drawn into public controversy.

(k) Our public relations policy is based on attraction rather than promotion; we need always maintain personal anonymity at the level of press, radio, and films.

(l) Anonymity is the spiritual foundation of all our Traditions, ever reminding us to place principles before personalities.

(6) Typical approach.
   (a) 90 meetings in first ninety days of recovery.
   (b) Taper off to 1–2 meetings per week.
   (c) Working the program includes:
      i) Meetings.
      ii) Readings.
      iii) Sponsorship.
      iv) Fellowship.
      v) Use of slogans.
      vi) Offering service.
   (d) Final process: "Give Away" what you've learned.

(7) Disadvantages.
   (a) Possible substitution of addiction to the program.
   (b) Spiritual focus unacceptable to some individuals.
   (c) Limited assistance to individuals with dual diagnoses.

e. Acupuncture.

Attempts to ameliorate withdrawal symptoms by the stimulation of the endogenous opioid system (Alterman, O'Brien, & McLellan, 1991).

f. Methadone Maintenance Treatment Program (MMTP).

(1) Most common form of narcotic substitution.

(2) Methadone kept at blood levels of 150 mg/ml (daily dose of 60 mg/day) and above are considered effective in stopping illicit opioid use.

(3) MMTP are frequently coupled with other services such as client contact, counseling, and urine monitoring (Alterman, O'Brien, & McLellan, 1991).

(4) May serve as a bridge to abstinence or naloxone therapy.

g. Individual and group counseling generally conducted by an addiction specific counselor.

2. Secondary.
   a. Psychotherapy.
      (1) Individual.
      (2) Family.
      (3) Group.
   b. Spiritual counseling.

Addictions: Nursing Diagnosis and Treatment

B. **Nursing Process**

1. Establish a plan of care based on nursing diagnosis.
    a. Using a case study approach or in a clinical practice setting, build a database of patient responses organizing them into phenomena of concern.
        (1) Biological responses.
        (2) Cognitive responses.
        (3) Psychosocial responses.
        (4) Spiritual responses.
    b. List nursing diagnoses relevant to addictions that are derived from database.
2. Set care goals specific to the individual. Prioritize nursing diagnosis relative to needs of patients, applicability to care setting, and level of practice. Set short-term goals and long-term goals.
3. Identify anticipated outcomes.
4. List criteria for identified outcomes.
5. Implement care, independent or in collaboration with peers or members of other disciplines.
    a. Minimum nursing interventions: Assessment and referral.
    b. Evaluation based on outcome criteria.

C. **Referral**

1. Guiding Principle: Simple ⟶ Complex.
2. Choosing referral as nursing intervention.
    a. The severity of the alcohol and other drug (AODA) problem, the readiness of the client, and the type of setting and services needed will help determine whether the client receives treatment in the original setting or is referred for treatment.
    b. Even when treatment services are available in the primary care setting, there may be a need to refer for specialized treatment services. Indicators include:
        (1) No change in physical, psychological, or behavioral symptoms after 90 days.
        (2) Care is too complex and time consuming.
        (3) Behavior is too disruptive for an ordinary clinical setting.
        (4) Suicidal tendencies.
    c. Objective of all parties in the referral process should be consistent.
        (1) Continuity of care.
        (2) Definition of goals.
        (3) Clear communication.
        (4) Understanding of responsibilities.
        (5) Sensitivity to the effects of the referral on the client.

3. Referral resources.
   a. Most practice settings have a protocol for the generalist nurse to make a referral.
   b. If there is no protocol, selecting a referral resource can be difficult, especially if the clinician is unfamiliar with local resources, if the community is so small that it has very limited resources, or if it is so large that it has a confusing array of resources of unknown quality.
   c. Choosing an appropriate professional or agency may be the most important service that a clinician can provide to a client with an alcohol and other drug problem.
   d. NIDA Drug Abuse Treatment and Referral Line: 800/662-HELP (4357).
   e. Regional Council on Alcoholism; AA Intergroup.
4. Establishing referral networks.
   a. Referrals may be made to a range of community services and resources.
      (1) Alcohol and other drug treatment and rehabilitation services.
      (2) Community mental health facilities.
      (3) Community social service and welfare agencies.
      (4) Community child development, evaluation, and testing services.
      (5) Hospital outpatient departments.
      (6) Independent nurse practitioners and visiting nurses.
      (7) Psychiatrists, psychologists, nurses, and social workers in private practice.
      (8) Community public school.
      (9) Court and probation systems.
5. Establishing contacts.
   a. Locating possible sources for referral may involve contacts with professional colleagues, mental health clinics, hospitals, medical schools, state and local medical associations, and state alcohol and drug abuse agencies.
   b. Establishing and maintaining personal contacts with the staff or referral agencies aids in the effective provision of comprehensive care. Where linkages are established, clear communication, responsibilities, and coordination are likely.
6. Criteria for evaluating referral resources.
   a. The program's record and success rate.
   b. Attitudes of program staff.
   c. Education and training of program staff.
   d. Licensure and accreditation of the program.
   e. Treatment of alcohol and drug dependence as primary disorders.
   f. Clients free of drugs early in the recovery process.
   g. Adequate provision for care of acute medical problems.

Addictions: Nursing Diagnosis and Treatment

      h. Extent to which the program will help expedite the client's entry into treatment.

      i. Use of a comprehensive treatment approach.

      j. Encouragement for families to participate in the treatment process.

      k. Active preparation of clients against relapse.

      l. Development of a plan for continuing care.

      m. Ability to respond to special issues and needs.

      n. Reasonable cost.

7. Preparing the client for referral.
    a. Give rationale for referral.
    b. Describe the referral resource.
    c. Provide support.
    d. Provide contact person.
    e. Discuss follow-up.
8. Provide appropriate information such as consultant's name or agency name and phone number.
9. Remain available, if possible, for supportive follow-up. By doing so, the nurse indicates a continuing interest in the client's well-being and also gathers feedback facilitating evaluation of referral effectiveness.

V. GENERALIST NURSING ROLES

A. Education on Addiction in the Adult Population

The generalist nurse is a registered nurse prepared at the baccalaureate, associate, or diploma level working in any health care setting. As such, the nurse will encounter clients of all ages who may be manifesting response patterns of abuse and addiction. Clients and families at risk for developing these patterns will also be met. Health teaching, as an integral part of comprehensive nursing care, may be done in any of these settings. This teaching may be a means of prevention or an adjunct to nursing care for other health problems.

Scope of health teaching at the generalist level:

1. Communication of the meaning of addiction and related concepts.
2. Information on common addictive substances including general classes of substances.
3. Communication appropriate to the level of the learner as to effects of addiction on the dimensions of the human system (psychosocial, biological, cognitive/perceptual, and spiritual/belief).
4. Communication of modalities of treatment and the implications of these for client and family.
5. Roles of nursing specialists and other personnel involved in treatment options.

Module II.3

B. Roles Implemented by the Nurse in the Acute and Chronic Care of the Addicted Individual and His/Her Family

1. Data collection on dimensions of the human system.
2. Documentation.
3. Contribution to the treatment team plan.
4. Safe and appropriate implementation of nursing functions, such as medication, administration, participation in milieu therapy, management of behavior program, assistance in self-care, and timely nursing assessments.
5. Therapeutic use of self-awareness of own attitudes, values, and responses and use of these qualities to engage, interact, and respond with the client.
6. Health educator.

C. Roles of the Nurse in the Long-Term Rehabilitative Care of the Addicted or Substance Abusing Client

1. As a change agent appropriate to the program in place.
2. As a case finder for human responses to the program which indicate changes.
3. As an observer of emerging patterns indicating need for interventions.
4. Caregiver within a nursing theoretical framework, identified as unique relative to other dimensions of care. For example, the present status of the person as acute, chronic, and rehabilitative simultaneously.
5. Health educator.

D. Relapse

1. Knowledge of risk factors for individuals and groups.
2. Knowledge of measures to control risk such as support programs and behavioral strategies.
3. Self-directed learner for updated trends in care in order to communicate accurate and appropriate education to clients.

E. Prevention

1. General prevention strategies for generalists and specialists in any setting.
   a. Education on addiction as it is manifested in relation to a substance or behavior, including recreational misuse of such substances as alcohol and drugs.
   b. Identification of individuals at high risk for the development of addictions; e.g., children of alcoholics and individuals who have been involved in a wide range of drug experimentation.
   c. Identification of early signs and symptoms of addiction.
   d. Activities to effect change, such as networking and support of legislation and policy directed toward reducing the incidence of addiction and its consequences on society.

Addictions: Nursing Diagnosis and Treatment

- e. Use of knowledge about alcohol, tobacco, food, and drug use and abuse in comprehensive health teaching of clients receiving nursing care.
- f. Use of knowledge of compulsive and dependent behaviors as the basis for health maintenance teaching.

2. Special strategies—Relapse prevention: The nurse is likely to meet a client in a *stressful situation*. Risk for relapse is increasing.
   - a. Identify situation in which client is most tempted to abandon positive behavior changes.
   - b. Identify feelings most likely to increase vulnerability for relapse.
   - c. Rehearse positive coping strategies for dealing with possible relapse situations; e.g., relaxation techniques.
   - d. Help client see that occasional relapses are normal.
   - e. In active relapse, approach the event constructively, as a learning experience.
   - f. If client is in early recovery, provide booster session focusing on positive gains observed by the client.
   - g. Elicit questions or concerns about relapse and facilitate appropriate educational intervention.
   - h. Become informed regarding reentry into treatment if relapse occurs.

3. Special strategies—Intervention with families: Generalist nurses.
   - a. Early identification of alcohol and other drug problems minimizes family distress. Educational efforts, accurate information, and an understanding of alcohol and other drugs counteract denial.
   - b. The generalist nurse can be the first person to break through the isolation and suppression of a family member—simply by outreach or by bringing up the subject.
   - c. Focus on family member presenting problem, not necessarily the abuser.
   - d. The generalist nurse can model attitudes about disclosure, treatment optimism, and communication patterns.
   - e. The generalist nurse can support and reinforce specialty interventions by data collection, administration of protocols, and exploration of existing resources.

MODULE II.3
ADDICTIONS: NURSING DIAGNOSIS AND TREATMENT

INSTRUCTOR'S GUIDE

Janet S. D'Arcangelo, MA, RN, C
Thomas Adamski, MEd, MSN, RNC, CRNA

Madeline A. Naegle, PhD, RN, FAAN
Project Director
Janet S. D'Arcangelo, MA, RN, C
Project Coordinator

Project SAEN
SUBSTANCE ABUSE
EDUCATION IN NURSING

CONTENTS

Component	Page
Module Description	258
Time Frame	258
Placement	258
Learner Objectives	259
Recommended Readings	260
Faculty Readings	260
Student Readings	260
Recommended Audiovisual and Other Resources	261
Overhead Masters	263
Handout Masters	299
Recommended Teaching Strategies and Sample Assignments	335
Test Questions and Answers	339
Bibliography	342

Module II.3

MODULE DESCRIPTION

This module facilitates the student's understanding of the addictive process and its manifestations in the adult client. Addiction to alcohol and drugs will be a primary focus, although appetitional disorders manifested in sexual overactivity, gambling, and eating disorders will be addressed. Nursing diagnoses related to psychological and physiologic dependence and behavioral disturbances associated with addiction will be presented. Nursing interventions will be discussed and evaluated according to anticipated outcomes and in relation to nursing role.

TIME FRAME

6 hours

PLACEMENT

Adult Health, Psychiatric-Mental Health Nursing, Community Health

Instructor's Guide

LEARNER OBJECTIVES

Upon successful completion of this module, the learner will:

1. Define central concepts of addiction abuse and dependence.

2. Describe the psychological dynamics and, where applicable, the physiological mechanisms central to addiction to drugs, alcohol, compulsive gambling, sexual activity, and eating disorders.

3. List nursing diagnoses which correspond to patterns manifested by the individual addicted to, or abusing drugs.

4. Describe treatment modalities for the individual abusing or addicted to substances or engaging in compulsive behavior.

5. Formulate and evaluate nursing interventions utilized with client and family when addiction and/or abuse are manifested.

6. Describe nursing roles implemented by the generalist practitioner of nursing in the prevention, treatment, and rehabilitation of the addicted client and family.

Module II.3

RECOMMENDED READINGS

FACULTY READINGS

American Psychiatric Association. (1987). *Diagnostic and statistical manual* (3rd ed., revised). Washington, DC: Author.

Bradshaw, J. (1988). *Bradshaw on: The family.* Deerfield Beach, FL: Health Communications, Inc.

Cadoret, R. J. (1986). An adoption study of genetic and environmental factors in drug abuse. *Archives of General Psychiatry, 43*(12), 1131–1136.

Magilvy, J. K., McMahon, M., Bachman, M., Roark, S., & Evenson, C. (1987). The health of teenagers: A focused ethnographic study. *Public Health Nursing, 4*(1), 35–42.

Vetter, H. J. (1985). Psychodynamic factors and drug addiction: Some theoretical and research perspectives. *Journal of Drug Issues, 15*(4), 447–461.

STUDENT READINGS

American Nurses' Association. (1988). *Standards of addictions nursing practice with selected diagnoses and criteria.* Kansas City, MO: Author.

American Nurses' Association, Drugs and Alcohol Nurses' Association, & National Nurses' Society on Addictions. (1987). *The care of clients with addictions: Dimensions of nursing practice.* Kansas City, MO: Author.

Bradshaw, J. (1988). *Bradshaw on: The family.* Deerfield Beach, FL: Health Communications, Inc.

Haack, M. (1986). The patient with chemical addiction. In J. D. Druham & S. B. Harden (Eds.), *The nurse psychotherapist in private practice* (pp. 173–186). New York: Springer.

Jack, L. (1989). *Nursing care planning with the addicted client.* Skokie, IL: National Nurses' Society on Addictions.

Naegle, M. (1989). Substance abuse. In L. Brickhead (Ed.), *Psychiatric mental health nursing: The therapeutic use of self* (pp. 427–464). Philadelphia: J. B. Lippincott.

Thurston, B. A. (1986). Substance abuse: The drug dependencies. In B. S. Johnson (Ed.), *Psychiatric-mental health nursing: Adaptation and growth.* New York: J. B. Lippincott.

Instructor's Guide

RECOMMENDED AUDIOVISUAL AND OTHER RESOURCES

1. **The Addicted Brain**

    This documentary takes viewers on a tour of the world's most prolific manufacturer and user of drugs—the human brain. The biochemistry of the brain is responsible for joggers' highs, for the compulsion of some people to seek thrills, for certain kinds of obsessive compulsive behavior, even for the drive to achieve power and dominance. This program explores the cutting edge of developments in the biochemistry of addiction and addictive behavior. (1990). 26 minutes. [VHS BD-1363. purchase ($199).] Available from Films for the Humanities & Sciences, P.O. Box 2053, Princeton, NJ 08543. 1-800-257-5126.

2. **Staying Off Cocaine: Avoiding Relapse**

    Reviews principles of relapse prevention with actual ex-addicts as spokespeople. (1987). **Reelization Productions, Woodstock, New York. 914/679-8363.**

3. **Bulimia**

    Narrated by Michael Learned, about Bulimia, risk factors, and consequences. Also includes presentation by a recovering bulimic and a demonstration of social pressures of thinness. (1987). 25 minutes. Available in VHS ½" or ¾", Beta I or II. Rental $80, Sale $385. Discount price available to Health Sciences Consortium members. **Contact Health Sciences Consortium, 201 Silver Cedar Court, Chapel Hill, NC 27514, 919/942-8731.**

4. **The Enigma of Anorexia Nervosa**

    A video program in three parts:

    Part I. Delusion and Discord

    History, description, and approaches to anorexia. (18 minutes).

    Part II. Clinical Intervention and Rehabilitation

    Describes signs/symptoms and clinical course including treatment plan (16 minutes).

    Part III. The Battle of Wills

    Dynamics and emotional issues of patients, family, and staff involved with eating disorders (24 minutes) (1986).

Module II.3

All available in ¾" VHS from **Carle Medical Communication, 510 West Main Street, Urbana, IL 61801, 217/384-4838.** Rental $50 each part, $135 set, Purchase $325 each part, $850 set.

5. Overeating: An American Obsession

This documentary about America's obsession with overeating combines facts with feelings by presenting information from nationally recognized experts who offer weight loss programs that work and compelling stories of people struggling to control their weight problem.

A unique aspect of the video is a section on childhood obesity. Color, 25 minutes, U-matic or VHS, Rental $65/3 days & $100/5 days, Purchase: $295. **Contact Carle Medical Communications, 110 West Main Street, Urbana, IL 61801-2700. Phone: 217/384-4838.**

6. Drug and Alcohol Rehabilitation

One in 10 Americans has a drinking problem, one in five has at least dabbled with drugs. This program focuses on the treatments in use to overcome these chemical dependencies, and on the four stages of treatment: detoxification, counseling, acceptance, and recovery. The program also covers two controversial therapies currently in use: aversion therapy for alcoholism, and methadone treatment for drug addiction. Viewers learn what the addict must do to avoid relapse, including taking it "one day at a time"—a basic tenent of self-help groups like Alcoholics Anonymous. (19 minutes, color). #LC1369, Purchase $149, Rental $75. **Films for the Humanities & Sciences, P.O. Box 2053, Princeton, NJ 08543-2053. Phone: (800)257-5126 or 609/452-1128.**

Instructor's Guide

OVERHEAD MASTERS

MODULE II.3   ADDICTIONS: NURSING DIAGNOSIS AND TREATMENT

1. The Episodic and Continuous Phenomenon of Addiction
2. Denial
3. Addiction: Neurochemical Aspects (A–D)
4. Substance Abuse Cycle
5. Dual Diagnosis
6. Guide to Treatment Referrals for Substance Aubse (A–E)
7. 12 Steps of Alcoholics Anonymous
8. 12 Traditions of Alcoholics Anonymous
9. Special Strategies: Relapse
10. Special Strategies: Families

Instructor's Guide

Module II.3—Overhead #1

THE EPISODIC AND CONTINUOUS PHENOMENON OF ADDICTION

Episodic....Episodic/Continuous....Continuous ...Continuous/Episodic

Life-threatening use

Level of severity represented by AMPLITUDE

Non-use

Pattern of use represented by FREQUENCY

Frequent/low severity

example: "recreational" cocaine user

Occasional/high severity

example: binge drinker

265

Instructor's Guide

Module II.3—Overhead #2

DENIAL

May be exhibited by numerous components of the abusing system.

- D Drug/Substance Abuser/Addict—Directly or indirectly.
- E Employers.
- N Nurses and other caregivers/health professionals.
- I Internal mechanisms defense against stress.
- A Advertising and other economic structures.
- L Loved ones—Family and friends of the abuser.

Module II.3—Overhead #3A

ADDICTION: STIMULATION OF THE BRAIN

Stimulation of the Brain → Nerve Action →

When an impulse arrives at the synapse, chemicals called transmitters enable the impulse to pass on to the next nerve cell.

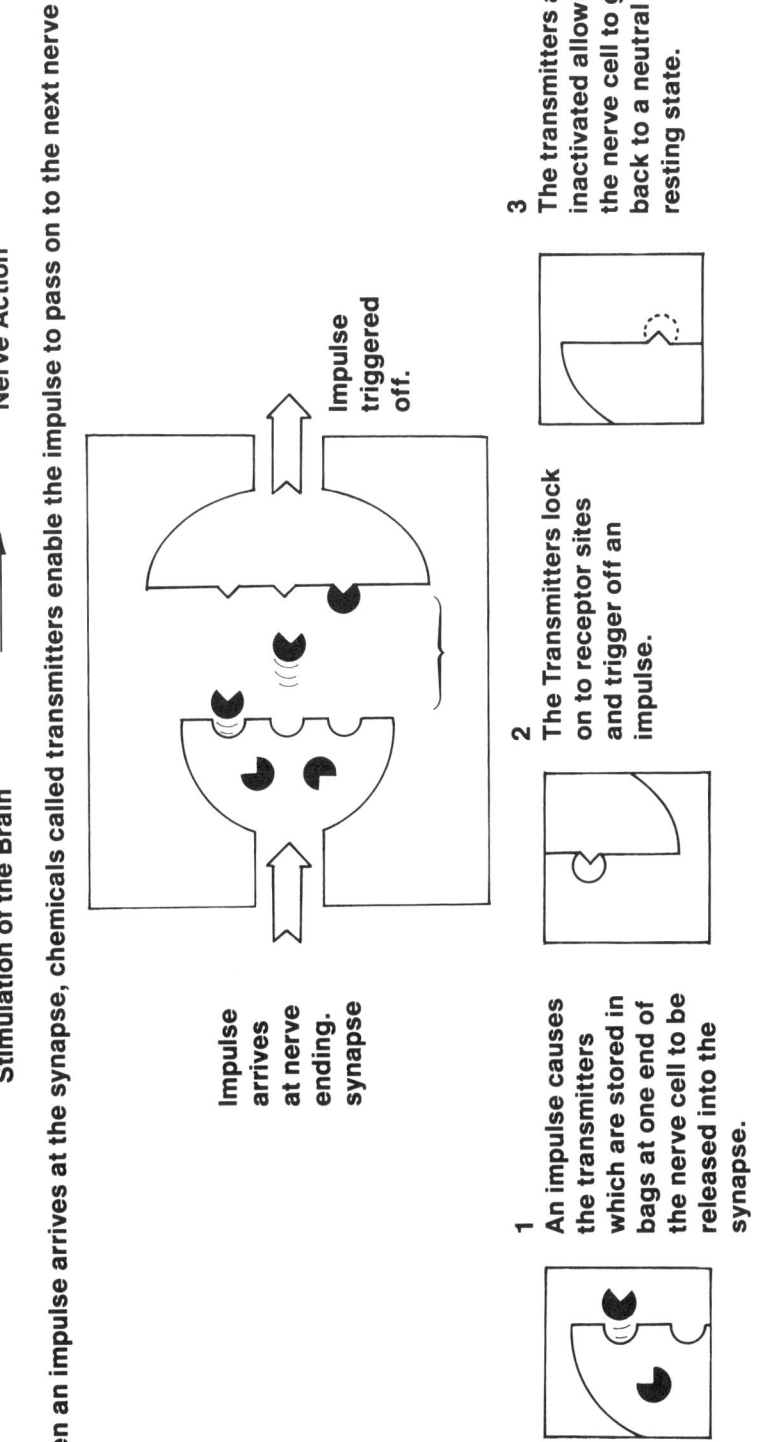

Impulse arrives at nerve ending. synapse

Impulse triggered off.

1 An impulse causes the transmitters which are stored in bags at one end of the nerve cell to be released into the synapse.

2 The Transmitters lock on to receptor sites and trigger off an impulse.

3 The transmitters are inactivated allowing the nerve cell to go back to a neutral resting state.

A NATURAL FEEDBACK SYSTEM DETERMINES AUTOMATIC PRODUCTION AND CESSATION OF NEUROTRANSMITTER

From: Pictorial Charts Educational Trust, 27 Kirchen Road, West Ealing London W13 OUD with permission for limited profit.

ADDICTION: DRUG EFFECTS

1. Nerves carry messages in the form of impulses. When the nerve endings are stimulated an impulse is generated which travels along to the end of the cell.

2. Chemicals are released into the synapse causing an impulse to be generated in the next cell.

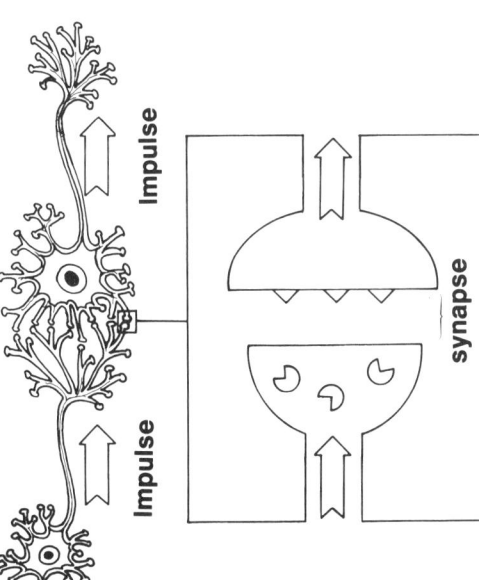

Impulse

synapse

The actual size of this gap is 0.00002 mm

Drugs

Drugs interfere with the chemicals which cross the synapses and affect the brain.

Stimulants

Increase the amount of transmitters released between nerve cells and speed up the activity of the brain (cocaine, amphetamines, caffeine, nicotine).

Hallucinogens

Overactivate many nerve cells causing visual illusions (LSD, cannabis, magic mushrooms, volatile solvents, aerosols).

Depressants

Reduce the amount of transmitters between some brain cells or blocks the action of other transmitters.

SEDATIVES: delay transmission of nerve impulses, calm people down (barbiturates, alcohol).

TRANQUILIZERS: slow down brain activity, induce sleep (valium, Librium).

PAINKILLERS: suppress parts of the brain responsible for the sense of pain (opiates such as morphine and heroin).

Module II.3—Overhead #3C

ALTERATION AT THE SYNAPSE: AMPHETAMINES

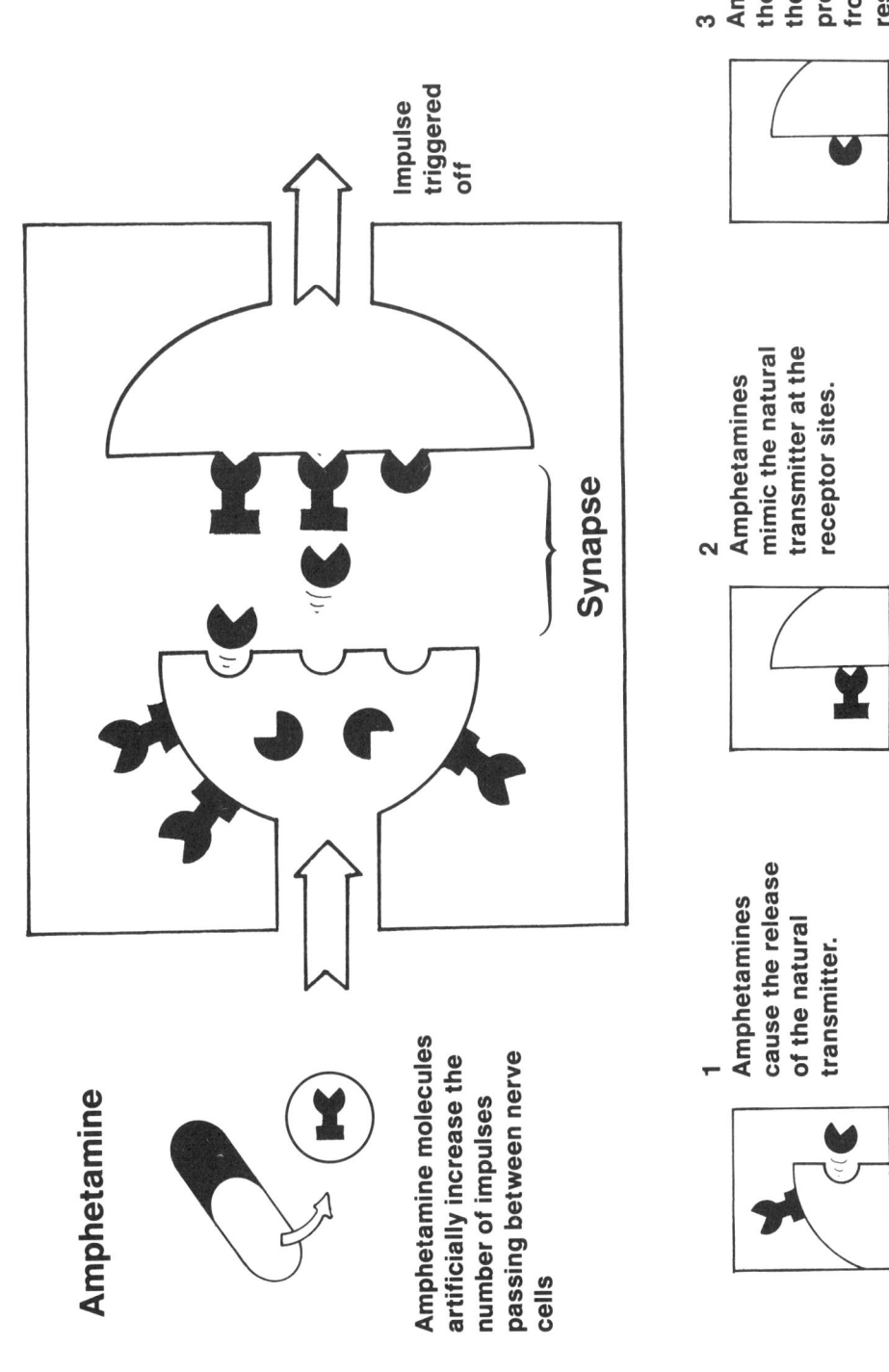

Amphetamine

Amphetamine molecules artificially increase the number of impulses passing between nerve cells

1 Amphetamines cause the release of the natural transmitter.

2 Amphetamines mimic the natural transmitter at the receptor sites.

3 Amphetamines stop the inactivation of the natural transmitter preventing the neuron from returning to resting state.

Instructor's Guide

Module II.3—Overhead #3D

ADDICTION: BASIC CONCEPTS

Tolerance

Tolerance refers to the way the body adapts to the repeated presence of a drug, meaning that higher doses are needed to maintain the same effect.

Cells learn to work in the presence of high levels of the drug which becomes part of the cell structure. The user needs the drug in order to act normally.

Dependence

Physical dependence exists when a user is tolerant to a drug and will experience physical withdrawal effects if usage is ended or reduced below a certain level

Psychological dependence refers to a craving to take more of a drug and an inability to function emotionally without.

Addiction

1. An overpowering desire to continue taking a drug.
2. A tendency to increase the dose.
3. A psychological and often a physical dependence on the effects of a drug.
4. A deterioration of the physical and emotional health of the individual.
5. The appearance of withdrawal effects when the drug is discontinued or reduced below a certain level.
6. A preoccupation with obtaining drugs, often at the expense of society.

Withdrawal

Withdrawal effects are the body's reactions to the sudden absence of a drug to which it has adapted.

Cells lose the ability to work in the absence of the drug because the natural transmitter is no longer available.

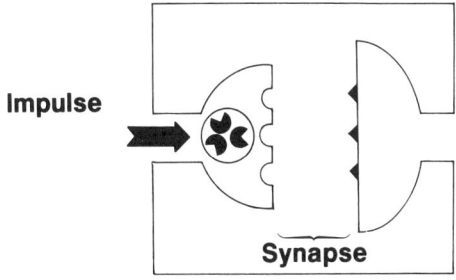

Module II.3—Overhead #4

SUBSTANCE ABUSE CYCLE

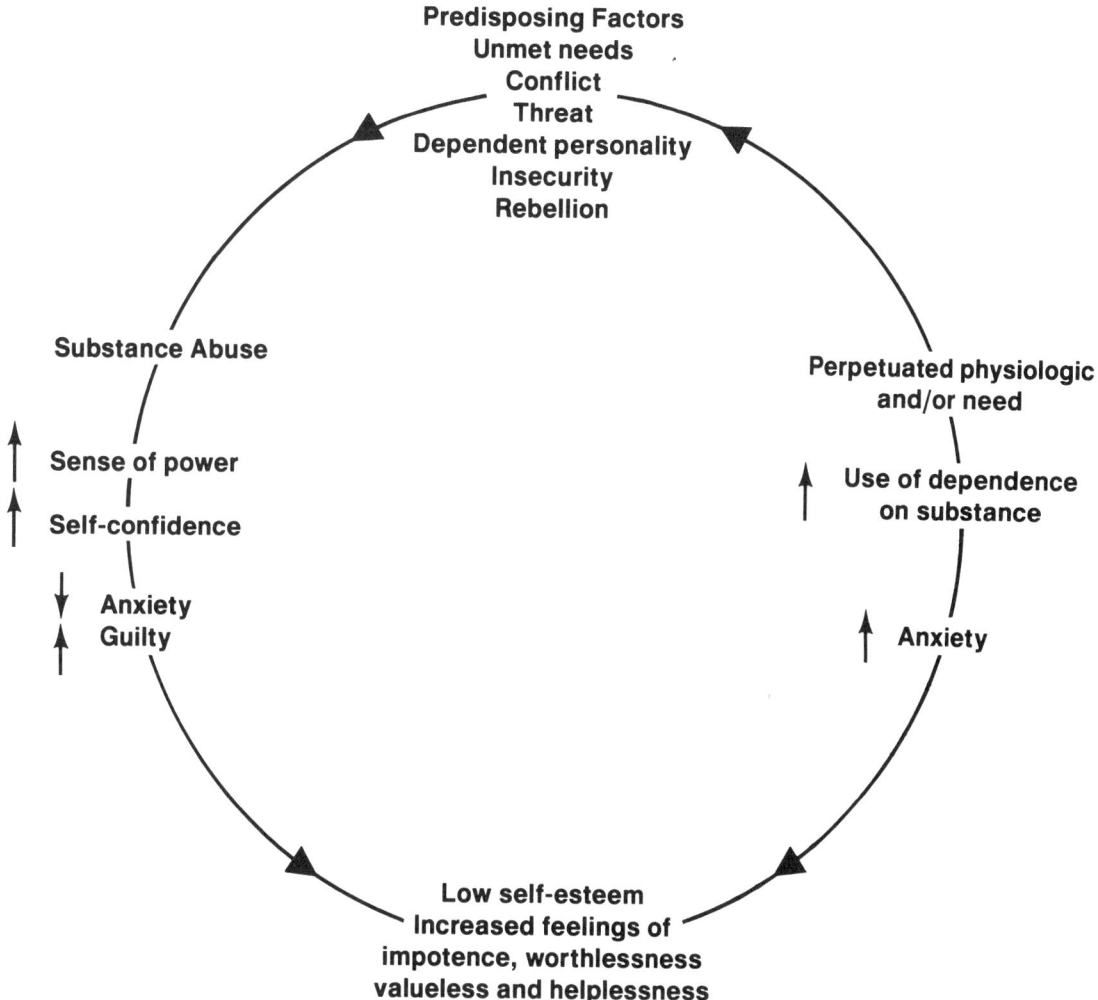

Module II.3—Overhead #5

DUAL DIAGNOSIS

One review of dual diagnosis literature produced the following distribution among psychiatric admissions:

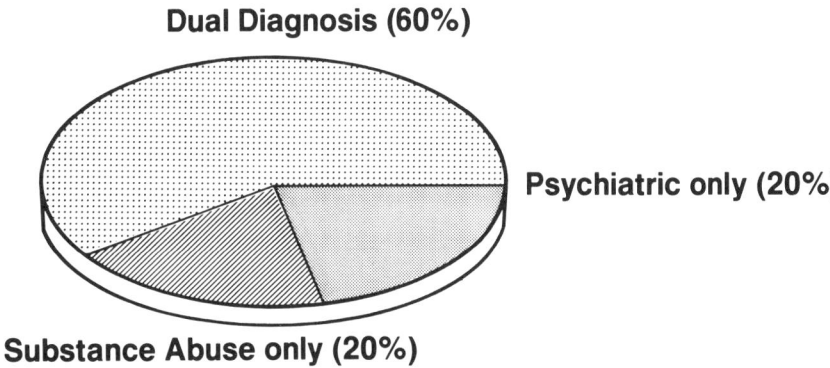

From: McKelvy, M. J., Kane, J. S., & Kellison, K. (1987) Substance abuse and mental illness: Double trouble. *Journal of Psychosocial Nursing and Mental Health Services, 25*(1), 20–25.

Module II.3—Overhead #6A

GUIDE TO TREATMENT REFERRALS FOR SUBSTANCE ABUSE

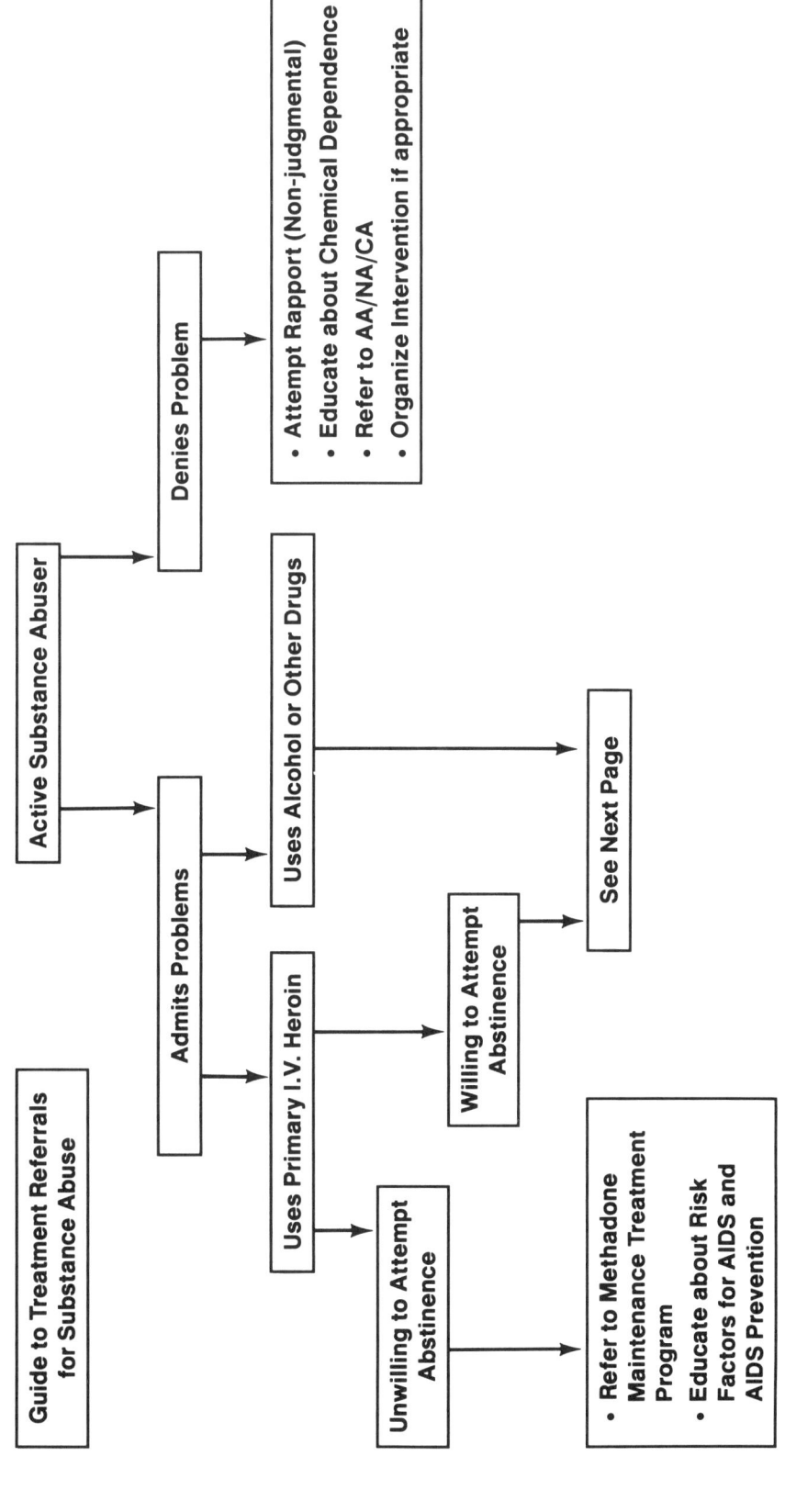

281

Module II.3—Overhead #6B

GUIDE TO TREATMENT REFERRALS FOR SUBSTANCE ABUSE

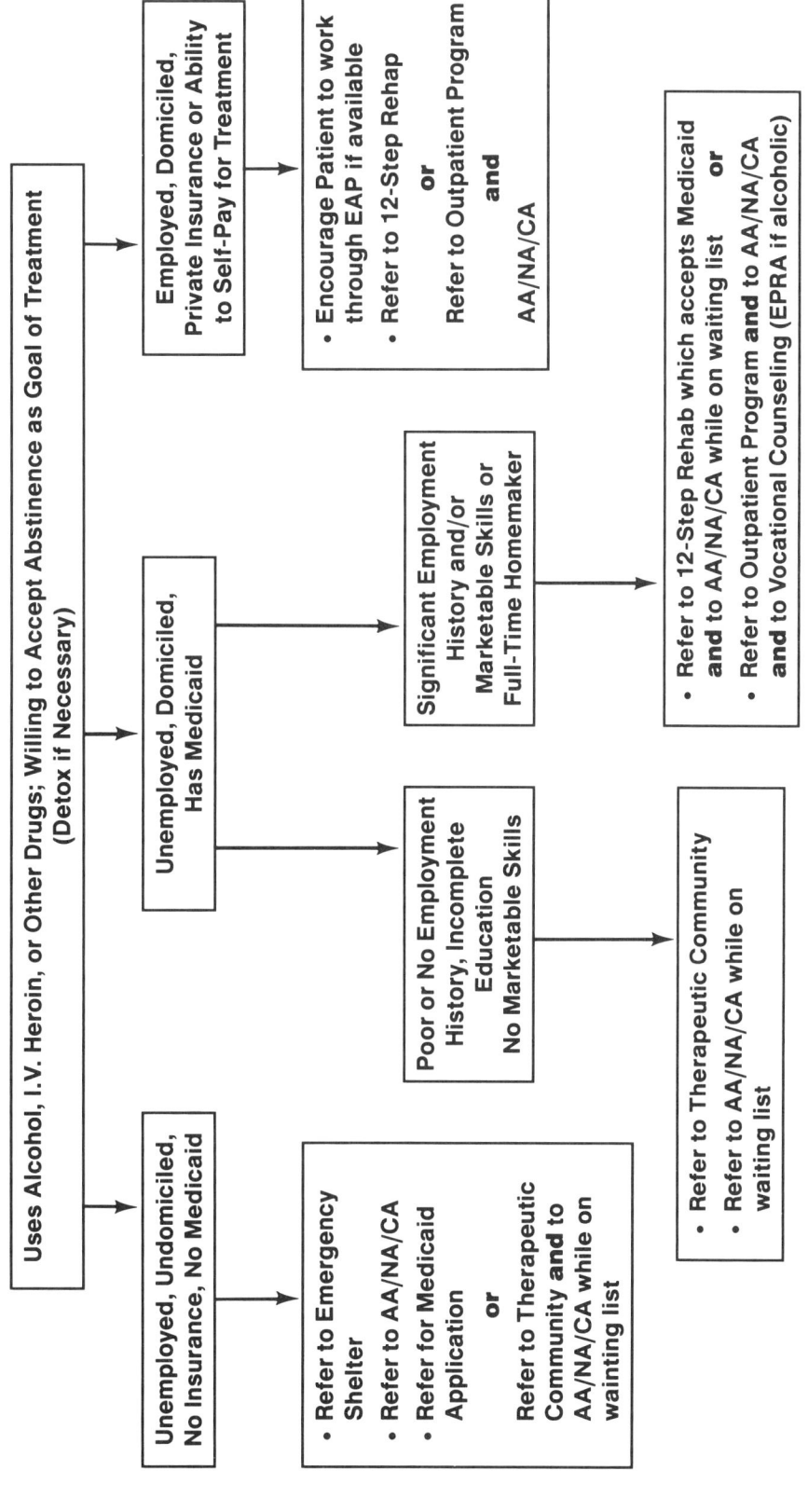

Instructor's Guide

Module II.3—Overhead #6C

GUIDE TO TREATMENT REFERRALS FOR SUBSTANCE ABUSE

Notes:

1. All known IVDUs should be referred for HIV counseling and testing as well as substance abuse treatment. Non-IV substance abusers should have HIV risk behaviors examined and referred for counseling and testing if appropriate.

2. Substance abusers with a significant psychiatric disorder (e.g., schizophrenia, uncontrolled bi-polar disorder) should have their psychiatric disorder stabilized as much as possible. Then they can be referred to a dual-diagnosis treatment center or to regular treatment if they are restored to an adequate functional level.

3. Virtually all abstinence based treatment programs (including therapeutic communities) strongly recommend continuing participation in self-help groups (AA/NA/CA) once the residential phase of treatment is completed.

4. Keep in mind that many substance abusers have recovered solely through participation in self-help groups.

Instructor's Guide

Module II.3—Overhead #6D

GUIDE TO TREATMENT REFERRALS FOR SUBSTANCE ABUSE

Glossary:

- **AA (Alcoholics Anonymous):** Self-help meetings based on a 12-step recovery program for alcoholics. AA has no dues or fees. The only requirement for membership is a desire to stop drinking. There are AA groups all over the nation (and the world) but the greater New York area has an especially high number of meetings. There are meetings in most neighborhoods and at virtually all times of day. Many (but not all) AA meetings in the New York area are tolerant of other drug problems in addition to alcohol.

- **NA (Narcotics Anonymous):** Self-help program styled after AA but for people with any drug problem (including alcohol).

- **CA (Cocaine Anonymous):** Self-help program styled after AA for people dependent on cocaine.

- **Therapeutic Community:** Approximately 18–24 month residential treatment programs which provide high school classes toward GED, vocational training, and highly structured socialization programs in addition to substance abuse treatment.

- **12-Steps Rehabs:** Approximately one month residential facilities, occasionally longer, based on the AA/NA programs which provide intensive rehabilitation for substance abuse but no high school or vocational training and usually minimal vocational counseling. They are ideal for those who are already employed or have a reasonable support system to return to after treatment.

Instructor's Guide

Module II.3—Overhead #6E

GUIDE TO TREATMENT REFERRALS FOR SUBSTANCE ABUSE

- **EAP (Employee Assistance Program):** Programs available through many employers which offer counseling and referral for a variety of personal problems including substance abuse. Since EAPs are familiar with employees' insurance coverage for various treatment programs, they often act as liaisons between employees and supervisors to protect the job while the employee receives treatment, and sometimes have special financial arrangements with particular treatment facilities.

- **MAP (Member Assistance Program):** Similar services to EAP but administered through the employee's labor union rather than through the employer.

- **EPRA (Employment Program for Recovering Alcoholics):** A free vocational rehabilitation program for recovering alcoholics which provides extensive vocational counseling and arranges employment "internships" in private industry which often result in job offers.

- **Intervention:** An organized attempt to engage an alcoholic or drug addict into treatment. Many treatment facilities have programs that will assist families in arranging an intervention. All those concerned with the substance abuser (family, friends, employers), and who are willing to participate, meet with a professional counselor who teaches them about the process. An appointment is then arranged with the substance abuser at which all concerned others are present in addition to the counselor. The substance abuser is then lovingly confronted with the consequences of the addiction on self and others and encouraged to enter a pre-arranged treatment program the same day. Usually "therapeutic leverage" (threatened loss of family support, job, marriage, etc.) is employed to move the substance abuser into treatment.

Module II.3—Overhead #7

THE 12 STEPS OF ALCOHOLICS ANONYMOUS

1. We admitted we were powerless over alcohol—that our lives had become unmanageable.

2. We came to believe that a Power greater than ourselves could restore us to sanity.

3. We made a decision to turn our will and our lives over to the care of God *as we understood Him.*

4. We made a searching and fearless moral inventory of ourselves.

5. We admitted to God, to ourselves, and to another human being the exact nature of our wrongs.

6. We were entirely ready to have God remove all these defects of character.

7. We humbly asked Him to remove our shortcomings.

8. We made a list of all persons we had harmed, and became willing to make amends to them all.

9. We made direct amends to such people wherever possible, except when to do so would injure them or others.

10. We continued to take personal inventory and when we were wrong promptly admitted it.

11. We sought through prayer and meditation to improve our conscious contact with God *as we understood Him,* praying only for knowledge of His will for us and the power to carry that out.

12. Having had a spiritual awakening as the result of these Steps, we tried to carry this message to others, and to practice these principles in all our affairs.

Instructor's Guide

Module II.3—Overhead #8

THE 12 TRADITIONS OF ALCOHOLICS ANONYMOUS

1. Our common welfare should come first; personal recovery depends upon AA unity.

2. For our group purpose there is but one ultimate authority—a loving God as He may express Himself in our group conscience. Our leaders are but trusted servants; they do not govern.

3. The only requirement for AA membership is a desire to stop drinking.

4. Each group should be autonomous except in matters affecting other groups or AA as a whole.

5. Each group has but one primary purpose—to carry its message to the alcoholic who still suffers.

6. An AA group ought never endorse, finance, or lend the AA name to any related facility or outside enterprise, lest problems of money, property, and prestige divert us from our primary purpose.

7. Every AA group ought to be full self-supporting, declining outside contributions.

8. Alcoholics Anonymous should remain forever nonprofessional, but our service centers may employ special workers.

9. AA, as such, ought never be organized; but we may create service boards or committees directly responsible to those they serve.

10. Alcoholics Anonymous has no opinion on outside issues; hence the AA name ought never be drawn into public controversy.

11. Our public relations policy is based on attraction rather than promotion; we need always maintain personal anonymity at the level of press, radio and films.

12. Anonymity is the spiritual foundation of all our Traditions, ever reminding us to place principles before personalities.

From: The Twelve Steps and Twelve Traditions. Reprinted with permission of Alcoholics World Services, Inc.

Module II.3—Overhead #9

SPECIAL STRATEGIES: RELAPSE

R   Relapse is a potential part of recovery.

E   Events can be a learning experience.

L   Look for positive gains antecedent to relapse.

A   Alternative/substitute actions to substance use, for example, going to 12-step meetings.

P   Practice alternative—12-step activity—"Give it back."

S   Situational factors are critical for triggering relapse. Look at situations (people, places, things).

E   Emotions/feelings greatly increase vulnerability in trigger situation—"Feelings are not facts."

Reach Out during Relapse.

Don't Reach In.

Instructor's Guide

Module II.3—Overhead #10

SPECIAL STRATEGIES: FAMILY

- F   Focus on member presenting problem.
- A   Assess education level, severity of denial.
- M   Model attitudes, effective communication.
- I   Isolation should be minimized.
- L   Look for strengths to reinforce, to create alternatives. Believe what you see.
- Y   Why? Discourage blaming among members.

Instructor's Guide

HANDOUT MASTERS

MODULE II.3 ADDICTIONS: NURSING DIAGNOSIS AND TREATMENT

1. Drug abuse terms: Glossary.
2. Denial
3. Common characteristics of dual-diagnosis clients.
4. Sogs, Score sheet.
5. Treatment of compulsive gambling.
6. Addictions nursing diagnoses.
7. NIDA Drug Abuse treatment and referral hotline.
8. Guideline for referrals.
9. Glossary of referral terms.
10. Self-help groups.
11. 12 steps.
12. 12 traditions.
13. Guideline admissions criteria for selected treatment services. Exemplar: State Medical Society of Wisconsin.
14. Nursing diagnosis: Fear—psychosocial.
15. Nursing diagnosis: Sexual dysfunction—biological.

Module II.3

Module II.3—Handout #1

DRUG ABUSE TERMS

This glossary contains street language regarding the drugs of abuse. The same term may have different meanings in different areas.

a-boot Under the influence of drugs.

Acapulco gold Mexican marijuana that contains about 1% or less of tetrahydrocannabinol (THC).

ace A marijuana cigarette.

acid LSD (Lysergic acid diethylamide).

acid head A user of LSD.

ad Refers to an addict.

all lit up Under the influence of a drug.

amys Amyl nitrite ampules.

angel dust Parsley leaves covered with phencyclidine, finely powdered hashish.

Are you anywhere? Do you use marijuana?

around the turn Having gone through withdrawal period.

artillery Equipment used for injecting and dissolving a powdered drug, or a solution of drugs.

baby Marijuana.

bad trip/bad acid An unpleasant reaction caused by a hallucinogenic drug, usually LSD; may be caused by taking a mixture of chemicals, resulting from an attempt at synthesis; emotions are dreadful and horrible; the images can be terrifying.

bag (1) A package of drugs, usually marijuana or heroin; (2) a person's favorite "thing" or drug.

bagman A person who supplies narcotics or other drugs; a pusher.

ball Absorption of stimulants and cocaine through the genitalia.

balloon A penny balloon that contains narcotics.

bambita Desoxyn or amphetamine derivative.

bammies A poor quality of marijuana.

bang The injection of narcotics, usually heroin.

banging Under the influence of drugs.

barb(s) Barbiturates.

barrels LSD tablets.

batted out Apprehended by law.

bean A capsule containing drugs.

beat the gong Smoke opium.

bedbugs Fellow addicts.

behind the iron house Staying in jail.

belongs On the habit.

belted Under the influence of a drug.

bending and bowing Under the influence of drugs.

bennies Benzedrine tablets (amphetamines).

Bernice Cocaine.

Bernie's flake Cocaine.

bhang Marijuana.

big bloke Cocaine.

big C Cocaine.

big D LSD.

big John Police, law.

big man A person who supplies drugs.

big O Opium.

bindle A package of narcotics (usually contains an ounce).

Module II.3—Handout #1 *(continued)*

bingle A supplier of drugs.

biz Utensils used in dissolving and injecting narcotics and other drugs.

black beauties Biphetamine capsules (amphetamines).

black magic LSD.

black stuff Opium.

blank Container of non-narcotic powder that is sold as heroin.

blast (1) Party; (2) a strong effect resulting from drug usage.

blasted Under the influence of a drug.

blow (1) To miss a vein when injecting; (2) to move from a place.

blow Charlie or snow Sniff cocaine.

blow horse Sniffing heroin.

blow (pot) Smoke a cigarette that contains marijuana.

blow your mind (1) To be high from a hallucinogenic drug; (2) to achieve a particular ecstatic mental level or high.

blue acid LSD.

blue angels, blue clouds, blue devils, blue heaven Amytal (amobarbital sodium) capsules.

blue cheer LSD, methamphetamine, and strychnine tablets.

blue heaven LSD.

blue morphine Numorphan tablets (no longer made).

blue velvet (1) A mixture of Terpin Hydrate and Codeine Elixir and Pyribenzamine (tripelennamine) (antihistamine); (2) a mixture of paregoric and antihistamine.

bluebirds Amytal (amobarbital sodium) capsules.

blues Amytal (amorbarbital sodium).

bo bo bush Marijuana.

bomb Heroin that is highly potent and relatively undiluted.

bombida Methamphetamine.

bombita An amphetamine injection, occasionally with heroin.

boost Robbery.

boxed Confined in jail.

boy Heroin.

brain Amphetamines.

bread Money.

broker A person who peddles dope to addicts.

brown dots LSD.

browns Multicolored capsules that are long-acting amphetamine sulfate.

bull (1) A federal narcotics agent; (2) a police officer.

bum trip A bad experience with psychedelics.

bummer Another word for a "bad trip."

burn transaction Selling a substance as a certain drug when actually it is something else; e.g., goldenrod for marijuana.

burned Getting cheated during a drug transaction.

bush Marijuana.

business Equipment used when injecting drugs.

businessman's trip Dimethyltryptamine (DMT).

busted Arrested for possession of drugs.

buttons Peyote buttons.

buy A purchase of drugs.

buzz Mild euphoric reaction to a drug.

C Cocaine.

C-joint A place where cocaine can be bought.

Module II.3

Module II.3—Handout #1 *(continued)*

cabbage head An individual who will use or experiment with any kind of drug.

caca (1) Heroin; (2) an inferior quality of hashish, heroin, or LSD; (3) imitation or counterfeit heroin.

cadet A new addict.

California sunshine LSD.

can A container that holds marijuana.

candy Barbiturates.

candy man A pusher.

cannabis Marijuana.

cap A gelatinous capsule that contains heroin or other drugs (usually 1 ounce or less).

Carrie Cocaine.

cartwheels Amphetamine tablets.

cashing a script Obtaining drugs by getting an illegal prescription filled.

catch up A process of withdrawal.

caught in a snow storm Being drugged by cocaine.

CB Doriden (glutethimide) tablet.

Cecil Cocaine.

charge A quick drug effect.

charged up Under the influence of drugs.

chicken powder Some amphetamine powder.

chief LSD.

chip Use small injections occasionally.

chipping Irregular use of small amounts of drugs.

chocolate chips LSD.

Cholley Cocaine.

Christmas trees Tuinal (secobarbital sodium and amobarbital sodium) or Eskatrol (dextroamphetamine sulfate and prochlorperazine).

Cibas Doriden (glutethimide).

Cibees Doriden (glutethimide).

clean Not using drugs any longer.

cleared up A withdrawal method.

clipped Getting arrested.

coasting Under the influence of drugs.

coast-to-coast Long-acting amphetamines.

coffee habit A beginner in the use of narcotics.

coke Cocaine.

cokie Cocaine addict.

cold turkey Sudden withdrawal from narcotics.

coming down Recovering from a drug experience or trip.

connect To make a purchase of drugs.

connection A drug supplier.

content lens LSD found on round gelatin flakes.

cooker Bottle cap or spoon needed for heating and dissolving heroin in preparation for injection.

cop To obtain drugs.

cop a deuceway To buy a $2 pack of narcotics.

cop man A supplier.

cop out (1) Running away; (2) to leave; (3) to inform; (4) not participating; (5) to defect.

cop-a-sneak To leave a place.

copilots Amphetamine tablets.

Corrine Cocaine.

cotton shot When water is added to cotton to attempt to get remaining heroin out.

crank Methamphetamine crystals.

crashing Withdrawing from drug experience.

Module II.3—Handout #1 *(continued)*

crashing pad Place where a user recovers from amphetamine use.

crinic, cris, Cristina Methamphetamine.

croaker A physician.

croaker joint A hospital.

crossroads Amphetamines tablets.

crusher A police officer.

crutch A device for holding a marijuana cigarette butt.

crystal Methamphetamine (Methedrine), cocaine.

crystal palace A room, location, or house where methamphetamine is injected.

cube juice Morphine.

cubehead A person who uses LSD frequently.

cupcakes LSD.

cut (1) To dilute a powder drug, usually a narcotic; (2) to dilute the potency of marijuana.

cut out To leave a certain place.

D Doriden (glutethimide) tablet.

dabble To use small amounts of drugs infrequently.

dead on arrival Phencyclidine base.

dealer (1) A person who supplies drugs; (2) a pusher.

deck A package of narcotics (usually an ounce).

dexies Dexedrine (dextroamphetamine sulfate) tablets or capsules (amphetamines).

diet pills Include amphetamine tablets or capsules.

dime bag $10 purchase, usually marijuana.

dirty Have drugs on you; can be arrested if searched.

do a bit To spend time in jail.

do righters Non-addicts.

DOA Phencyclidine base.

doin' Using some kind of drug, such as "He is doin' cocaine."

dollies Dolophine (methadone) tablets.

DOM STP (2,5-dimethoxy-4-methylamphetamine).

domes LSD tablets.

domino To complete a purchase of drugs.

doojee Heroin.

dope Includes any narcotics, sometimes extended to other drugs.

dope fiend A heroin addict.

doper Someone who uses drugs regularly.

double trouble Tuinal (secobarbital sodium and amobarbital sodium) capsule.

down, downer, downie (1) Barbiturates; (2) tranquilizers.

down it To swallow a pill or capsule.

dream Cocaine.

dried up Off drugs, especially heroin.

dripper Eyedropper.

drop To take a capsule or tablet orally.

drop acid To take LSD.

drop out To leave a place.

dujie Heroin.

dummy (1) A purchase in which there are no narcotics; (2) a poor quality of merchandise.

dust Heroin, cocaine.

dust of angels Phencyclidine base.

dynamite (1) A high quality of heroin and cocaine taken together; (2) a strong drug.

eighth Heroin ($1/8$ ounce) that is diluted with some inert powder.

emsel Morphine.

Module II.3—Handout #1 (continued)

eye openers Amphetamines.
factory The equipment used when injecting drugs.
fall To be arrested.
fall out When an addict nods or falls asleep on and off after injecting.
far out (1) Out of touch with reality; (2) under the influence of drugs.
Feds Federal agents.
fine stuff Marijuana that is finely cut or manicured.
fix An injection of a drug.
fixed Under the influence of a drug.
flake Cocaine.
flash A euphoric feeling following an injection.
flashback When a previous drug user hallucinates without taking the drug again.
flats LSD tablets.
flea powder Poor-quality heroin or heroin that is greatly diluted.
flip Become psychotic.
floating Under the influence of drugs.
flying high Under the influence of marijuana.
fold up A withdrawal procedure.
folding stuff Money.
foolish powder Heroin.
footballs Amphetamine tablets or capsules that are oval-shaped.
freak A regular user of a particular drug; e.g., acid freak.
freakout An experience that is unpleasant and frightful, resulting from the use of a drug.
freeze When a sale is turned down.
fresh and sweet A person coming out of jail.

front of the bread The money is put up first for a drug purchase.
fu Marijuana.
Fuzz (1) A policeman; (2) a detective.
Fuzzy tail Police.
gage Marijuana.
garbage A poor-quality drug.
gazer A federal agent.
GBs Seconal (secobarbital), Tuinal (secobarbital and amobarbital), or Doriden (glutethimide).
gear Refers to drugs in general.
gee head A person who uses paregoric.
geetis Money.
geezer A needle shot of any type of narcotic.
get beat To buy a package that does not contain any heroin.
get a gift To obtain some narcotics.
get high To smoke a cigarette containing marijuana.
get off To inject or use drugs.
get the wind To leave a place or area.
gimmicks Equipment with which a person injects drugs.
girl Cocaine.
give wings Give the first heroin injection to a friend.
glad rag A handkerchief or cloth saturated with substances to be inhaled.
glass eyes A narcotic addict.
glued Arrested.
gluey An individual who sniffs glue vapors.
G-man A federal agent.
go in sewer Inject a drug into a vein.
gold A Mexican marijuana that has 1% or less of tetrahydrocannabinol (THC).

Module II.3—Handout #1 *(continued)*

gold dust Cocaine.

good go Purchase a fair amount of narcotics for the money.

good trip Psychedelic drugs that cause good emotional feelings and pleasant imagery.

goods (1) Narcotics; (2) includes any drugs.

goofball Barbiturate.

gorilla pills Doriden (glutethimide).

gow head Addict.

gram The cube form of hashish.

grape parfait LSD.

grass Marijuana.

green domes LSD tablets.

greenies The mixture of barbiturates and amphetamines found in a green heart-shaped tablet.

griefo Marijuana.

gun (1) Eyedropper; (2) syringe; (3) hypodermic needle.

H Heroin.

hack Physician.

hairy Heroin.

half spoon Half a teaspoon of heroin.

hand-to-hand Paying for drugs when they are delivered.

hang-up (1) A personal problem or personality problem; (2) a withdrawal.

happy dust Cocaine.

hard narcotics Includes all addicting narcotics.

hard stuff Includes all addicting narcotics; e.g., heroin, morphine.

harness bull Police.

Harry Heroin.

hash Hashish.

hassle The procedure of buying drugs, preparing them, and taking the injection.

Hawaiian sunshine LSD.

hay Marijuana.

head A person who depends on drugs.

hearts Amphetamine tablets that are heart-shaped.

heat The police.

heaven dust Cocaine.

heavenly blue Morning glory seeds.

heavy man Someone who possesses narcotics.

hemp Marijuana.

high Under the influence of drugs.

hit To make a purchase of drugs.

hitting the pipe, hitting the steam Smoking opium.

hitting the stuff Under the influence of drugs.

hitting up The act of injecting drugs.

hocus Morphine.

hog Vegetable material that has phencyclidine in it.

holding To have drugs in one's possession.

hooked Dependent on drugs.

hop Opium.

hop head A narcotic addict, mainly an opium addict.

hoppie A narcotic addict.

horner One who sniffs narcotics.

horse Heroin.

hot (1) Sought by police; (2) stolen articles, merchandise.

hotshot A fatal injection of heroin, that may have been intentional.

hot sticks Marijuana cigarettes.

hustle (1) Prostitution; (2) any activity used to obtain money for heroin.

hustler Prostitute.

hype Addict.

Module II.3—Handout #1 (continued)

ice-cream habit   Non-regular drug user.
iced   In jail.
I'm beat   I need a marijuana cigarette.
I'm holding   I am carrying drugs.
I'm way down   I need a marijuana lift.
in high   Under the influence of drugs.
in a jam   Wanted by the police.
Indian bay, Indian hay   Marijuana.
into   Involved with a drug; e.g., "She is into acid."
jab   (1) To inject a drug; (2) a hypodermic shot.
jag   (1) Under the influence of drugs; (2) under the influence of amphetamines.
jay   Marijuana cigarette.
jelly beans   Tuinal (secobarbital sodium and amobarbital sodium).
jive   Marijuana.
jive sticks, joints   Marijuana cigarettes.
jolly beans   Pep pills.
Jones   A habit.
joy popping   (1) Subcutaneously injecting a drug; (2) irregular drug habit.
joy powder   Cocaine.
jump skid   To leave a place.
junk   (1) Heroin; (2) can denote any drug.
junker, junkie   Addict (heroin).
kee   A kilogram of a drug, usually heroin.
keif   Hashish.
kick   To get rid of a habit.
kick the habit   To stop using narcotics or drugs in general.
kick sticks   Marijuana cigarettes.
kicking   A withdrawal process.
kicking the gong   To be around an area where narcotics are sold.
kilo   A kilogram of drugs equivalent to 2.2 pounds.

kit   Equipment used when injecting drugs.
knocking on the door   When an addict is trying to stay away from other addicts while attempting to quit a habit.
LA turnouts   Various-colored capsules that are long-acting amphetamine sulfate.
lay out   (1) Equipment for injecting drugs; (2) opium smoker's outfit.
laying on the hip   Smoking opium.
laying the hypo   Receiving or taking a shot of narcotics.
LBJ-336-JB-336   Methyl piperidyl benzilate (hallucinogen).
leader   User of cocaine.
leaping   Under the influence of drugs.
lemonade   Poor-quality heroin or any merchandise.
lettuce   Money.
lid   A measure of marijuana in a sale.
lid poppers   Amphetamines.
lid proppers   Amphetamines.
lie down   To smoke opium.
light artillery   A hypodermic addict.
Lipton tea   Poor-quality merchandise.
lit up   Under the influence of drugs.
load   A quantity of 25 bags of heroin.
loco weed   Marijuana.
log   Marijuana cigarette.
long green   Money.
love drug   (1) MDA (methylene dioxyamphetamine); (2) methaqualone (soapers).
love weed   Marijuana.
LSD   Lysergic acid diethylamide.
m   Morphine.
machinery   Utensils used when injecting drugs.

Module II.3—Handout #1 *(continued)*

magic mushroom A mushroom containing psilocybin.

magic pumpkin seed An STP (2,5-dimethoxy-4-methylamphetamine) tablet shaped like a pumpkin seed.

mainlining Shooting or injecting a drug directly into a vein.

maintaining Keeping a particular level of a drug effect.

make a croaker To trick a physician into giving narcotics.

make a meet To make a buy.

make a reader To get a physician to fill out a prescription.

make the turn A withdrawal process.

man (1) Policeman; (2) detective.

manicure Removal of seeds, dirt, and stems from dried marijuana.

Mary Jane, Mary Warner Marijuana.

merchandise Narcotics or any drug in general.

mese Mescaline (hallucinogenic drug from the peyote cactus).

meth (1) Methamphetamine; (2) methadone; (3) methedrine; (4) methaqualone.

meth head A regular user of methamphetamine.

meth run Constant intravenous injection of methamphetamine.

Mexican horse Mexican (brown) heroin.

Mexican reds Secobarbital capsules.

mezz Marijuana.

Mickey Chloral hydrate.

Mickey Finn The mixture of chloral hydrate plus alcohol.

micro dots LSD.

mikes Micrograms (millionths of a gram).

mind benders, mind blowers Hallucinogens.

Miss Emma Morphine.

MJ Marijuana.

monkey A drug habit in which there is a physical dependence.

monster Methamphetamine.

mootos Marijuana cigarettes.

mor-a-grifa Marijuana.

morph, morphie, morpho Morphine.

mouth worker A narcotic addict who swallows his drugs.

Mr. Whiskers Federal agents

mud Asthmador mixed with a carbonated cola beverage.

muggles Marijuana cigarettes.

mule A supplier of drugs.

mutah Marijuana.

nail Needle.

nailed Arrested.

narc, narco Federal, state, or local narcotic officer.

needle The syringe for injecting drugs.

needle freak A person who enjoys using a needle.

nibies Nembutal (pentobarbital sodium).

nickels bag (1) A $5 purchase of marijuana; (2) a measure of heroin.

nimby Nembutal (pentobarbital sodium).

noise Heroin.

nose candy Cocaine.

OD An overdose of drugs or narcotics, resulting in death or a coma.

OJ Opium joint, a marijuana cigarette that has been dipped or smeared in opium.

on ice In jail.

on the beam Feeling good.

on the blues Using Numorphan (oxymorphone hydrochloride).

Module II.3—Handout #1 (continued)

on the bricks, on the ground Out of jail.

on the nod The cycle of dozing and awaking when using heroin.

oranges wedges LSD.

oranges Heart-shaped amphetamine tablets containing Dexedrine (dextroamphetamine sulfate).

out of it Non-addict.

outfit Equipment used when injecting drugs.

over the lump The completion of withdrawal.

Owsley's acid LSD.

pad A person's habitat or room.

Pam freak Person who inhales aerosolized products.

Panatella A large, strong marijuana cigarette.

panic man Addict who has lost his source of drugs.

paper (1) A package of drugs (usually a quantity of 1 ounce); (2) prescription.

PCP Phencyclidine.

PCPA *p*-Chlorophenylalnine.

peace (1) LSD tablets; (2) STP (2,5-dimethoxy-4-methylamphetamine).

peace pill Phencyclidine.

peace tablet LSD tablets.

peaches Benzedrine (amphetamine sulfate) tablets.

peanuts Barbiturates.

pearly gates Morning glory seeds.

peddler Dealer in drugs.

pee Heroin powder.

pep pills Amphetamine capsules or tablets.

Pepsi Cola habit A small habit.

Peter Chloral hydrate.

pickup To buy drugs.

piece (1) A measure of narcotics; (2) a holder of drugs.

pig Policeman.

piki A person who smokes opium.

pillhead A person who often uses drugs, usually amphetamines and barbiturates.

pillows Sealed polyethylene bags that contain drugs.

pin yen Opium.

pinks Seconal (secobarbital sodium) capsules.

pipe (1) To look; (2) an opium utensil.

plant A place to hide drugs.

play around Irregular use of drugs.

pod Marijuana.

pop To inject drugs, usually below the skin.

poppers Amyl nitrite ampules.

pot Marijuana or hashish.

pothead Marijuana user.

product IV Combination capsules of PCP and LSD.

purple barrels, purple haze, purple ozone LSD.

purple rock A mixture of caffeine, barbiturates, heroin, and strychnine.

push shorts (1) To cheat a buyer of drugs; (2) to sell short amounts of drugs.

pusher A person who peddles drugs, narcotics, marijuana.

R and R, ripple and reds Taking secobarbital capsules when drinking Ripple wine.

rainbows Tuinal (secobarbital sodium and amobarbital sodium) capsules.

red birds, red devils, red lilies, reds Secobarbital capsules.

red rock Mixture of heroin and strychnine, barbiturates, and caffeine.

Module II.3—Handout #1 *(continued)*

reefer Marijuana cigarette.
riding the wave Under the influence of narcotics.
roach A marijuana cigarette butt.
roach clip A device that holds a marijuana cigarette butt.
robe Robitussin A-C cough syrup (guaifenesin and codeine phosphate).
robo, romo Codeine.
rope Marijuana.
roses Benzedrine (amphetamine sulfate) tablets.
run Continuing the injection of methamphetamine.
Sam Federal agent.
satch cotton Cotton used to strain drugs before injection.
sativa Marijuana.
scag Heroin.
scene Place where a person can buy drugs.
schmack (1) Heroin; (2) cocaine.
schoolboy Codeine.
score To purchase drugs.
scrap iron A bootleg drink made with a hypochlorite solution, alcohol, and mothballs.
scratch Prescription.
script Physician's prescription.
script writer A person who forges prescriptions.
seccy, seggy Seconal (secobarbital sodium) capsules.
seeds Morning glory seeds.
serenity, tranquility, and pace STP (2,5-dimethoxy-4-methylamphetamine).
sex juice An aphrodisiac.
sharps Needles.
shit (1) Heroin; (2) poor-quality heroin, hashish, or LSD; (3) drugs.

shoot up To inject drugs.
shooting The injection of drugs.
shooting gallery Location, room, or house where drugs are injected.
short go To take a small portion of narcotics.
shot down Under the influence of drugs.
shrink Psychiatrist.
sizzling Sought by police.
skee Opium.
skid (1) Heroin; (2) to leave a place.
skin popping The injecting of a narcotic underneath the skin.
slammed In jail.
sleepers, sleeping pills Barbiturates.
sleigh ride Under the influence of drugs.
smack (1) Heroin; (2) cocaine.
smash Marijuana that has been cooked with acetone, the oil residue of which is added to hashish.
smears LSD.
smoke (1) Wood alcohol; (2) marijuana.
snappers Amyl nitrite ampules.
sniffer A narcotic addict who takes drugs through his nose.
sniffing Inhaling solvents, cleaning fluid, etc.
snort The inhalation of cocaine or heroin through the nose.
snorter A person who sniffs drugs through his nose.
snow Cocaine crystals.
snowbird Cocaine addict.
soapers Methaqualone (sleeping pill).
sound Benactyzine.
spaghetti sauce Robitussin A-C cough syrup (guaifenesin and codeine phosphate).

Module II.3—Handout #1 *(continued)*

speed Amphetamines, usually methedrine.

speed demon Methamphetamine user.

speed freak Frequent methamphetamine user.

speedball A mixture of heroin and cocaine that is taken intravenously.

spike Hyperdermic needle.

splash Amphetamine powder.

splim Marijuana.

split To leave a place.

splivins Amphetamine powder.

spoon (1) A measure of heroin; (2) the spoon used for dissolving heroin over heat.

spots Dextroamphetamine.

square An individual who does not use drugs.

squirrels LSD.

star dust Cocaine.

stash A safe place to keep drugs.

station worker A user of narcotics who injects into his arms or legs.

stick Marijuana.

stinking Under the influence of drugs.

stoned (1) Under the influence of drugs; (2) a relaxed, pleasant state of mind.

stoolie Informer.

stoppers Barbiturates.

straight (1) Not using any drugs; (2) not having any drugs in one's possession.

strawberry field LSD.

street market Black market.

strung out An amphetamine overdose.

stuff Narcotics.

stumblers (1) Barbiturates; (2) tranquilizers.

sunshine LSD.

superman pills Amphetamines.

sweet Lucy Marijuana.

swing man A supplier of drugs.

syrup Codeine.

TMA A combination of mescaline, LSD, and tetrahydrocannabinol.

T-man A federal agent.

take a powder, take the wind To leave a certain area.

taking a main Injecting directly into a vein.

tar Opium.

taste A small amount of narcotics.

tea Marijuana.

tea pad The place where a group of people smoke marijuana.

tea party A party where mostly everyone is smoking marijuana.

teed up Intoxicated by a large quantity of drugs.

Texas tea Marijuana.

the bag The bag used to sniff airplane glue or cleaning fluid.

the confidence drug Amphetamine.

the one A material like hashish, supposedly natural tetrahydrocannabinol.

thing A person's particular interest, often refers to a specific drug.

three-day-habit The irregular use of drugs.

TNT Heroin.

to be off A process of withdrawal.

toak (toke) A drag off a marijuana cigarette.

toke pipe A short-stem pipe used for smoking marijuana.

tooies Tuinal (secobarbital sodium and amobarbital sodium) capsules.

Module II.3—Handout #1 *(continued)*

tools Equipment used when injecting drugs.

toy A small container of drugs.

tracks Needle scars that result from frequent injecting of drugs.

tranquility STP (2,5-dimethoxy-4-methylamphetamine).

travel agent LSD pusher.

trey A purchase worth $3.

trip A hallucinogenic drug experience.

tripping out Under the influence of any hallucinogen.

truck drivers Amphetamine tablets.

tuies Tuinal (secobarbital sodium and amobarbital sodium).

turkey The absence of drugs or narcotics.

turkey trots Scars and marks left from the use of a hypodermic needle.

turn off To quit using drugs.

turn on (1) To introduce a person to the use of drugs; (2) any stimulating experience caused by the use of drugs.

turn up To feel the influence of a drug.

turned on Under the influence of drugs.

turps Terpins Hydrate and Codeine Elixir (a cough syrup).

twenty-five LSD.

twist A marijuana cigarette.

twisted Intense sedation caused by the use of drugs.

uncle, Uncle Sam Federal narcotics agent.

unkie Morphine.

upper, ups Amphetamine tablets.

viper's weed Marijuana.

wake ups, washed ups Amphetamines.

washed up A withdrawal process.

wasted Under the influence of drugs.

wedges (1) Dexedrine (dextroamphetamine sulfate) tablets; (2) LSD tablets.

weed Marijuana.

weekend habit The irregular use of drugs.

wen shee Gum opium.

whickers Federal agents.

white junk Heroin.

white lightning LSD.

white merchandise, white snuff Morphine.

whites Amphetamines.

whiz bang A combination of morphine and cocaine, or heroin and cocaine, used by the old addicts.

window glass A square gelatin flake that contains LSD.

work the leather To leave an area.

works Equipment used when injecting drugs.

yellow birds Nembutal (pentobarbital sodium).

yello dimples LSD.

yellow jackets, yellow submarines, yellows Nembutal (pentobarbital sodium) capsules.

yen hook The utensil used when smoking opium.

yen shee The ashes from opium.

yen sleep A period of restlessness and drowsiness during a withdrawal process.

Module II.3

Module II.3—Handout #2

DENIAL

Nurse-client interactions which enable denial.

   a. Inefficient assessment techniques.

   b. Communication of biased attitude.

   c. Ignorance.

   d. Lack of referral, follow-up.

   e. Failure to explore motivational state.

Techniques of diminishing denial.

   a. Awareness of phenomenon of denial.

   b. Providing key alternative—in order to stop denying, clients need tools to deal with reality.

   c. Increase client awareness of present behavior and its effect on self and others.

   d. Education on the disease process or the health implication of alcohol and other substance abuse.

   e. Pointing out negative consequences.

   f. Working with families and significant others.

Instructor's Guide

Module II.3—Handout #3

COMMON CHARACTERISTICS OF DUAL-DIAGNOSIS CLIENTS

In addition to the individual's substance use and psychiatric issues.

1. High anxiety.
2. Dysphoria.
3. Alexithymia.
4. Low self-esteem/negative self-concept.
5. Unresolved grief/loss issues.
6. Poor physical health.
7. Loneliness/isolation.
8. Immaturity (developmental).
9. Ambivalence.
10. Primitive defense mechanisms.
11. Boundary problems.
12. Identity confusion.
13. Poor communication skills.
14. Social impairment.
15. History of abuse/neglect/trauma.
16. Familial alcoholism/drug use.

These characteristics tend to appear in all diagnostic categories but, of course, not in all clients.

Module II.3

Module II.3—Handout #4

SOUTH OAKS GAMBLING SCREEN (SOGS)

Name: _____

Date: _____

1. Please indicate which of the following types of gambling you have done in your lifetime. For each type, mark one answer: "not at all," "less than once a year," or "once a week or more."

	Not At All	Less Than Once A Week	Once A Week Or More	
a.	___	___	___	Played cards for money.
b.	___	___	___	Bet on horses, dogs or other animals (at OTB, the track or with a bookie).
c.	___	___	___	Bet on sports (parlay cards, with bookie or at Jai Alai).
d.	___	___	___	Played dice games (including craps, over and under or other dice games) for money.
e.	___	___	___	Went to casino (legal or otherwise).
f.	___	___	___	Played the numbers or bet on lotteries.
g.	___	___	___	Played bingo.
h.	___	___	___	Played the stock and/or commodities market.
i.	___	___	___	Played slot machines, poker machines or other gambling machines.
j.	___	___	___	Bowled, shot pool, played golf or some other game of skill for money.

2. What is the largest amount of money you have ever gambled with on any one day?

   ___ never have gambled   ___ more than $100 up to $1000

   ___ $1 or less   ___ more than $1000 up to $10,000

   ___ more than $1 up to $10   ___ more than $10,000.

   ___ more than $10 up to $100

Instructor's Guide

Module II.3—Handout #4 *(continued)*

3. Do (did) your parents have a gambling problem?

   _____ Both my father and mother gamble(d) too much.

   _____ My father gambles (or gambled) too much.

   _____ My mother gambles (gambled) too much.

   _____ Neither one gambles too much.

4. When you gamble, how often do you go back another day to win back money you lost?

   _____ Never.

   _____ Some of the time (less than half the time I lose).

   _____ Most of the time I lose.

   _____ Every time I lose.

5. Have you ever claimed to be winning money gambling but weren't really? In fact, you lost?

   _____ Never (or never gamble).

   _____ Yes, less than half the time I lost.

   _____ Yes, most of the time.

6. Do you feel you have ever had a problem with gambling?

   _____ No.

   _____ Yes, in the past but not now.

   _____ Yes.

Check "yes" or "no" for each:

		Yes	No
7.	Did you ever gamble more than you intended to?	( )	( )
8.	Have people criticized your gambling?	( )	( )
9.	Have you ever felt guilty about the way you gamble or what happens when you gamble?	( )	( )
10.	Have you ever felt like you would like to stop gambling but didn't think you could?	( )	( )
11.	Have you ever hidden betting slips, lottery tickets, gambling money, or other signs of gambling from your spouse, children, or other important people in your life?	( )	( )
12.	Have you ever argued with people you live with over how you handle money?	( )	( )
13.	(If you answered yes to question 12): Have money arguments ever centered on your gambling?	( )	( )

Module II.3

Module II.3—Handout #4 *(continued)*

		Yes	No
14.	Have you ever borrowed from someone and not paid them back as a result of your gambling?	( )	( )
15.	Have you ever lost time from work (or school) due to gambling?	( )	( )
16.	If you borrowed money to gamble or to pay gambling debts, who or where did you borrow from? (check "yes" or "no" for each)	( )	( )
	a. From household money.	( )	( )
	b. From your spouse.	( )	( )
	c. From other relatives or in-laws.	( )	( )
	d. From banks, loan companies or credit unions.	( )	( )
	e. From credit cards.	( )	( )
	f. From loan sharks ("Shylocks").	( )	( )
	g. You cashed in stocks, bonds or other securities.	( )	( )
	h. You sold personal or family property.	( )	( )
	i. You borrowed on your checking account (passed bad checks).	( )	( )
	j. You have (had) a credit line with a bookie.	( )	( )
	k. You have (had) a credit line with a casino.	( )	( )

Instructor's Guide

Module II.3—Handout #4 *(continued)*

SOUTH OAKS GAMBLING SCREEN SCORE SHEET

Scores on the SOGS are determined by adding up the number of questions which show an "at risk" response:

Questions 1, 2, & 3 not counted.

_____ Question 4:   Most of the time I lose.
         or   Every time I lose.

_____ Question 5:   Yes, less than half the time I lose.
         or   Yes, most of the time.

_____ Question 6:   Yes, in the past but not now.
         or   Yes.

_____ Question 7:   Yes.

_____ Question 8:   Yes.

_____ Question 9:   Yes.

_____ Question 10: Yes.

_____ Question 11: Yes.

_____ Question 12: Not counted.

_____ Question 13: Yes.

_____ Question 14: Yes.

_____ Question 15: Yes.

_____ Question 16a: Yes.

_____ Question   b: Yes.

_____ Question   c: Yes.

_____ Question   d: Yes.

_____ Question   e: Yes.

_____ Question   f: Yes.

_____ Question   g: Yes.

_____ Question   h: Yes.

_____ Question   i: Yes.

(Questions 16 j & k not included here.)

Total = _____ (There are 20 questions which are counted.)

0 = no problem   1–4 = some problem

5 or more = probable pathological gambler

Module II.—Handout #5

TREATMENT OF COMPULSIVE GAMBLING

Phase	Goals	Methods
Intervention	Initial problem definition. Establishment of initial motivation. Completed referral to assessment and treatment.	Breaking through denial and rationalization via sympathetic, nonjudgmental confrontation (individual, group, or family setting).
Assessment	Formal Diagnosis. Identification of patient and family problems. Initiation of treatment.	Personal and family history. Examination of current health, family, legal, social, and financial status.
Initial Treatment	Establishment of abstinence. Development of continuing motivation. Education about compulsive gambling and other addictions. Learning to handle stress without gambling. Attention to urgent problems.	Self-help groups. Psychotherapy. Counseling: individual, spiritual, group, legal, marital, financial, family. Psychodrama. Physical healthcare. Vocational rehabilitation.
Continuing Care	Prevention of relapse. Continued development of healthy patterns of handling emotions and life problems.	All methods mentioned for initial treatment.
Long Term Follow up	Prevention of relapse. Reinforcement of healthy living patterns.	Self-help. Psychotherapy and counseling as needed.

From: Blume, S. B. (1988). Current trends explored in compulsive gambling. *The Psychiatric Times* (December 1988), p. 29.

Instructor's Guide

Module II.3—Handout #6

NANDA DIAGNOSES COMMON TO ADDICTIONS NURSING

Nursing Diagnosis

- Sensory-perceptual alterations.
- Potential for injury.
- Self-care deficit.
- Potential for infection.
- Sleep pattern disturbance.
- Alteration in nutrition: Less than body requirements.
- Alteration in comfort: Pain.
- Altered growth and development: Biological.
- Knowledge deficit.
- Verbalization of knowledge deficit.
- Alteration in thought process.
- Non-compliance.
- Impaired communication.

Examples of Defining Characteristics

- Fluctuation in mental status, confusion, disorientation.
- Blackouts, hallucinations.
- Ataxia; history of flashbacks; history of seizures.
- Intolerance to activity; diminished self-esteem; discomfort.
- Homeless lifestyle; practice of unsafe sex; severe withdrawal syndrome.
- Sleep pattern reversal; mild, fleeting nystagmus.
- Report of inadequate dietary intake; change in appetite; dental caries.
- Distracted behavior, moaning, crying, pacing.
- Guarding behavior, positioning; alter muscle tone.
- Infants of alcoholic mothers; newborn exhibiting drug-induced sedation; retardation of brain growth.
- Use of denial in acknowledging addictions process.
- Inaccurate perception of health status.
- Mood swings, restlessness; impairment of recent memory; lack of insight.
- Continuing pattern of addiction; verbalization of non-compliance; inability to set goals.
- Inability to express feelings; slurring of speech; inappropriate speech patterns.

Module II.3—Handout #6 *(continued)*

- Ineffective individual coping.
- Alterations in self-concept.
- Anxiety (specific level of anxiety).
- Behavioral characteristics; restlessness.
- Dysfunctional family process.
- Altered parenting.
- Altered growth and development: Psychosocial.
- Potential for violence.
- Spiritual distress.
- Ineffective coping with feelings of defeat; replacing one addiction with another; ineffective choices and actions.
- Body image disturbance; self-esteem: social withdrawal; role performance: role conflict.
- Subjective feelings of discomfort.
- Affective characteristics; alarmed; cognitive characteristics.
- Social isolation; forgetfulness; seeking isolation from others; expressing feelings of loneliness; non-verbal behaviors.
- Disturbed social communication; dependency; loss of family support system.
- Continued substance abuse while breast-feeding; verbalization of role frustration; lack of parental attachment behavior.
- Lack of trust in adults; fear of losing control.
- Harsh self-criticism.
- Threats of anger, or rage; aggressive behavior; rigid body language.
- Distress in human spirit secondary to addiction; i.e., guilt, shame, grief.

Instructor's Guide

Module II.3—Handout #7

NIDA DRUG ABUSE TREATMENT AND REFERRAL HOTLINE

800-662-HELP

- Hours: Eastern Time
  M–F 9am–3pm
  S,S 12n–3am

- An entry-level hotline.

- Administered by National Institute of Drug Abuse (NIDA).

- Government funded; part of U.S. Public Health Service.

- Hotline answered by an information specialist prepared to ask questions and give the caller further directions; health professionals, addicts, family members, and the general public will be guided to the appropriate resources.

- Information is given about local treatment programs, support groups, and other hotlines.

- Main resource for the hotline is the National Directory of Drug Abuse and Alcoholism Treatment and Prevention Programs. This document, updated periodically, is available at public libraries. It can be ordered from the Government Printing Office, Stock # 017-024-01252-1 ADM-85-321, Superintendent of Documents, North Capitol Street, Washington, DC 20402.

Module II.3—Handout #8

GUIDELINES FOR REFERRALS

Guiding Principle: Simple ⟶ Complex

1. The severity of the alcohol and other drugs problem, the readiness of the client, and the type of setting and services needed will help determine whether the client receives treatment in the original setting or is referred for treatment.

2. Even when treatment services are available in the primary care setting, there may be a need to refer for specialized treatment services. Indicators include no change in physical, psychological, or behavioral symptoms after 90 days; case is too complex and time consuming; behavior is too disruptive for an ordinary clinical setting; and suicidal tendencies.

3. Objectives of all parties in the referral process.

    a. Continuity of care.

    b. Definition of goals.

    c. Clear communication.

    d. Understanding of responsibilities.

    e. Sensitivity to the effects of the referral on the client.

4. Referral Resources.

    a. Most practice settings will have a protocol for the general nurse to make a referral.

    b. If not, selecting a referral resource can be difficult, especially if the clinician is unfamiliar with local resources, if the community is so small that it has very limited resources, or if it is so large that it has a confusing array of resources of unknown quality.

    c. Nonetheless, choosing an appropriate professional or agency may be the most important service that a clinician can provide to a client with an alcohol or other drug problem.

5. Establishing referral networks.

    a. Referrals may be made to a range of community services and resources.

    - Alcohol and other drug treatment and rehabilitation services.
    - Community mental health facilities.
    - Community social service and welfare agencies.

Module II.3—Handout #8 *(continued)*

- Community child development, evaluation, and testing services.
- Hospital outpatient departments.
- Independent nurse practitioners and visiting nurses.
- Psychiatrists, psychologists, and social workers in private practice.
- Community public school systems.
- Court and probation systems.

　b. Establishing contacts.

- Locating possible sources for referral may involve contacts with professional colleagues, mental health clinics, hospitals, medical schools, State and local medical associations, and State alcohol and drug abuse agencies.
- Establishing and maintaining personal contacts with the staff or referral agencies aids in the effective provision of comprehensive care. Where linkages are established, clear communication, responsibilities, and coordination are likely to occur.

6. Criteria for evaluating referral resources.

　a. The program's record and success rate.

　b. Attitudes of program staff.

　c. Education and training of program staff.

　d. Licensure and accreditation of the program.

　e. Treatment of alcohol and drug dependence as primary disorders.

　f. Patients free of drugs early in the recovery process.

　g. Adequate provision for care of acute medical problems.

　h. Extent to which the program will help expedite the client's entry into treatment.

　i. Use of a comprehensive treatment approach.

　j. Encouragement of families to participate in the treatment process.

　k. Active preparation of clients against relapse.

　l. Development of a plan for continuing care.

　m. Ability to respond to special issues and needs.

　n. Reasonable cost.

Module II.3—Handout #8 (continued)

7. Preparing the client for referral.
   a. Give rationale for referral.
   b. Describe the referral resource.
   c. Provide support.
   d. Provide contact person.
   e. Discuss follow up.
8. Provide appropriate information such as consultant's name or agency name and phone number.
9. Remain available, if possible, for supportive follow up. By doing so, the nurse indicates a continuing interest in the client's well-being and also gathers feedback that will facilitate evaluation of referral effectiveness.

Instructor's Guide

Module II.3—Handout #9

GLOSSARY OF REFERRAL TERMS

- AA (Alcoholics Anonymous): Self-help meetings based on a 12-step recovery program for alcoholics. AA has no dues or fees. The only requirement for membership is a desire to stop drinking. There are AA groups all over the nation (and the world) but the greater N.Y. area has an especially high number of meetings. There are meetings in most neighborhoods and at virtually all times of day. Many (but not all) AA meetings in the N.Y. area are tolerant of other drug problems in addition to alcohol.

- NA (Narcotics Anonymous): Self-help program styled after AA but for people with any drug problem (including alcohol).

- CA (Cocaine Anonymous): Self-help program styled after AA for people dependent on cocaine.

- Therapeutic Community: Approximately 18–24 month residential treatment programs which provide high school classes toward GED, vocational training, and highly structured socialization programs in addition to substance abuse treatment.

- 12-Steps Rehabs: Approximately 1 month residential facilities, occasionally longer, based on the AA/NA programs which provide intensive rehabilitation for substance abuse but no high school or vocational training and usually minimal vocational counseling. They are ideal for those who are already employed or have a reasonable support system to return to after treatment.

- EAP (Employee Assistance Program): Programs available through many employers which offer counseling and referral for a variety of personal problems including substance abuse. EAP's are familiar with their employees' insurance coverage for various treatment programs, often act as liaisons between employees and supervisors to protect the job while the employee receives treatment, and sometimes have special financial arrangements with particular treatment facilities.

- MAP (Member Assistance Program): Similar services to EAP but administered through the employee's labor union rather than through the employer.

- EPRA (Employment Program for Recovering Alcoholics): A free vocational rehabilitation program for recovering alcoholics which provides extensive vocational counseling and arranges employment "internships" in private industry which often result in job offers.

- Intervention: An organized attempt to engage an alcoholic or drug addict into treatment. Many treatment facilities have programs that will assist families in arranging an intervention. All those concerned with the substance abuser (family, friends, employers) who are willing to participate meet with a professional counselor who teaches them about the process. An appointment is then arranged with the substance abuser at which all concerned others are present in addition to the

Module II.3

Module II.3—Handout #9 *(continued)*

counselor. The substance abusers are then lovingly confronted with the consequences of their addiction on themselves and others and encouraged to enter a pre-arranged treatment program the same day. Usually "therapeutic leverage" (threatened loss of family support, job, marriage, etc.) is employed to move the substance abuser into treatment.

Instructor's Guide

Module II.3—Handout #10

SELF-HELP GROUPS

Group	Population Served	Purpose
• Alcoholics Anonymous (AA)	• Individuals who desire to stop drinking.	• AA is a voluntary worldwide fellowship. Members seek sobriety, freedom from alcohol through the practice of the 12 Steps.
• Narcotics Anonymous (NA)	• Individuals who desire to refrain from the use of narcotics.	• NA is voluntary fellowship. Members seek a drug-free life style through the practice of the 12 Steps.
• Al-Anon	• Friends and relatives of individuals with drinking problems.	• Through a 12-Step fellowship, relatives and friends work toward a sense of distance, perspective and personal sanity, as they deal with those who have drinking problems.
• Nar-Anon	• Relatives and friends of narcotic addicts.	• Recovery from behaviors which respond to the drug-addicted individuals. Goals include self-care, self-development, detachment from the drug addict.
• Ala-Teen	• Adolescents and young people whose lives have been affected by the addiction of someone close to them.	• Development of perspectives on personal life and self-related responsibilities.
• Adult Children of Alcoholics (ACOA)	• Adult children of alcoholics and otherwise dysfunctional families.	• Insight into personal behaviors developed in response to life with a dysfunctional parent/ family.
• Families Anonymous	• For persons whose lives have been affected by the use of mind altering substances and related behavior of a relative or friend.	• Insight into personal behavior; understanding of addiction.

Module II.3

Module II.3—Handout #11

THE 12 STEPS OF ALCOHOLICS ANONYMOUS

1. We admitted we were powerless over alcohol—that our lives had become unmanageable.
2. We came to believe that a Power greater than ourselves could restore us to sanity.
3. We made a decision to turn our will and our lives over to the care of God *as we understood Him*.
4. We made a searching and fearless moral inventory of ourselves.
5. We admitted to God, to ourselves, and to another human being the exact nature of our wrongs.
6. We were entirely ready to have God remove all these defects of character.
7. We humbly asked Him to remove our shortcomings.
8. We made a list of all persons we had harmed, and became willing to make amends to them all.
9. We made direct amends to such people wherever possible, except when to do so would injure them or others.
10. We continued to take personal inventory and when we were wrong promptly admitted it.
11. We sought through prayer and meditation to improve our conscious contact with God *as we understood Him*, praying only for knowledge of His will for us and the power to carry that out.
12. Having had a spiritual awakening as the result of these Steps, we tried to carry this message to others, and to practice these principles in all our affairs.

From: The Twelve Steps and Twelve Traditions. Reprinted with permission of Alcoholics World Services, Inc.

Instructor's Guide

Module II.3—Handout #12

THE 12 TRADITIONS OF ALCOHOLICS ANONYMOUS

1. Our common welfare should come first; personal recovery depends upon AA unity.
2. For our group purpose there is but one ultimate authority—a loving God as He may express Himself in our group conscience. Our leaders are but trusted servants; they do not govern.
3. The only requirement for AA membership is a desire to stop drinking.
4. Each group should be autonomous except in matters affecting other groups or AA as a whole.
5. Each group has but one primary purpose—to carry its message to the alcoholic who still suffers.
6. An AA group ought never endorse, finance, or lend the AA name to any related facility or outside enterprise, lest problems of money, property, and prestige divert us from our primary purpose.
7. Every AA group ought to be full self-supporting, declining outside contributions.
8. Alcoholics Anonymous should remain forever nonprofessional, but our service centers may employ special workers.
9. AA, as such, ought never be organized; but we may create service boards or committees directly responsible to those they serve.
10. Alcoholics Anonymous has no opinion on outside issues; hence the AA name ought never be drawn into public controversy.
11. Our public relations policy is based on attraction rather than promotion; we need always maintain personal anonymity at the level of press, radio and films.
12. Anonymity is the spiritual foundation of all our Traditions, ever reminding us to place principles before personalities.

From: The Twelve Steps and Twelve Traditions. Reprinted with permission of Alcoholics World Services, Inc.

Module II.3

Module II.3—Handout #13

STATE MEDICAL SOCIETY OF WISCONSIN, GUIDELINE ADMISSION CRITERIA FOR CHEMICAL DEPENDENCY TREATMENT SERVICES

Guideline Admission Criteria
For Chemical Dependency Treatment Services

The State Medical Society Committee on Alcoholism and Other Drug Abuse has developed, with the approval of the SMS Board of Directors, guideline admission criteria for the following chemical dependency treatment services:

(1) Detoxification.
(2) Inpatient evaluation and rehabilitation.
(3) Outpatient treatment.

Detoxification

Admission to the hospital depends on the presence of one or more of the following:

1. Presence of a clustering of withdrawal symptoms (not all inclusive).
    a. Tremulousness (inner/outer shakes).
    b. Insomnia.
    c. Irritability/restlessness.
    d. Vague somatic complaints.
    e. Nausea, vomiting, diarrhea.
    f. Diaphoresis.
    g. Headaches.
    h. Abnormal vital signs.
    i. Mental confusion/fluctuating orientation.
    j. Hallucinations, hallucinosis.
    k. Psychoses.
    l. Seizures.
    m. Delirium treatments.
    n. Stupor.
    o. Rhinorrhea.
2. Presence of associated medical problems.
3. Suspected alcohol and drug dependency.
4. History of withdrawal syndrome.
5. History of prolonged intoxication.
6. Signs and symptoms that may be due to specific chemical dependency, not listed above, but recognized by the physician.

Instructor's Guide

Module II.3—Handout #13 *(continued)*

Inpatient Evaluation and Rehabilitation

Admission to the inpatient program depends on medical stability, the absence of acute withdrawal symptoms which may interfere with rehabilitation (and/or completion of detoxification), and the presence of one or more of the following:

1. Need for environmental control.

2. Need for 24-hour behavioral monitoring and confrontation.

3. Counterproductive medical or psychosocial situation.

4. Presence of a clustering of the following:

    a. Neurological psychological symptoms.

    (1) Denial.

    (2) Anguish.

    (3) Mood fluctuations.

    (4) Over-reaction to stress.

    (5) Lowered stress tolerance.

    (6) Impaired ability to concentrate.

    (7) Limited attention span.

    (8) High level of distractibility.

    (9) Extreme negative emotions.

    (10) Extreme anxiety.

    (11) Extreme depression.

    b. Reversible memory impairments.

    c. Thought process impairments.

    (1) Impairment in abstract thinking.

    (2) Limitations in ability to conceptualize.

    (3) Periodic episodes of mental confusion.

5. Previous outpatient treatment has failed.

6. Multiple drug dependency.

Module II.3

Module II.3—Handout #13 *(continued)*

Outpatient Treatment

Admission to outpatient treatment depends on one or more of the following:

1. Patient does not fit criteria for detoxification, specifically, patient does not present acute withdrawal symptoms (refer to detoxification criteria).
2. Patient does not fit criteria for inpatient evaluation and rehabilitation program.
3. Patient has ability to remain sober for at least five days.
4. Patient is willing to take Antabuse if medically recommended.
5. Patient is willing to attend AA.
6. Patient is willing to have family involvement.

From: Wisconsin State Medical Society, Committee on Alcohol and Other Drug Abuse. Guideline admission criteria for chemical dependency treatment services. *Wisconsin Medical Journal,* 80:11,5, 1981.

Instructor's Guide

Module II.3—Handout #14

NURSING DIAGNOSIS: FEAR—PSYCHOSOCIAL

Defining Characteristics.

- Dread related to a real or threatened external danger as evidenced by the use of denial, noncompliance, anxiety, hopelessness, and helplessness.
- Low self-esteem, guilt, and feelings of inadequacy related to social disapproval.
- Inability to articulate specific fears evidenced by increased anxiety.

Process Criteria: The nurse.

- Identifies potential areas of high risk when the individual is fearful.
- Destigmatizes the individual's behavior by teaching about the addiction process.
- Teaches the individual problem-solving skills.
- Encourages the individual, family, and significant others to participate in therapeutic groups to begin to share feelings more openly.

Outcome Criteria: The individual.

- Relates how addictions are related to the fears experienced.
- Recognizes the environmental stimuli that reinforce healthful behaviors.

Outcome Criteria: The family or significant other.

- Demonstrate greater ability to communicate their own fears in a group and with the individual.

Module II.3

Module II.3—Handout #15

NURSING DIAGNOSIS: SEXUAL DYSFUNCTION—BIOLOGICAL

Defining Characteristics.

- Actual or perceived limitation imposed by disease or therapy.
- Alteration in libido.
- Report of inability to achieve desired sexual satisfaction.

Process Criteria: The nurse.

- Assesses physiological and psychological etiology of problem in collaboration with sexual dysfunction expert.
- Teaches effect of addictions on the reproductive system and libido.
- Refers to appropriate resources for follow-up care.
- Teaches strategies that can be used to create an environment that promotes desired intimacy.

Outcome Criteria: The individual.

- Verbalizes the role of an addictions-free life-style in relation to sexual functioning.
- Verbalizes strategies to enhance sexual functioning and satisfaction.

Instructor's Guide

RECOMMENDED TEACHING STRATEGIES AND SAMPLE ASSIGNMENTS

RECOMMENDED TEACHING STRATEGIES

- Lecture
- Field trips to community agencies
- Clinical placement in facilities specializing in the treatment of addicted client(s)
- Case studies
- Simulated client interviews

SAMPLE ASSIGNMENTS

Sample Assignment #1

Combine aspects of DSM-III-R, nursing process, and addictions nursing diagnoses to design a cogent care plan for a patient you care for in a clinical setting.

Sample Assignment #2

CASE VIGNETTE

Ramona Hendrick

Ramona Hendrick is a 40-year-old housewife, mother of three children ages 18, 15, and 12, who is in her second year of recovery from addiction to Valium. Her husband encouraged her to seek additional counseling several months ago when he became increasingly distressed with the quality of their marriage and concerned about Ramona's general fearfulness which the family often perceives as irrational. Ramona reports that she and her spouse have distanced sexually and have not had sexual intercourse for six months although they enjoyed a satisfying sexual relationship in the early years of their marriage. Ramona is becoming increasingly home-bound as she finds grocery shopping and being in crowds extremely anxiety-provoking. She relies on her two older children to complete this task. She refused to attend a parent-teacher conference for her 12-year-old child stating that the teachers would judge her as an incompetent parent because of her addiction. Her husband accompanied her for her initial interview to the nursing counseling service in their community.

Module II.3

Role-Play—Nurse's Script

Your task in this role play is to:

1. Identify the psychological dynamics central to addiction to drugs and sexual activity in this client.
2. Explore nursing roles implemented by generalist practitioners of nursing in the treatment and rehabilitation of this addicted client and her family in the past and as currently indicated.
3. Formulate nursing diagnoses which correspond to patterns manifested by this individual recovering from drug addiction.
4. Formulate nursing interventions utilized with the client and her family; e.g., by:
   a. Teaching the effect of addictions on the reproductive system and libido.
   b. Teaching strategies that can be used to create an environment that promotes desired intimacy.
   c. Identifying potential areas of high risk when the client is fearful.
   d. Encouraging the client and her family to participate in therapeutic groups to begin to share feelings more openly.

Sample Assignment #3

DENIAL ACTIVITY

Instruction: The following is a list of statements about denial. Please indicate with a check (✓) in the appropriate column the statements which enable denial or are techniques for diminishing denial.

Statements	Enable	Technique
Education on the disease process or the health implications.		
Lack of referral or follow-up.		
Awareness of the phenomenon of denial.		
Working with families and significant others.		
Inefficient assessment techniques.		
Pointing out negative consequences.		
Ignorance.		
Increasing client awareness of present behavior and its effect on self and others.		
Failure to explore motivational state.		
Providing key alternative—in order to stop denying, clients need tools to deal with reality.		
Communication of biased attitudes.		

Instructor's Guide

Sample Assignment #4

MATCHING COLUMN

The following are the possible answers to descriptions in 1–8. There is one answer.

- (a) Primary Prevention.
- (b) Secondary Prevention.
- (c) Intervention.
- (d) Non-intensive outpatient.
- (e) Intensive outpatient.
- (f) Aftercare Treatment.
- (g) Short-term Residential Treatment.
- (h) Long-term Residential Treatment.
- (i) Dual Diagnosis Residential Treatment.
- (j) 12–Step groups.

1. Here, participants might be attending group counseling sessions 3 or 4 nights a week. 1. _____
2. This type of program might be best for a person who is chemically dependent and depressed. 2. _____
3. This type of program would be targeted towards teens who are "at risk" for chemical dependency. 3. _____
4. This type of program would probably be a common denominator to any alcohol or drug treatment program. 4. _____
5. This type of program would be targeted to all people. 5. _____
6. This type of program might be best for a person who has already completed a residential program. 6. _____
7. This type of program might be best for a person who has relapsed after three or four residential programs. 7. _____
8. This type of program might include weekly family therapy sessions. 8. _____

Answers:

1. e.
2. i.
3. b.
4. j.
5. a.
6. f.
7. h.
8. d.

Module II.3

Sample Assignment #5

What do the following abbreviations stand for?

1. COA
2. AA
3. ACOA
4. ADD
5. NA
6. DMS-III-R
7. DD
8. CAC
9. TC
10. MICA
11. d.o.c.
12. CARN

Answers

1. Child of Alcoholic.
2. Alcoholics Anonymous.
3. Adult Child of Alcoholic.
4. Attention Deficit Disorder.
5. Narcotics Anonymous.
6. Diagnostic & Statistical Manual, 3rd edition, revised.
7. Dual Diagnosis.
8. Certified Alcoholism Counselor.
9. Therapeutic Community.
10. Mentally Ill Chemical Abuser.
11. drug of choice.
12. Certified Addiction—Registered Nurse.

TEST QUESTIONS AND ANSWERS

TEST QUESTIONS

1. An appropriate evaluation criterion for the nursing care of a person with a long history of alcoholism would be:
   a. recognition of the reasons for drinking.
   b. total abstinence from drinking.
   c. increasingly long periods of abstinence.
   d. social drinking with control.

2. An evaluation criterion for the nursing care of a woman who is addicted to sedatives and stimulants is that the patient will:
   a. recognize the situations in which she uses drugs.
   b. verbalize that she is dependent on drugs.
   c. understand the reasons she became addicted to drugs.
   d. discuss her addictive behavior with others openly.

3. Physical dependence on a substance such as heroin is evident when the substance is unavailable and the individual:
   a. experiences extremely high levels of anxiety.
   b. constantly craves the substance.
   c. exhibits physiological symptoms of withdrawal.
   d. expresses anger at unavailability of the substance.

4. In relation to substance abuse, to which of the following does the term "tolerance" refer?
   a. Individual's need for increased amounts of alcohol or drugs in order to achieve the desired effect.
   b. Family's acceptance or indifference to a member's drug- or alcohol-dependency problem.
   c. Government's failure to act responsibly in controlling availability of alcohol and drugs.
   d. Individual's compulsive use of alcohol or drugs to achieve a sense of well-being.

5. Which one of the following nursing diagnostic statements is *most* specific to an adult with psychological dependence on alcohol or drugs?
   a. Convulsions related to inaccessibility of addictive substances.
   b. Hallucinations related to disrupted sensory perceptions from substance use.

c. Confabulation related to prolonged and excessive use of alcohol or drugs.

d. Anxiety related to inaccessibility of substance on which an individual is dependent.

6. Which criterion is necessary for the diagnosis of all cases of substance dependence?

    a. Evidence of tolerance to the drug or withdrawal syndrome.

    b. A pattern of dysfunctional use.

    c. Impairment in social or occupational functioning.

    d. A duration of one month of signs of the abuse pattern.

7. Group therapy is frequently the method of choice for treatment of alcoholic clients because:

    a. it provides for confrontation by peers.

    b. it assists in preventing dependency on the care giver.

    c. alcoholic clients accept exposure of denial more readily from other alcoholics.

    d. all of the above.

8. Which aspect of the Addictions Standards of Practice describes the environmental context necessary for the achievement of any given standard?

    a. rationale.

    b. structure criteria.

    c. process criteria.

    d. outcome criteria.

9. Which one of the following defenses interferes the *most* with a person recognizing and accepting drug addiction as a problem?

    a. Denial.

    b. Preservation.

    c. Suppression.

    d. Regression.

10. Mr. Jones, a 36-year-old salesman, is attending his first meeting of Alcoholics Anonymous because he finally realized and admitted that he is an alcoholic. The most effective treatment of alcoholism is accomplished by:

    a. admission to an alcoholic unit in a general hospital.

    b. individual or group psychotherapy.

    c. the daily administration of disulfiram (Antabuse).

    d. active membership in AA.

11. The most important factor in Mr. Jones' rehabilitation is:

    a. his emotional or motivational readiness.

    b. the qualitative level of his physical state.

    c. his family's accepting attitude.

    d. the availability of community resources.

Instructor's Guide

ANSWER KEY

1. c
2. b
3. c
4. a
5. d
6. a
7. d
8. b
9. a
10. d
11. a

BIBLIOGRAPHY

MODULE II.3 ADDICTIONS: NURSING DIAGNOSIS AND TREATMENT

Alterman, A. I., O'Brien, C. P., & McLellan, A. T. (1991). Differential therapeutics for substance abuse. In R. J. Frances & S. I. Miller, *Clinical textbook of addictive disorders* (pp. 369–390). New York: Guilford.

American Nurses' Association, & Drug & Alcohol Nursing Association. (1987). *The care of clients with addictions: Dimensions of nursing practice.* Kansas City, MO: Author.

American Nurses' Association. (1988). *Standards of addictions nursing practice with selected diagnoses and criteria.* Kansas City, MO: Author.

American Psychiatric Association. (1987). *Diagnostic and statistical manual* (3rd ed., revised). Washington, DC: Author.

Barbarin, O. (1979). Recidivism in drug addiction: A behavioral analysis. *Addictive Behaviors, 4*(2), 121–132.

Bennett, G., Vourakis, C., & Wolf, D. (1983). *Substance abuse: Pharmacological, developmental and clinical perspectives.* New York: John Wiley.

Blume, S. B. (1988). Current trends explored in compulsive gambling. *The Psychiatric Times* (December, 1988), 28–29.

Blume, S. B., & Nobel, J. (October 2, 1991). Science Times Section. New York Times.

Bradshaw, J. (1988). *On: The Family: A Revolutionary Way of Self Discovery.* Deerfield Beach, FL.: Health Communications, Inc.

Brick, J. (1987). Drugs and the brain: An introduction to neuropharmacology. *Center of Alcohol Studies Pamphlet Series.* New Brunswick, NJ: Alcohol Research Documentation, Inc.

Brill, L. (1977). The treatment of drug abuse: Evolution of a perspective. *American Journal of Psychiatry, 134*(2), 157–160.

Burkhalter, P. (1975). *Nursing care of the alcohol and drug abuser.* New York: McGraw-Hill Co.

Cadoret, R. J. (1986). An adoption study of genetic and environmental factors in drug abuse. *Archives of General Psychiatry, 43*(12), 1121–1136.

Carnes, P. (1983). *Out of the shadows: Understanding sexual addiction.* Minneapolis: CompCare Publishers.

Childress, A. R., McLellan, A. T., & O'Brian, C. (1985). Behavioral therapies for substance abuse. *International Journal of American Psychiatric Association: Addictions, 20*(6&7), 947–969.

Cohen, S. (1988). *The chemical brain: The neurochemistry of addictive disorders.* Irvine, CA: Care Institute.

Custer, R. L. (1984). Profile of the pathological gambler. *Journal of Clinical Psychiatry, 45,* 35–38.

DeLem, G. (1987). Alcohol use among drug abusers: Treatment outcomes in a therapeutic community. *Alcoholism: Clinical and Experimental Research, 11*(5), 430–436.

Dole, V. (1988). Implications for methadone maintenance for theories of narcotic addiction. *Journal of American Medical Association, 260,* 20.

Donovan, J. M. (1986). An etiologic model of alcoholism. *American Journal of Psychiatry, 148*(1), 1–11.

Douglas, D. B. (1986). Alcoholism as an addiction: The disease concept reconsidered. *Journal of Substance Abuse Treatment, 3*(2).

Drew, L. R. H. (1968). Alcoholism as a self limiting disease. *Journal of Studies on Alcoholism, 29,* 956–967.

Estes, M. & Heinemann, N. E. (1980). *Alcoholism: Development, consequences and interventions.* St. Louis: C. V. Mosby.

Fleming, J. P. & Kellam, S. G. (1982). Early predictions of age at first use of alcohol, marijuana and cigarettes. *Drug & Alcohol Dependence, 9*(4), 285–303.

Flood, M. (1989). Addictive eating disorders. In J. Zerveckh (Ed.), *Nursing Clinics of North America, 24*(1), 45–53.

Frances, R. & Franklin, J. (1989). *Concise guide to alcoholism and addiction treatment.* New York: AAPI Press.

Galanter, M. (1983). Psychotherapy for alcohol and drug abusers: An approach based on learning theory. *Journal of Psychiatric Treatment and Evaluation, 5*(6), 551–556.

Galanter, M. (Ed.). (1984). *Recent developments in alcoholism* (Vols. I & II). New York: Plenum.

Galanter, M., Castaneda, R., & Ferman, J. (1988). Substance abuse among general psychiatric patients: Place of presentation, diagnosis and treatment. *American Journal of Drug and Alcohol Abuse, 14,* 211–235.

Haack, M. (1986). The patient with chemical addiction. In J. D. Durham & S. B. Harden (Eds.), *The nurse psychotherapist in private practice* (pp. 173–186). New York: Springer.

Haber, K. A., Hoskins, P. P., Leach, A. M., & Sideleau, B. F. (1987). *Comprehensive psychiatric nursing.* New York: McGraw-Hill.

Halmi, K. A. (1982). The state of research on anorexia nervosa and bulimia. *Psychiatric Developments, 1,* 247.

Halmi, K. A. (1983). Pragmatic information on eating disorders. *Psychiatric Clinics of North America, 5*(2), 371–377.

Hasin, D., Grant, B., & Endicott, J. (1988). Treated and untreated suicide attempts in substance abuse patients. *Journal of Nervous and Mental Diseases, 176*(5), 289–294.

Jack, L. (Ed.). (1989). *Nursing care planning with the addicted client.* Skokie, IL: National Nurses Society on Addictions.

Jack, L. (Ed.). (1990). *The care curriculum of addictions nursing.* Skokie, IL: National Nurses Society on Addictions.

Johnson, C., & Flack, A. (1985). Family characteristics of 105 patients with bulimia. *American Journal of Psychiatry, 142,* 1321–1324.

Kagan, D. M., & Squires, R. L. (1983). Dieting, compulsive eating and feelings of failure among adolescents. *International Journal of Eating Disorders, 3,* 15–26.

Kaplan, C. (1978). The psychoanalytic theory of addiction: A re-evaluation by use of a statistical model. *American Journal of Psychoanalysis, 38*(4), 317–326.

Kaplan, H. I., & Sadock, B. J. (1988). *Synopsis of psychiatry.* Baltimore, MD: Williams & Wilkins.

Lesieur, H. R., Blume, S. B., & Zoppa, R. M. (1986). Alcoholism, drug abuse and gambling. *Alcoholism Clinical and Experimental Research, 10,* 33–38.

Lesieur, H. R., & Blume, S. B. (1988). The South Oaks Gambling Screen (SOGS): A new instrument for the identification of pathological gamblers. *American Journal of Psychiatry, 144,* 1184–1188.

Lettieri, D. (1978). *Drugs and suicide: When other coping strategies fail.* Beverly Hills, CA: Sage.

Levin, J. D. (1987). *Treatment of alcoholism and other addictions: A self-psychology approach.* Northvale, NJ: Jason Aronon, Inc.

Litman, G., Eiser, J., & Taylor, C. (1979). Dependence, relapse and extinction: A theoretical critique and a behavioral examination. *Journal of Clinical Psychology, 35*(1), 192–199.

Magilvy, J. K., McMahon, M., Bachman, M., Roark, S., & Evenson, C. (1987). The health of teenagers: A focused ethnographic study. *Public Health Nursing, 4*(1), 35–42.

Maisto, S. A. & Caddy, R. (1981). Self-control and addictive behavior: Present status and prospects. *The International Journal of the Addictions, 16,* 109–133.

Marlatt, G. & Nathan, P. (1978). *Behavioral approaches to alcoholism.* New Brunswick, NJ: Rutgers University Center for Alcohol Studies.

Matthew, R. & Korman, M. (1981). Abuse of inhalants: Motivation and consequences. *Psychological Reports, 49*(2), 519–526.

McClelland, D. C., Davis, W., Kalin, R. and Wanner, E. (1972). *The Drinking Man: Alcohol and Human Motivation.* New York: The Free Press.

McCormick, R. A. (1984). Affective disorders among pathologic gamblers seeking treatment. *American Journal of Psychiatry, 141,* 215–218.

McKelvy, M. J., Kane, J. S., & Kellison, K. (1987). Substance abuse and mental illness: Double trouble. *The Journal of Psychosocial Nursing and Mental Health Services, 25*(1), 20–25.

Mello, N. K. (1977). Stimulus self-administration: Some implications for the prediction of drug abuse liability. In T. Thompson & K. R. Unna (Eds.), *Predicting dependence liability of stimulant and depressant drugs.* Baltimore, MD: University Park Press.

Mello, N. (1979). An examination of some etiologic theories of alcoholism. *Academic Psychology Bulletin, 4*(4), 467–474.

Mendelsohn, J. & Mello., N. (Eds.). (1979). *The diagnosis and treatment of alcoholism.* New York: McGraw-Hill.

Meyer, R. (Ed.). (1986). *Psychopathology and addictive disorders.* New York: Guilford.

Meyer, R., Babor, T., & Mirkin, P. (1983). Typologies in alcoholism: An overview. *International Journal of the Addictions, 18*(2), 235–249.

Milby, J. B. (1981). *Addictive behavior and its treatment.* New York: Springer.

Milkman, H., & Sunderwirth, S. (1982). Addictive processes. *Journal of Psychoactive Drugs, 14,* 177–192.

Miller, W. (Ed.). (1980). *The addictive behaviors.* New York: Pergamon Press.

Millman, R. (1986). Considerations on the psychotherapy of the substance abuser. *Journal of Substance Abuse Treatment, 3,* 103–109.

Millman, R., Cushman, P., & Lowinson, J. (Eds.). (1981). *Research developments in drug and alcohol use.* New York: New York Academy of Sciences.

Mintz, N. E. (1982). Bulimia: A new perspective. *Clinical Social Work Journal, 10,* 289–302.

Naegle, M. (1989). Substance abuse. In L. Birckhead (Ed.), *Psychiatric mental health nursing: The therapeutic use of self.* Philadelphia, PA: J. B. Lippincott.

Naegle, M. (1988). Theoretical perspectives on the etiology of substance abuse. *Holistic Nursing Practice, 2*(4), 1–13.

O'Brien, C. P., Childress, A. R., Arndt, I. O., McLellan, A. T., Woody, G. E., & Maany, I. (1988). Pharmacological and behavioral treatments of cocaine dependence: Controlled studies. *Journal of Clinical Psychiatry, 49,* 17–22.

Orford, J. (1985). *Excessive appetites: A psychological view of addictions.* Chichester: John Wiley.

Pasquali, E. A., Arnold, H. M., & DeBasio, N. (1989). *Mental health nursing: A holistic approach* (3rd ed.). St. Louis, MO: Mosby.

Peele, S. (1989). *The diseasing of America.* Lexington, MA: Lexington Books.

Regier, D. A., Farmer, M. E., Rae, D. S., et al. (1990). Comorbidity of mental disorders with alcohol and the other drug abuse: Results from the Epidemiological Catchment Area (ECA) study. *Journal of the American Medical Association, 264,* 2511–2518.

Robinson, J. (1968). Psychosocial aspects of addiction. *American Journal of Public Health, 58*(11), 2142–2155.

Saleebey, D. (1985). A social psychological perspective on addiction: Themes and disharmonies. Special Issue: Social thought on alcoholism. *Journal of Drug Issues, 15*(1), 17–28.

Salmon, R. & Salmon, S. (1977). The causes of heroin addiction. *International Journal of Addictions, 12*(5), 679–696.

Schuckit, M. (1988). Pathological gambling. Is it a valid diagnosis? *Drug Abuse and Alcoholism Newsletter, 17*(9), 1–4.

Module II.3

Shaffer, H. (1983). Integrating theory, research and clinical practice: A perspective for the treatment of the addictions. *Bulletin of the Society of Psychoanalysis, 2*(1), 34–41.

Spitz, H. & Rosecan, J. (Eds.). (1987). *Cocaine abuse: New directions in treatment and research.* New York: Brunner/Mazel, Inc.

Stall, R. (1984). Disadvantages of eclecticism in the treatment of alcoholism: The problems of recidivism. *Journal of Drug Issues, 14*(3), 437–448.

Stuart, G. W., & Sundeen, S. J. (1991). *Pocket guide to psychiatric nursing* (2nd ed.). St. Louis, MO: Mosby.

Stuart, G. W., & Sundeen, S. J. (1991). *Principles and practice of psychiatric nursing* (4th ed.). St. Louis, MO: Mosby.

Stunkard, A. J. (1980). Obesity. In A. M. Freedman, H. I. Kaplan, & B. J. Sadock (Eds.), *Comprehensive textbook of psychiatry* (3rd ed.). Baltimore, MD: Williams & Wilkins.

The Addicted Brain (video), (1990). Princeton, NJ: Films for the Humanities and Sciences.

Townsend, M. C. (1991). *Nursing diagnosis in psychiatric nursing.* Philadelphia, PA: F. A. Davis.

Thurston, B. A. (1986). Substance abuse: The drug dependencies. In B. S. Johnson (Ed.), *Psychiatric-mental health nursing: Adaptation and growth.* New York: J. B. Lippincott.

Vaccani, J. M. (1989). Borderline personality and alcohol abuse. *Archives of Psychiatric Nursing, 3*(2), 113–119.

Vetter, H. J. (1985). Psychodynamic factors and drug addiction: Some theoretical and research perspectives. *Journal of Drug Issues, 15*(4), 447–461.

Wallace, B. C. (1987). Cocaine dependence treatment on an in-patient detoxification unit. *Journal of Substance Abuse Treatment, 4*(2), 85–91.

Waldholz, M. (1991, July 14). New studies lend support to 'Alcohol Gene' finding. *Wall Street Journal*, B1, 5.

West, R. J., & Russell, M. A. (1985). Dependence on nicotine chewing gum. *Journal of American Medical Association, 256*(23), 3214–3215.

Whitfield, C. (1982). *The patient with alcoholism and other drug problems.* Chicago: Yearbook Medical Publishers.

Wolkowitz, O., Roy, A., & Doran, A. (1985). Pathologic gambling and other risk-taking pursuits. Special Issues: Self-destructive behavior. *Psychiatric Clinics of North America, 8*(2), 311–322.

Wurmser, L. (1978). *The hidden dimension: Psychodynamics in compulsive drug use.* New York: Jason Aronson.

Yoder, B. (1990). *The recovery resource book.* New York: Simon and Schuster.

MODULE II.4
NURSING CARE IN ACUTE INTOXICATION

Margaret Compton, MS, RN

Madeline A. Naegle, PhD, RN, FAAN
Project Director
Janet S. D'Arcangelo, MA, RN, C
Project Coordinator

Project SAEN
SUBSTANCE ABUSE
EDUCATION IN NURSING

CONTENT OUTLINE

I. Signs and Symptoms of Acute Intoxication
   A. Definition of Intoxication
   B. Central Nervous System Depressants
   C. Central Nervous System Stimulants
   D. Narcotics
   E. Hallucinogens
      1. LSD, Mescaline, Psilocybin
      2. Phencyclidine (PCP)
   F. Volatile Inhalants
   G. Marijuana
II. Nursing Intervention
   A. Assessment
      1. Body systems
      2. Brief mental status exam
      3. Brief history of drug intake
      4. Data collection
   B. Establish Nursing Diagnoses: ANA Addictions Nursing and NANDA Nursing Diagnoses
      1. Anxiety
      2. Sensory-perceptual alteration
      3. Alteration in thought processes
      4. Alteration in respiratory function
      5. Alteration in self-concept
      6. Potential for violence
      7. Potential for self-harm
      8. Potential for poisoning
   C. Nursing Intervention
      1. Implement nursing regimens to address physiological needs
      2. Implement nursing regimens to address psychological needs
      3. Evaluate potential for long-term care

Module II.4

CONTENTS

I. SIGNS AND SYMPTOMS OF ACUTE INTOXICATION

A. Definition of Intoxication

Human responses, usually less than 24 hours, are related directly to the ingestion of psychoactive drugs. Specific effects and duration of intoxication will vary among drugs, individual users, and settings in which drug use takes place. All psychoactive drugs produce a disinhibition, euphoria, or feeling of well-being. Physiological effects are most commonly evident in the central nervous and cardiopulmonary systems.

Intoxication effects are typically dose-related, and toxic or overdose responses can be manifested at larger doses. Common psychological toxic effects of most drugs of abuse include psychotic symptoms (see Handout # 1, DSM-III-R Diagnostic Criteria for Intoxication).

B. Central Nervous System Depressants (ETOH, Barbiturates, Sedative-Hypnotics)

1. Actions:
   a. Cause a descending depression of CNS functioning via enhancing the action of inhibitory neurotransmitters, beginning at level of cerebral hemispheres, progressing to limbic and cerebellar sites, and finally to brainstem; inhibit ascending conduction from the reticular activating system.
   b. Depressants used concurrently produce extreme synergistic effects; also commonly used in conjunction with central nervous system stimulants.
   c. Continued use of CNS depressants results in the development of tolerance; withdrawal response evident upon cessation of use.
2. Effects:
   a. Intoxication responses (see Handout # 2, DSM-III-R Diagnostic Criteria for Sedative, Hypnotic, or Anxiolytic Intoxication):
      (1) General slowing of mental functions; poor comprehension, memory disturbances, reduced judgment, drowsiness, limited attention span.
      (2) Impaired motor coordination; slurred speech, ataxia, increased reaction time, hyperreflexia.
      (3) Euphoric mood; labile mood; decreased anxiety.
      (4) Disinhibition.
      (5) Cranial nerve dysfunction—nystagmus, diplopia.
      (6) Decreased heart rate, blood pressure, respirations.
   b. Toxic/Overdose responses:
      (1) Depressed level of consciousness, confusion to obtunded to comatose.
      (2) Decreased/absent response to painful stimuli.
      (3) Marked respiratory depression; slow, noisy respirations, apnea, respiratory arrest; pulmonary edema, aspiration pneumonia, atelectasis.

Nursing Care in Acute Intoxication

- (4) Amnesic disorder.
- (5) Specific to ETOH overdose:
  - (a) Fluid and electrolyte imbalances.
  - (b) Hepatic encephalopathy.
  - (c) Acute upper GI hemorrhage.

C. **Central Nervous System Stimulants**

1. Actions:
   a. Create euphoria by increasing the extracellular concentration of catecholamines within the central and autonomic nervous systems.
   b. Direct cardiovascular actions as a potent cardiac stimulator and vasoconstrictor.
   c. Cocaine additionally acts as a local anesthetic.
   d. Continued use of CNS stimulants results in the development of tolerance; withdrawal response evident with cessation of drug use.
2. Effects:
   a. Intoxication responses (see Handout # 3, DSM-III-R Diagnostic Criteria for Amphetamine or Similarly Acting Sympathomimetic Intoxication):
      (1) Psychological disinhibition; decreased anxiety, impaired judgment, impulsivity, hypersexuality.
      (2) Clear sensorium without confusion/hallucinations, decreased fatigue, heightened curiosity, increased interest in the environment, increased feeling of competence, increased self-esteem.
      (3) Psychomotor activation, tremulousness.
      (4) Increased heart rate, blood pressure.
      (5) Decreased appetite.
      (6) Mydriasis.
   b. Toxic/Overdose responses:
      (1) Hyperactivity.
      (2) Anxiety, confusion, hallucinations, paranoia.
         (a) Can progress to acute psychotic reactions including delirium, panic attacks, extreme paranoid delusions with violent and assaultive behaviors.
      (3) Seizures and coma.
      (4) Diaphoresis, hyperpyrexia.
      (5) Tachycardia with cardiac arrhythmia, pulmonary edema, cardiac arrest.
      (6) Hypertensive crisis with extreme vasoconstriction.
         (a) Can lead to myocardial infarction, cerebral stroke, placental infarction, spontaneous abortion, fetal cerebrovascular accident.

Module II.4

D. **Narcotics**

1. Actions:
   a. Bind to opiate receptors in various areas of the central and autonomic nervous systems, resulting in euphoria and analgesia.
   b. Brainstem depression.
   c. Peripheral vasodilation.
   d. Decreased gastrointestinal motility.
   e. Continued use of narcotics results in the development of tolerance; withdrawal response evident upon cessation of use.

2. Effects:
   a. Intoxication responses (see Handout # 4, DSM-III-R Diagnostic Criteria for Opioid Intoxication):
      (1) Euphoria with altered sensory perception, poor comprehension, memory disturbances.
      (2) Drowsiness, decreased social interaction.
      (3) Miosis.
      (4) Mild hypotension with tachycardia, decreased respirations.
   b. Toxic/Overdose responses:
      (1) Depressed level of consciousness, obtunded to comatose.
      (2) Depressed respirations leading to apnea and respiratory arrest; pulmonary edema, aspiration pneumonia or atelectasis may also develop.
      (3) Bradycardia, marked hypotension and shock.
      (4) Gastrointestinal atony.

E. **Hallucinogens**

1. LSD, Mescaline, Psilocybin:
   a. Actions:
      (1) Act at multiple receptor sites within the CNS resulting in CNS stimulation and depression; induce euphoria and perceptual alterations. General sympathetic effects noted on cardiovascular system.
      (2) Continued hallucinogen use does not result in tolerance.
   b. Effects:
      (1) Intoxication responses (see Handout # 5, DSM-III-R Diagnostic Criteria for Hallucinogen Hallucinosis).
         (a) Euphoria with transcendent experience qualities; perceptual alterations (primarily visual), increased sensory sensitivity, synesthesias, altered thought associations, hypersuggestibility, distractibility, labile mood, body image changes, sense of depersonalization, altered judgment ability.
         (b) Increased heart rate, mild hypertension, mild temperature increases, flushed face.

Nursing Care in Acute Intoxication

- (c) Pupil dilation.
- (d) Mild incoordination, hyperreflexia, fine tremor, restlessness.
- (e) Nausea.

(2) Toxic/Overdose responses:

- (a) Acute dysphoric reaction with anxiety, panic, hypervigilance, paranoid delusions.

2. Phencyclidine (PCP):
   a. Action:
   (1) Similar to actions of other hallucinogens; acts upon multiple CNS receptor sites with general sympathomimetic actions on body systems.
   (2) Symptoms of CNS depression at high doses.
   (3) Tolerance not reported with continued PCP use.
   b. Effects:
   (1) Intoxication responses (see Handout # 6, DSM-III-R Diagnostic Criteria for Phencyclidine [PCP] or Similarly Acting Arylcyclohexylamine Intoxication):
   - (a) Mild agitation, excitement, poor judgment.
   - (b) Increased heart rate and blood pressure.
   - (c) Decreased response to painful stimuli.
   - (d) Ataxia, dysarthria, hyperreflexia.
   - (e) Diaphoresis.
   - (f) Pupillary constriction with blank staring appearance.

   (2) Toxic/Overdose responses:
   - (a) Muscle rigidity; tonic-clonic movements, seizures, status epilepticus.
   - (b) Tachycardia with cardiac arrhythmias.
   - (c) Tachypnea, Cheyne-Stokes respirations.
   - (d) Hyperthermia.
   - (e) Nystagmus.
   - (f) Late toxic responses include delirium, psychosis with alterations in body image, aggressive/bizarre behavior, auditory and visual hallucinations, violence, hostility; CNS depression, coma, catatonic syndrome, absent corneal and gag reflexes; respiratory depression, apnea.

F. Volatile Inhalants (Aerosols, Paint Thinner, Gasoline, Plastic/Model Cement)

1. Actions:
   a. Act as a CNS depressant by inhibiting neuronal firing.

Module II.4

    b. Continued use of inhalants results in the development of tolerance; withdrawal response is not consistent upon cessation of use.

2. Effects:

    a. Intoxication responses (see Handout # 7, DSM-III-R Diagnostic Criteria for Inhalant Intoxication):

        (1) Euphoria, dizziness, excitation, pleasant exhilaration, visual and auditory hallucinations.

        (2) Sneezing (most likely due to local effects of inhaling drug).

        (3) Nausea and vomiting.

    b. Toxic/Overdose responses:

        (1) Confusion, loss of self-control, loss of consciousness, seizures.

        (2) Headache, tinnitus, blurred vision, diplopia, nystagmus.

        (3) Muscle incoordination, slurred speech, decreased reflexes.

        (4) Cardiac arrhythmias, pulmonary edema.

        (5) Suicide attempts.

G. Marijuana

1. Actions:

    a. Specific site of action unknown, although specific THC receptors have been theorized to exist within the CNS to produce euphoria.

    b. Has antiemetic properties.

    c. Decreased intraocular pressure.

    d. Continued use of marijuana results in the development of tolerance; withdrawal response not evident upon cessation of use.

2. Effects:

    a. Intoxication responses (see Handout # 8, DSM-III-R Diagnostic Criteria for Cannabis Intoxication):

        (1) Altered time sense, decreased inability to concentrate, passivity, lassitude, impaired short-term memory, drowsiness or hyperactivity, altered sensory perception.

        (2) Tachycardia with orthostatic hypotension.

        (3) Conjunctival infection, nystagmus.

        (4) Increased appetite.

        (5) Dry mouth.

    b. Toxic/Overdose response:

        (1) Anxiety or panic reactions (especially in first time users), depersonalization, paranoid delusions.

Nursing Care in Acute Intoxication

II. **NURSING INTERVENTION**

   A. **Assessment**

   1. Body systems:
      a. Cardiovascular system:
         (1) Heart rate, rhythm, heart sounds, presence of murmurs.
            (a) Presence of arrhythmias on ECG, periodic episodes.
         (2) Peripheral pulses; strength and regularity.
         (3) Blood pressure, orthostatic changes.
         (4) Jugular distention.
         (5) Skin color, temperature.
      b. Respiratory system:
         (1) Respirations rate, rhythm.
         (2) Chest percussion.
         (3) Adventitious or decreased breath sounds.
         (4) Secretions, cough.
         (5) Presence of cyanosis, evidence of hypoxia.
      c. Neurological system:
         (1) Rapid eye test (see Handout # 9). Increasingly used in ER's and by police to detect intoxication.
         (2) Level of consciousness.
         (3) Cranial nerve exam.
            (a) Presence of corneal, gag reflexes.
         (4) Deep tendon and stretch reflexes.
         (5) Cerebellar exam including gait, coordination, presence of tremor.
         (6) Sensory exam and response to painful stimuli.
         (7) Autonomic evidence of sympathetic stimulation.
   2. Brief mental status exam:
      a. General appearance and behavior.
      b. Level of consciousness and orientation.
      c. Emotional status.
      d. Attention level.
      e. Language/speech.
      f. Memory.
      g. Content of thought; presence of hallucinations or delusions.
      h. Suicidal, homicidal, or violent ideation.

Module II.4

3. Brief history of drug intake:
   a. Ascertain drug(s), amount, route and time used:
      (1) Ensure confidentiality; promote atmosphere to maximize honest communication.
      (2) Utilize reports of others; i.e., those who brought the patient to medical attention.
      (3) Utilize alternate sources of information (mental exam, physical assessment, urine/blood toxicology reports, collateral histories from family and/or friends) to enhance veracity of self-reports.
4. Data collection:
   a. Urine/blood toxicology reports.

B. Establish Nursing Diagnoses

ANA Addictions Nursing Diagnoses and NANDA Nursing Diagnoses: Common in nursing practice when caring for clients experiencing intoxication or toxic effects of drugs.

1. *Anxiety* related to perceived threat to biological or personal integrity, as evidenced by delusional thoughts, paranoid thoughts, restlessness, social impaired attention span, hypervigilance, isolation.
2. *Sensory-perceptual alteration* related to drug effects on CNS functioning, as evidenced by confusion, disorientation, hallucinations, delusions, inability to process sensory information.
3. *Alteration in thought processes* related to drug effects on CNS functioning, as evidenced by disorientation, delusions, hallucinations, altered attention span, impaired judgment, impaired memory.
4. *Alteration in respiratory function* secondary to depression of brainstem function, as evidenced by abnormal or absent breath sounds, decreased respiratory rate and depth, abnormal respiratory rhythm, decreased gag reflex, fatigue, cyanosis.
5. *Alteration in self-concept* related to inability to distinguish between self and non-self, as evidenced by distorted body perception, altered ability to recognize body in relation to environment, feelings of depersonalization, lack of clear psychological boundaries.
6. *Potential for violence* related to perceived threat to personal integrity, poor impulse control and/or feelings of helplessness, as evidenced by anger, hostility and rage, aggressive behavior, rigid body language, suspiciousness, delusional patterns of thinking related to anger.
7. *Potential for self-harm* related to suicidal ideation, as evidenced by verbalized suicidal thoughts, acute agitation, poor impulse control, impaired judgment.
8. *Potential for poisoning* related to drug overdose, as evidenced by toxic symptoms, extreme CNS depression, extreme respiratory depression, recent history of toxic amount of drug intake.

Nursing Care in Acute Intoxication

C. **Nursing Intervention**

1. Implement nursing regimens to address physiological needs:
    a. Perform cardiovascular, respiratory, and neurological nursing assessments as appropriate; watch for patterns of change over time.
    b. Monitor vital signs.
    c. Monitor toxicology reports.
    d. Implement seizure precautions.
    e. Monitor intake and output.
    f. Administer pharmacological agents as ordered to counteract toxic effects of drugs (i.e., Narcan) and monitor effects.
    g. Implement nursing interventions to enhance removal of drug from body (i.e., gastric lavage, urinary excretion).

2. Implement nursing regimens to address psychological needs:
    a. Orient client to reality as necessary.
    b. Stay with patient as possible.
    c. Create an accepting and supportive environment; attempt to be nonjudgmental in all interactions.
    d. Restrain only as necessary.
    e. Administer pharmacological agents as ordered and monitor effects.
    f. Assess for potential for violence and take actions to avoid escalation in levels of agitation, anxiety.
    g. Implement suicide precautions as necessary.

3. Evaluate potential for long-term care:
    a. Assess severity of client's drug use problem.
    b. Assess client's potential for accepting referrals.
    c. Involve family/significant others in plan of care.
    d. Obtain consultation as necessary.
    e. Assess for presence of concomitant health problems and provide appropriate health teaching.
    f. Refer to community or institutional resources as necessary.
    g. Prepare/monitor for withdrawal syndrome as necessary.

MODULE II.4
NURSING CARE IN ACUTE INTOXICATION

INSTRUCTOR'S GUIDE

Margaret Compton, MS, RN

Madeline A. Naegle, PhD, RN, FAAN
Project Director
Janet S. D'Arcangelo, MA, RN, C
Project Coordinator

Project SAEN
SUBSTANCE ABUSE
EDUCATION IN NURSING

CONTENTS

Component	Page
Module Description	362
Time Frame	362
Placement	362
Learner Objectives	363
Recommended Readings	364
Faculty Readings	364
Student Readings	364
Recommended Audiovisual and Other Resources	366
Overhead Masters	367
Handout Masters	391
Recommended Teaching Strategies and Sample Assignments	401
Test Questions and Answers	403
Bibliography	406

Module II.4

MODULE DESCRIPTION

This module assists the student in developing an understanding of physiological and psychological patterns associated with ingestion of alcohol and other drugs. Nursing interventions to address physiological and psychological crisis states resulting from the ingestion of drugs in various classes will be presented.

TIME FRAME

3 hours

PLACEMENT

Adult Health; Acute Adult Illness; Psychiatric-Mental Health

Instructor's Guide

LEARNER OBJECTIVES

Upon successful completion of this module, the learner will:

1. Describe signs and symptoms of intoxication from alcohol and other drugs.
2. List nursing diagnoses which correspond to the human responses precipitated by acute intoxication.
3. Identify clinical skills utilized in acute care of the intoxicated client.
4. Formulate and evaluate nursing interventions with human responses in acute intoxication.
5. Describe anticipated outcomes of nursing interventions with the intoxicated client.
6. Utilize consultation and client referral as appropriate.

Module II.4

RECOMMENDED READINGS

FACULTY READINGS

American Nurses' Association, & National Nurses Society on Addictions. (1988). *Standards of addictions nursing practice with selected diagnoses and criteria.* Kansas City, MO: Author.

American Psychiatric Association. (1987). *DSM-III-R: Diagnostic and statistical manual of mental disorders* (3rd ed., revised). Washington, DC: American Psychiatric Association.

Anderson, W. H., & Kuchnli, J. C. (1981). Diagnosis and early management of acute psychosis. *New England Journal of Medicine, 305,* 112–116.

Chychula, N. M. (1984). Screening for substance abuse in a primary care setting. *Nurse Practitioner, 12,* 15–24.

Di Sclafani, A., II, Hall, R. C. W., & Gardner, E. R. (1981). Drug induced psychosis: Emergency department diagnosis and management. *Psychosomatics, 22,* 845–855.

Glassroth, J., Adams, G. D., & Schnoll, S. (1987). The impact of substance abuse on the respiratory system. *Chest, 91*(4), 596–602.

Jaffee, J. H. (1989). Drug dependence: Opioids, non-narcotics, nicotine (tobacco), and caffeine. In H. I. Kaplan & B. J. Sadock (Eds.), *Comprehensive textbook of psychiatry, Volume I* (5th ed., pp. 642–686). Baltimore: Williams & Wilkins.

Khantzian, E. J., & McKenna, G. J. (1979). Acute toxic and withdrawal reactions associated with drug use and abuse. *Annals of Internal Medicine, 90,* 361–372.

Lipkin, G. B., & Cohen, R. (1986). *Effective approaches to patients' behavior.* New York: Springer Co.

Tennant, F. (1988). The rapid eye test to detect drug abuse. *Postgraduate Medicine, 84*(1), 108–111.

STUDENT READINGS

American Nurses' Association, & National Nurses Society on Addictions. (1988). *Standards of addictions nursing practice with selected diagnoses and criteria.* Kansas City, MO: Author.

American Psychiatric Association. (1987). *DSM-III-R: Diagnostic and statistical manual of mental disorders* (3rd ed., revised). Washington, DC: American Psychiatric Association.

Instructor's Guide

Anderson, W. H., & Kuchnli, J. C. (1981). Diagnosis and early management of acute psychosis. *New England Journal of Medicine, 305,* 112–116.

Estes, N., & Heinemann, M. E. (1982). *Alcoholism: Development, consequences and interventions.* St. Louis, MO: C. V. Mosby.

Hutchinson, S. A. (1988). Applying the nursing process for clients with psychoactive substance use disorders. In H. S. Wilson & C. R. Kneisl (Eds.), *Psychiatric nursing* (3rd ed., pp. 348–395). Menlo Park, CA: Addison-Wesley.

Lipkin, G. B., & Cohen, R. (1986). *Effective approaches to patients' behavior.* New York: Springer Co.

Piscarik, G. (1981). The violent patient. *Nursing, 11*(9), 63–65.

Schenk, E. A. (1987). Substance abuse. In W. Phipps, B. Long, & N. Woods (Eds.), *Medical-surgical nursing: Concepts and practice.* St. Louis, MO: C. V. Mosby.

Module II.4

RECOMMENDED AUDIOVISUAL AND OTHER RESOURCES

AUDIOVISUAL RESOURCES

1. **Drug Emergencies**

   Demonstrates interpersonal and medical skills for overdose from alcohol and PCP, cocaine and cannabis. Videotape, 3/4", 20 minutes. **Available on loan ($5.00) from National Library of Medicine, Collection Access Section, 8600 Rockville Pike, Bethesda, Maryland 20894.** For purchase, contact **Network for Continuing Medical Education, One Harmon Place, Secaucus, New Jersey 07094.**

2. **Care of Substance Abuse Patients**

   Demonstrates the handling by emergency personnel of various drug abusing individuals before their transfer to a hospital. **Available from Great Plains Instructional TV Library, University of Nebraska, P.O. Box 80669, Lincoln, Nebraska 68501.**

3. **The Inebriated Patient**

   Outlines nursing management of acute intoxication for depressants. **Available from American Journal of Nursing Company, Educational Service Division, 555 West 57th Street, New York, New York 10019-2961. Phone: 1-800-223-2282 or (212) 582-8820.** Rental #7538V ($60) or purchase #7538S ($275).

Instructor's Guide

OVERHEAD MASTERS

MODULE II.4 NURSING CARE IN ACUTE INTOXICATION

1. Intoxication
2. Diagnostic Criteria for Intoxication
3. Diagnostic Criteria for Sedative, Hypnotic, or Anxiolytic Intoxication
4. Diagnostic Criteria for Amphetamine or Similarly Acting Sympathomimetic Intoxication
5. Diagnostic Criteria for Opioid Intoxication
6. Diagnostic Criteria for Hallucinogen Hallucinosis
7. Diagnostic Criteria for Phencyclidine (PCP) or Similarly Acting Arylcyclohexylamine Intoxication
8. Diagnostic Criteria for Inhalant Intoxication
9. Diagnostic Criteria for Cannabis Intoxication
10. Drug-Induced Psychosis: Presenting Features, Emergency Diagnosis, and Treatment
11. Nursing Diagnosis Common for the Patient Experiencing Acute Intoxication

Instructor's Guide

Module II.4—Overhead #1

INTOXICATION

Human responses, usually short-lived (less than 24 hours), directly related to the ingestion of a psychoactive drug.

Specific effects and duration of intoxication will vary between drug, individual users, and settings in which drug use takes place.

All psychoactive drugs produce disinhibition, euphoria, or feeling of well-being.

Physiological effects are most commonly evident in the central nervous and cardiopulmonary systems.

Intoxication effects are typically dose-related, and toxic or overdose responses can be manifested at larger doses. Common psychological toxic effects of most drugs of abuse include psychotic symptoms.

Module II.4—Overhead #2

DIAGNOSTIC CRITERIA FOR INTOXICATION

1. Development of a substance-specific syndrome due to recent ingestion of a psychoactive substance. (*Note:* More than one substance may produce similar or identical syndromes.)

2. Maladaptive behavior during the waking state due to the effect of the substance on the central nervous system (e.g., belligerence, impaired judgment, impaired social or occupational function).

3. The clinical picture does not correspond to any of the other specific organic mental syndromes, such as delirium, organic delusional syndrome, organic hallucinosis, organic mood syndrome, or organic anxiety syndrome.

From: DSM-III-R: Diagnostic and statistical manual of mental disorders (3rd ed., revised). Copyright American Psychiatric Association, Washington, DC, 1987. Used with permission.

Instructor's Guide

Module II.4—Overhead #3

DIAGNOSTIC CRITERIA FOR SEDATIVE, HYPNOTIC, OR ANXIOLYTIC INTOXICATION

1. Recent use of sedative, hypnotic, or anxiolytic substance.
2. Maladaptive behavioral changes (e.g., disinhibition of sexual or aggressive impulses, mood lability, impaired judgment, impaired social or occupational function).
3. At least one of the following signs:
    a. Slurred speech.
    b. Incoordination.
    c. Unsteady gait.
    d. Impairment in attention or memory.
4. Not due to any physical or other mental disorder.

From: DSM-III-R: *Diagnostic and statistical manual of mental disorders* (3rd ed., revised). Copyright American Psychiatric Association, Washington, DC, 1987. Used with permission.

Module II.4—Overhead #4

DIAGNOSTIC CRITERIA FOR AMPHETAMINE OR SIMILARLY ACTING SYMPATHOMIMETIC INTOXICATION

1. Recent use of amphetamine or a similarly acting sympathomimetic.

2. Maladaptive behavioral changes (e.g., fighting, grandiosity, hypervigilance, psychomotor agitation, impaired judgment, impaired social or occupational functioning).

3. At least two of the following signs within one hour of use:

    a. Tachycardia.

    b. Pupillary dilation.

    c. Elevated blood pressure.

    d. Perspiration or chills.

    e. Nausea or vomiting.

4. Not due to any physical or other mental disorder.

From: DSM-III-R: *Diagnostic and statistical manual of mental disorders* (3rd ed., revised). Copyright American Psychiatric Association, Washington, DC, 1987. Used with permission.

Instructor's Guide

Module II.4—Overhead #5

DIAGNOSTIC CRITERIA FOR OPIOID INTOXICATION

1. Recent use of an opioid.

2. Maladaptive behavioral changes (e.g., initial euphoria followed by apathy, dysphoria, psychomotor retardation, impaired judgment, impaired social or occupational functioning).

3. Pupillary constriction (or pupillary dilation due to anoxia from severe overdose) and at least one of the following signs:

    a. Drowsiness.

    b. Slurred speech.

    c. Impairment in attention or memory.

4. Not due to any physical or other mental disorder.

Note: When the differential diagnosis must be made without a clear-cut history, testing with an opioid antagonist, or toxicologic analysis of body fluids, it may be qualified as "provisional."

From: DSM-III-R: Diagnostic and statistical manual of mental disorders (3rd ed., revised). Copyright American Psychiatric Association, Washington, DC, 1987. Used with permission.

Instructor's Guide

Module II.4—Overhead #6

DIAGNOSTIC CRITERIA FOR HALLUCINOGEN HALLUCINOSIS

1. Recent use of a hallucinogen.

2. Maladaptive behavioral changes (e.g., marked anxiety or depression, ideas of reference, fear of losing one's mind, paranoid ideation, impaired judgment, impaired social or occupational functioning).

3. Perceptual changes occurring in a state of full wakefulness and alertness (e.g., subjective intensification of perceptions, depersonalization, illusions, hallucinations, synesthesias).

4. At least two of the following signs:

    a. Pupillary dilation.

    b. Tachycardia.

    c. Sweating.

    d. Palpitations.

    e. Blurring of vision.

    f. Tremors.

    g. Incoordination.

5. Not due to any physical or other mental disorder.

From: DSM-III-R: Diagnostic and statistical manual of mental disorders (3rd ed., revised). Copyright American Psychiatric Association, Washington, DC, 1987. Used with permission.

Instructor's Guide

Module II.4—Overhead #7

DIAGNOSTIC CRITERIA FOR PHENCYCLIDINE (PCP) OR SIMILARLY ACTING ARYLCYCLOHEXYLAMINE INTOXICATION

1. Recent use of phencyclidine or a similarly acting arylcyclohexylamine.

2. Maladaptive behavioral changes (e.g., belligerence, assaultiveness, impulsiveness, unpredictability, psychomotor agitation, impaired judgment, impaired social or occupational functioning).

3. Within an hour (less when smoked, insufflated ["snorted"] or used intravenously), at least two of the following signs:

    a. Vertical or horizontal nystagmus.

    b. Increased blood pressure or heart rate.

    c. Numbness or diminished responsiveness to pain.

    d. Ataxia.

    e. Dysarthria.

    f. Muscle rigidity.

    g. Seizures.

    h. Hyperacusis.

4. Not due to any physical or other mental disorder (e.g., phencyclidine [PCP] or similarly acting arylcyclohexylamine delirium).

From: DSM-III-R: *Diagnostic and statistical manual of mental disorders* (3rd ed., revised). Copyright American Psychiatric Association, Washington, DC, 1987. Used with permission.

Instructor's Guide

Module II.4—Overhead #8

DIAGNOSTIC CRITERIA FOR INHALANT INTOXICATION

1. Recent use of an inhalant.
2. Maladaptive behavioral changes (e.g., belligerence, assaultiveness, apathy, impaired judgment, impaired social or occupational functioning).
3. At least two of the following signs:
   a. Dizziness.
   b. Nystagmus.
   c. Incoordination.
   d. Slurred speech.
   e. Unsteady gait.
   f. Lethargy.
   g. Depressed reflexes.
   h. Psychomotor retardation.
   i. Tremor.
   j. Generalized muscle weakness.
   k. Blurred vision or diplopia.
   l. Stupor or coma.
   m. Euphoria.
4. Not due to any physical or other mental disorder.

From: DSM-III-R: *Diagnostic and statistical manual of mental disorders* (3rd ed., revised). Copyright American Psychiatric Association, Washington, DC, 1987. Used with permission.

Instructor's Guide

Module II.4—Overhead #9

DIAGNOSTIC CRITERIA FOR CANNABIS INTOXICATION

1. Recent use of cannabis.

2. Maladaptive behavioral changes (e.g., euphoria, anxiety, suspiciousness or paranoid ideation, sensation of slowed time, impaired judgment, social withdrawal).

3. At least two of the following signs developing within 2 hours of cannabis use:

    a. Conjunctival infection.

    b. Increased appetite.

    c. Dry mouth.

    d. Tachycardia.

4. Not due to any physical or other mental disorder.

From: DSM-III-R: Diagnostic and statistical manual of mental disorders (3rd ed., revised). Copyright American Psychiatric Association, Washington, DC, 1987. Used with permission.

Module II.4—Overhead #10

DRUG-INDUCED PSYCHOSIS: PRESENTING FEATURES, EMERGENCY DIAGNOSIS, AND TREATMENT

1. Sensory distortion, hypersensitivity of all senses, euphoria, hallucinations, pseudohallucinations

   Physical examination

   | Sympathetic excess hallucinogens: STP, mescaline, nutmeg | Minimal changes EpineIndole-type hallucinogens: LSD, psilocybin |

   Treatment

   Controlled environment, support and reassurances (talking down). Administer Haldol for behavior control

2. Agitation with blank stare, anxiety, stupor, aggression, panic, bizarre behavior

   Physical examination

   Elevated blood pressure and heart rate, vertical and horizontal nystagmus, analgesia to pinprick, muscular rigidity, salivation, vomiting

   Phencyclidine (PCP)

   Treatment

   Minimal intervention (no talking down)
   Sensory deprivation with observation at a distance
   Administer Haldol for psychosis
   Administer no phenothiazines
   Administer Diazepam for seizures
   Administer Antihypertensives

From: Di Sclafani, A., Hall, R., & Gardner, E. (1981). *Psychosomatics, 22*(10), 845–855.

Module II.4—Overhead #11

NURSING DIAGNOSES COMMON FOR THE PATIENT EXPERIENCING ACUTE INTOXICATION

Anxiety related to perceived threat, to biological or personal integrity, as evidenced by delusional thoughts, paranoid thoughts, restlessness, interpersonal withdrawal, impaired attention span, hypervigilance.

Sensory-perceptual alteration related to drug effects on CNS functioning, as evidenced by confusion, disorientation, hallucinations, delusions, inability to process judgment, impaired memory.

Alteration in thought processes related to drug effects on CNS functioning, as evidenced by disorientation, delusions, hallucinations, altered attention span, impaired judgment, impaired memory.

Alteration in respiratory function related to depression of brainstem functioning, as evidenced by abnormal or absent breath sounds, decreased respiratory rate and depth, abnormal respiratory rhythm, decreased gag reflex, fatigue, cyanosis.

Alteration in self-concept related to inability to distinguish between self and non-self, as evidenced by distorted body perception, altered ability to recognize body in relation to environment, feelings of depersonalization, lack of clear psychological boundaries.

Potential for violence related to perceived threat to personal integrity, poor impulse control and/or feelings of helplessness, as evidenced by threats of anger, hostility and rage, aggressive behavior, rigid body language, suspiciousness, delusional patterns of thinking related to anger.

Potential for self-harm related to suicidal ideation, as evidenced by verbalization of suicidal thoughts, acute agitation, poor impulse control, impaired judgment.

Potential for poisoning related to drug overdose, as evidenced by toxic symptoms, extreme CNS depression, extreme respiratory depression, recent history of toxic amount of drug intake.

Instructor's Guide

HANDOUT MASTERS

MODULE II.4 NURSING CARE IN ACUTE INTOXICATION

1. Diagnostic Criteria for Intoxication
2. Diagnostic Criteria for Sedative, Hypnotic, or Anxiolytic Intoxication
3. Diagnostic Criteria for Amphetamine or Similarly Acting Sympathomimetic Intoxication
4. Diagnostic Criteria for Opioid Intoxication
5. Diagnostic Criteria for Hallucinogen Hallucinosis
6. Diagnostic Criteria for Phencyclidine (PCP) or Similarly Acting Arylcyclohexylamine Intoxication
7. Diagnostic Criteria for Inhalant Intoxication
8. Diagnostic Criteria for Cannabis Intoxication
9. The Rapid Eye Test

Module II.4—Handout #1

DIAGNOSTIC CRITERIA FOR INTOXICATION

1. Development of a substance-specific syndrome due to recent ingestion of a psychoactive substance. (*Note:* More than one substance may produce similar or identical syndromes.)

2. Maladaptive behavior during the waking state due to the effect of the substance on the central nervous system (e.g., belligerence, impaired judgment, impaired social or occupational function).

3. The clinical picture does not correspond to any of the other specific organic mental syndromes, such as delirium, organic delusional syndrome, organic hallucinosis, organic mood syndrome, or organic anxiety syndrome.

From: DSM-III-R: Diagnostic and statistical manual of mental disorders (3rd ed., revised). Copyright American Psychiatric Association, Washington, DC, 1987. Used with permission.

Instructor's Guide

Module II.4—Handout #2

DIAGNOSTIC CRITERIA FOR SEDATIVE, HYPNOTIC, OR ANXIOLYTIC INTOXICATION

1. Recent use of sedative, hypnotic, or anxiolytic substance.

2. Maladaptive behavioral changes (e.g., disinhibition of sexual or aggressive impulses, mood lability, impaired judgment, impaired social or occupational function).

3. At least one of the following signs:

    a. Slurred speech.

    b. Incoordination.

    c. Unsteady gait.

    d. Impairment in attention or memory.

4. Not due to any physical or other mental disorder.

From: DSM-III-R: Diagnostic and statistical manual of mental disorders (3rd ed., revised). Copyright American Psychiatric Association, Washington, DC, 1987. Used with permission.

Module II.4—Handout #3

DIAGNOSTIC CRITERIA FOR AMPHETAMINE OR SIMILARLY ACTING SYMPATHOMIMETIC INTOXICATION

1. Recent use of amphetamine or a similarly acting sympathomimetic.
2. Maladaptive behavioral changes (e.g., fighting, grandiosity, hypervigilance, psychomotor agitation, impaired judgment, impaired social or occupational functioning).
3. At least two of the following signs within one hour of use:
   a. Tachycardia.
   b. Pupillary dilation.
   c. Elevated blood pressure.
   d. Perspiration or chills.
   e. Nausea or vomiting.
4. Not due to any physical or other mental disorder.

From: DSM-III-R: Diagnostic and statistical manual of mental disorders (3rd ed., revised). Copyright American Psychiatric Association, Washington, DC, 1987. Used with permission.

Instructor's Guide

Module II.4—Handout #4

DIAGNOSTIC CRITERIA FOR OPIOID INTOXICATION

1. Recent use of an opioid.

2. Maladaptive behavioral changes (e.g., initial euphoria followed by apathy, dysphoria, psychomotor retardation, impaired judgment, impaired social or occupational functioning).

3. Pupillary construction (or pupillary dilation due to anoxia from severe overdose) and at least one of the following signs:

    a. Drowsiness.

    b. Slurred speech.

    c. Impairment in attention or memory.

4. Not due to any physical or other mental disorder.

Note: When the differential diagnosis must be made without a clear-cut history, testing with an opioid antagonist, or toxicologic analysis of body fluids, it may be qualified as "provisional."

From: *DSM-III-R: Diagnostic and statistical manual of mental disorders* (3rd ed., revised). Copyright American Psychiatric Association, Washington, DC, 1987. Used with permission.

Module II.4

Module II.4—Handout #5

DIAGNOSTIC CRITERIA FOR HALLUCINOGEN HALLUCINOSIS

1. Recent use of a hallucinogen.
2. Maladaptive behavioral changes (e.g., marked anxiety or depression, ideas of reference, fear of losing one's mind, paranoid ideation, impaired judgment, impaired social or occupational functioning).
3. Perceptual changes occurring in a state of full wakefulness and alertness (e.g., subjective intensification of perceptions, depersonalization, illusions, hallucinations, synesthesias).
4. At least two of the following signs:
    a. Pupillary dilation.
    b. Tachycardia.
    c. Sweating.
    d. Palpitations.
    e. Blurring of vision.
    f. Tremors.
    g. Incoordination.
5. Not due to any physical or other mental disorder.

From: DSM-III-R: Diagnostic and statistical manual of mental disorders (3rd ed., revised). Copyright American Psychiatric Association, Washington, DC, 1987. Used with permission.

Instructor's Guide

Module II.4—Handout #6

DIAGNOSTIC CRITERIA FOR PHENCYCLIDINE (PCP) OR SIMILARLY ACTING ARYLCYCLOHEXYLAMINE INTOXICATION

1. Recent use of phencyclidine or a similarly acting arylcyclohexylamine.

2. Maladaptive behavioral changes (e.g., belligerence, assaultiveness, impulsiveness, unpredictability, psychomotor agitation, impaired judgment, impaired social or occupational functioning).

3. Within an hour (less when smoked, insufflated ["snorted"] or used intravenously), at least two of the following signs:

    a. Vertical or horizontal nystagmus.

    b. Increased blood pressure or heart rate.

    c. Numbness or diminished responsiveness to pain.

    d. Ataxia.

    e. Dysarthria.

    f. Muscle rigidity.

    g. Seizures.

    h. Hyperacusis.

4. Not due to any physical or other mental disorder (e.g., Phencyclidine [PCP] or similarly acting arylcyclohexylamine delirium).

From: DSM-III-R: Diagnostic and statistical manual of mental disorders (3rd ed., revised). Copyright American Psychiatric Association, Washington, DC, 1987. Used with permission.

Module II.4

Module II.4—Handout #7

DIAGNOSTIC CRITERIA FOR INHALANT INTOXICATION

1. Recent use of an inhalant.
2. Maladaptive behavioral changes (e.g., belligerence, assaultiveness, apathy, impaired judgment, impaired social or occupational functioning).
3. At least two of the following signs:
   a. Dizziness.
   b. Nystagmus.
   c. Incoordination.
   d. Slurred speech.
   e. Unsteady gait.
   f. Lethargy.
   g. Depressed reflexes.
   h. Psychomotor retardation.
   i. Tremor.
   j. Generalized muscle weakness.
   k. Blurred vision or diplopia.
   l. Stupor or coma.
   m. Euphoria.
4. Not due to any physical or other mental disorder.

From: DSM-III-R: *Diagnostic and statistical manual of mental disorders* (3rd ed., revised). Copyright American Psychiatric Association, Washington, DC, 1987. Used with permission.

Instructor's Guide

Module II.4—Handout #8

DIAGNOSTIC CRITERIA FOR CANNABIS INTOXICATION

1. Recent use of cannabis.
2. Maladaptive behavioral changes (e.g., euphoria, anxiety, suspiciousness or paranoid ideation, sensation of slowed time, impaired judgment, social withdrawal).
3. At least two of the following signs developing within 2 hours of cannabis use:
   a. Conjunctival infection.
   b. Increased appetite.
   c. Dry mouth.
   d. Tachycardia.
4. Not due to any physical or other mental disorder.

From: DSM-III-R: Diagnostic and statistical manual of mental disorders (3rd ed., revised). Copyright American Psychiatric Association, Washington, DC, 1987. Used with permission.

Module II.4—Handout #9

THE RAPID EYE TEST FOR DRUG ABUSE

Component	Method	Common findings
General Observation	Observe eye in room light.	Redness of sclera. Ptosis. Retracted upper lid (walleye or bugeye) with sclera visible above iris, causing blank stare or exophthalmic appearance. Glazing film over cornea; excessive tearing of one or both eyes; swelling of eyelids.
Pupil Size	In room light, determine whether pupil diameter is wider or narrower than one side of iris, less than 3.0 mm, or greater than 6.5 mm.	Dilation. Constriction.
Pupil Reaction	Flash light into each pupil.	Slow, sluggish, or absent responses.
Nystagmus	Hold your finger in a vertical position, tell to follow your finger as you move it from side to side, in a circle (rotation), and up and down (vertical).	Failure to hold gaze. Jerkiness of movements.
Convergence	Hold your finger in a vertical position about one foot from subject's nose; tell subject to (1) follow your finger as you move it to about 1" in front of his/her nose and (2) hold this position for 5 seconds.	Inability to track or hold the crosseyed position.
Corneal Reflex	Touch cornea with strand of cotton or thread.	Decreased rate of blinking.

From: Tennant, F. (1988). The rapid eye test to detect drug abuse. *Postgraduate Medicine, 84*(1), 108–111.

RECOMMENDED TEACHING STRATEGIES AND SAMPLE ASSIGNMENTS

RECOMMENDED TEACHING STRATEGIES

- Lecture
- Clinical placement
- Case studies
- Media

CASE VIGNETTE

Cassandra Brown

Cassandra is a 17-year-old high school junior with a dual diagnosis of anorexia nervosa and cocaine addiction. She is currently hospitalized because of her family's concern about her weight loss and her hostile attitude. Although she had remained clean of drug or alcohol use for the six months following treatment at a drug rehabilitation facility, Cassandra relapsed. She last used cocaine ten hours ago. The nursing staff is focused on building an alliance with her despite her verbally abusive attitude. They are extremely concerned about her emaciated appearance as she is well below normal weight for her age and height. She is tremulous, restless, and nauseated. Dinner is being served on the unit when she approaches her one-to-one nursing staff attendant to shout obscenities and demands that the "foul smelling garbage be removed from this dump immediately." She proceeds to belittle the nurse's aide, who is in tears as she approaches the charge nurse for assistance.

Cassandra Brown—Nurse's Script

Role-Play Teaching Format

1. Describe the signs and symptoms of intoxication from cocaine.
2. List appropriate nursing diagnoses which correspond to the human responses.
3. Explore your clinical skill in accepting this client's marked suffering and assisting the nursing aide.

Module II.4

4. Begin nursing interventions with this acutely distressed client; e.g., by:

    - Creating a mealtime atmosphere that is quiet and without distractions for this client as well as others.

    - Providing an outlet for the client's feelings, encouraging the verbal expression of feelings.

    - Exploring the client's past experiences around mealtime in a matter-of-fact manner.

    - Monitoring the client's weight and the safety of both the client and others on the unit.

Instructor's Guide

TEST QUESTIONS AND ANSWERS

TEST QUESTIONS

1. In general, *all* psychoactive drug intoxication produces:
    a. respiratory depression.
    b. disinhibited euphoria.
    c. autonomic activation.
    d. motor incoordination.
2. CNS depressants and narcotics are similar in their ability to produce:
    a. brainstem depression.
    b. decreased GI motility.
    c. hypotension with tachycardia.
    d. fluid and electrolyte imbalances.
3. Tolerance is evident with all of the following drugs *except*:
    a. barbiturates.
    b. amphetamines.
    c. volatile inhalants.
    d. phencyclidine.
4. Toxic effects of CNS stimulants include all of the following *except*:
    a. upper GI hemorrhage.
    b. panic attacks.
    c. coma.
    d. cerebral infarction.
5. Which of the following statements about Narcan is *true?*
    a. It can reverse the CNS effects of both depressants and narcotics.
    b. Its emetic actions help to remove drugs from the body.
    c. It is active in reversing drug effects for 48–72 hours.
    d. It precipitates acute withdrawal in the narcotic addict.
6. Decreased level of consciousness and coma are toxic effects of which of the following drugs?
    a. LSD.
    b. PCP.

c. Volatile inhalants.

d. Marijuana.

7. In the rapid eye test, each of the following ocular assessments are made *except:*

    a. visual fields.

    b. corneal reflex.

    c. pupil size.

    d. tearing or discharge.

8. When caring for the patient at risk for violence, each of the following are appropriate nursing interventions *except:*

    a. Discontinue treatment if patient's agitation or hostility appears to be escalating.

    b. Do not isolate yourself with the patient.

    c. Use touch as a means to reassure/calm patient.

    d. Assess environment for presence of objects which patient could use to harm self or others.

9. When caring for the patient experiencing drug-induced psychosis, which of the following nursing interventions is most appropriate?

    a. Apply physical restraints to keep the patient from harming self or others.

    b. Leave patient undisturbed in dark, quiet room.

    c. Calm and frequently reorient patient to reality.

    d. Utilize confrontation strategies to help patient appreciate deleterious effects of drug.

10. When planning the nursing care of a patient recovering from acute drug intoxication, monitoring for withdrawal symptoms is necessary for patients abusing the following drugs *except:*

    a. barbiturates.

    b. cocaine.

    c. volatile inhalants.

    d. narcotics.

Instructor's Guide

ANSWER KEY

1. b
2. a
3. d
4. a
5. d
6. b
7. a
8. c
9. c
10. c

Module II.4

BIBLIOGRAPHY

MODULE II.4 NURSING CARE IN ACUTE INTOXICATION

American Nurses' Association, & National Nurses Society on Addictions. (1988). *Standards of addictions nursing practice with selected diagnoses and criteria.* Kansas City, MO: Author.

American Psychiatric Association. (1987). *DSM-III-R: Diagnostic and statistical manual of mental disorders* (3rd ed., revised). Washington, DC: Author.

Anderson, W. H., & Kuchnli, J. C. (1981). Diagnosis and early management of acute psychosis. *New England Journal of Medicine, 305,* 112–116.

Ansbaugh, P. (1977). Emergency management of intoxicated patients with head injuries. *Journal of Emergency Nursing, 3*(3), 9–13.

Aronow, R. (1978). Phencyclidine overdose: An emerging concept of management. *Journal of American College Emergency Physicians, 7,* 56–59.

Aronson, T. A., & Craig, T. J. (1986). Cocaine precipitation of panic disorder. *American Journal of Psychiatry, 143*(5), 643–645.

Barnes, G. (1979). Solvent abuse: A review. *International Journal of the Addictions, 14,* 1–26.

Baselt, R. (Ed.). (1987). *Abused drug monograph series.* Abbott Park, IL: Abbott Diagnostics.

Chychula, N. M. (1984). Screening for substance abuse in a primary care setting. *Nurse Practitioner, 12,* 15–24.

Cohen, S. (1989). The hallucinogens. In American Psychiatric Association, *Treatments of psychiatric disorders, Volume 2* (pp. 1203–1209). Washington, DC: Author.

Cohen, S., & Gallant, D. M. (1982). *Diagnosis of drug and alcohol abuse.* Rockville, MD: National Institute on Drug Abuse.

Corales, R. L. (1980). Phencyclidine abuse mimicking head injury. *Journal of American Medical Association, 243*(22), 2323–2324.

Cucco, R. A., Yoo, O. H., Cregler, L., & Chang, J. C. (1987). Nonfatal pulmonary edema after "freebase" cocaine smoking. *American Review of Respiratory Disease, 136,* 179–181.

Daghestini, A. N., & Schnoll, S. H. (1989). Phencyclidine abuse and dependence. In American Psychiatric Association, *Treatments of psychiatric disorders, Volume 2* (pp. 1209–1218). Washington, DC: Author.

Di Sclafani, A., II, Hall, R. C. W., & Gardner, E. R. (1981). Drug induced psychosis: Emergency department diagnosis and management. *Psychosomatics, 22,* 845–855.

Estes, N., & Heinemann, M. E. (1982). *Alcoholism: Development, consequences and interventions.* St. Louis, MO: C. V. Mosby.

Galanter, M. (1989). Treatment of alcoholism: Introduction. In American Psychiatric Association, *Treatments of psychiatric disorders,* Volume 2 (pp. 1063–1065). Washington, DC: Author.

Gawin, F. H., & Ellinwood, E. H. (1989). Stimulants. In American Psychiatric Association, *Treatments of psychiatric disorders,* Volume 2 (pp. 1218–1241). Washington, DC: Author.

Gawin, F. H., & Ellinwood, E. H. (1988). Cocaine and other stimulants: Actions, abuse treatment. *New England Journal of Medicine, 318*(18), 1173–1182.

Gillham, M. D., Southworth, K., & Dollabite, J. (1986). Nutritional treatment for the alcoholic patient. *Critical Care Quarterly, 8*(4), 20–28.

Glassroth, J., Adams, G. D., & Schnoll, S. (1987). The impact of substance abuse on the respiratory system. *Chest, 91*(4), 596–602.

Golbe, L. I., & Merkin, M. D. (1986). Cerebral infarction in a user of freebase cocaine ("crack"). *Neurology, 36,* 1602–1603.

Hornbacker, A. E. (1986). Hematologic disorders in the critically ill alcoholic. *Critical Care Quarterly, 8*(4), 29–39.

Hutchinson, S. A. (1988). Applying the nursing process for clients with psychoactive substance use disorders. In H. S. Wilson & C. R. Kneisl (Eds.), *Psychiatric nursing* (3rd ed., pp. 348–395). Menlo Park, CA: Addison-Wesley.

Isner, J. M., Estates, N. A. M., Thompson, P. D., Costanzo-Nordin, M. R., Subramanian, R., Miller, G., Katsas, G., Sweeney, K., & Sturner, W. Q. (1986). Acute cardiac events temporally related to cocaine abuse. *New England Journal of Medicine, 315*(23), 1438–1443.

Jaffee, J. H. (1985). Drug addiction and drug abuse. In L. Goodman & A. G. Gillman (Eds.), *The pharmacological bases of therapeutics* (7th ed., pp. 532–581). New York: MacMillan Publishing Company.

Jaffee, J. H. (1989). Drug dependence: Opioids, non-narcotics, nicotine (tobacco), and caffeine. In H. I. Kaplan & B. J. Sadock (Eds.), *Comprehensive textbook of psychiatry,* Volume 1 (5th ed., pp. 642–686). Baltimore, MD: Williams & Wilkins.

Jaffee, J. H., & Kleber, H. D. (1989). Opioids: General issues and detoxification. In American Psychiatric Association, *Treatments of psychiatric disorders,* Volume 2 (pp. 1309–1332). Washington, DC: Author.

Johnson, D. (1986). Fluid and electrolyte dysfunction in alcoholism. *Critical Care Quarterly, 8*(4), 53–62.

Kellerman, A. L., Fihn, S. D., LoGerfo, J. P., & Copass, M. K. (1987). Impact of drug screening in suspected overdose. *Annals of Emergency Medicine, 16*(11), 1206–1216.

Khantzian, E. J., & McKenna, G. J. (1979). Acute toxic and withdrawal reactions associated with drug use and abuse. *Annals of Internal Medicine, 90,* 361–372.

Module II.4

Leiken, J. B., & Hryhorczuk, D. O. (1987). PCP or cocaine intoxication? *Annals of Emergency Medicine, 16*(2), 235–236.

Lipkin, G. B., & Cohen, R. (1986). *Effective approaches to patients' behavior.* New York: Springer Co.

Millman, R. (1989). Cannabis abuse and dependence. In American Psychiatric Association, *Treatments of psychiatric disorders, Volume 2* (pp. 1241–1261). Washington, DC: Author.

Myers, J. A., & Earnest, M. P. (1984). Generalized seizures and cocaine abuse. *Neurology, 34,* 675–676.

Nicholl, A. M. (1983). The inhalants: An overview. *Psychosomatics, 21,* 914–921.

Piscarik, G. (1981). The violent patient. *Nursing, 11*(9), 63–65.

Rada, R. (1981). The violent patient: Rapid assessment and management. *Psychosomatics, 22,* 101–109.

Resnick, H. L. P., & Ruben, H. L. (1975). *Emergency psychiatric care.* Bowie, MD: The Charles Press.

Ricci, J. A. (1987). Alcohol-induced upper GI hemorrhage: Case studies and management. *Critical Care Nursing, 7*(56), 58–68.

Richards, M. L. (1979). Phencyclidine psychosis. *Drug Intelligence Clinical Pharmacology, 13,* 336–339.

Rounsaville, B. J. (1989). Clinical assessment of drug abusers. In American Psychiatric Association, *Treatments of psychiatric disorders, Volume 2* (pp. 1183–1192). Washington, DC: Author.

Schenck, E. A. (1987). Substance abuse. In W. Phipps, B. Long, & N. Woods (Eds.), *Medical-surgical nursing: Concepts and practice.* St. Louis, MO: C. V. Mosby.

Smith, D. E., Landry, M. J., & Wesson, D. R. (1989). Barbiturate, sedative, hypnotic agents. In American Psychiatric Association, *Treatments of psychiatric disorders, Volume 2* (pp. 1294–1309). Washington, DC: Author.

Tennant, F. (1988). The rapid eye test to detect drug abuse. *Postgraduate Medicine, 84*(1), 108–111.

Weinstein, S. P., Gottheil, E., Smith, R. H., & Migrala, K. A. (1986). Cocaine users seen in medical practice. *American Journal of Drug and Alcohol Abuse, 12*(4), 341–354.

Westermeyer, J. (1987). The psychiatrist and solvent-inhalant abuse: Recognition, assessment and treatment. *American Journal of Psychiatry, 144*(7), 903–907.

Woods, J. R., Plessinger, M. A., & Clark, K. E. (1987). Effect of cocaine on uterine blood flow and fetal oxygenation. *JAMA, 257*(7), 957–961.

MODULE II.5
NURSING CARE
IN WITHDRAWAL

Margaret Compton, MS, RN

Madeline A. Naegle, PhD, RN, FAAN
Project Director
Janet S. D'Arcangelo, MA, RN, C
Project Coordinator

Project SAEN
SUBSTANCE ABUSE
EDUCATION IN NURSING

CONTENT OUTLINE

I. The Withdrawal Syndrome

II. Signs and Symptoms of Drug Withdrawal

    A. Physiological Mechanisms of Drug Dependence Withdrawal from Classes of Drugs

    B. Psychological States Associated with Withdrawal

III. Nursing Intervention

    A. Assessment for Impending or Actual Withdrawal Syndrome

    B. Establish Nursing Diagnoses

    C. Intervention

Module II.5

CONTENTS

I. THE WITHDRAWAL SYNDROME

   A. Definition

      1. A constellation of physiological and psychological responses which follow abrupt cessation or reduced intake of a substance upon which an individual is dependent.

         a. Withdrawal is one of the diagnostic criteria for psychoactive substance dependence as described in the DSM-IIIR (American Psychiatric Association, 1987).

         b. Related DSM-IIIR diagnostic criteria: An individual will seek substance in an effort to relieve or avoid *withdrawal syndrome* symptoms.

      2. Physiologically, withdrawal represents a homeostatic response to the physiological changes induced by chronic use of a substance. In that substances are psychoactive, changes are consistently noted in neurophysiological systems.

      3. Withdrawal symptoms vary greatly across classes of substances. Marked physiological signs are common with opiates and Central Nervous System (CNS) depressants. Such signs are less obvious or well-documented with CNS stimulants and hallucinogens as well as nicotine, but intense subjective symptoms can occur upon withdrawal from heavy use of these substances.

         a. Morbidity associated with withdrawal or likelihood of relapse does not directly relate to intensity of physical withdrawal.

         b. Typically, withdrawal symptoms are somewhat opposite in nature from the direct effects of the substance.

         c. Withdrawals from all classes of substances are similar in producing symptoms of acute anxiety and protracted depression.

         d. Polydrug use—the use of more than one drug—is increasingly the norm rather than the exception; any withdrawal syndrome may be accompanied by a second set of symptoms, or can be masked by intoxication of another substance.

      4. In that the substance abuser is frequently known to be self-medicating a behavioral disorder that antedates drug exposure, the withdrawal syndrome evokes evidence of a previously masked set of psychiatric symptoms, such as phobias, anxiety, neurosis, or borderline personality.

II. SIGNS AND SYMPTOMS OF DRUG WITHDRAWAL

   A. Physiological Mechanisms of Drug Dependence Withdrawal from Classes of Drugs

      1. CNS depressants (ETOH, barbiturates, sedative-hypnotics):

         a. Most dangerous of withdrawal syndromes; abrupt withdrawal is *never* advocated or therapeutically indicated.

Nursing Care in Withdrawal

- b. In contrast to the CNS depression caused by depressant ingestion, abstinence is associated with systemic adrenergic hyperactivity manifested at levels of cerebral cortex, limbic system, and brainstem.
    - (1) It has been hypothesized that chronic depressant intake results in rebound increased CNS stimulation without the depressant effects of the drug. Uncontrolled CNS over-stimulation predominates.
- c. Physiological manifestations:
    - (1) Withdrawal syndrome may be mild to severe depending on chronicity of depressant dependence and degree of tolerance established.
    - (2) Onset of syndrome will vary with half-life of depressant; i.e., within 6–8 hours for ETOH, 24–36 hours for phenobarbital.
    - (3) Symptoms do not follow a specific sequence, but commonly progress in severity as follows:
        - (a) Tremulousness, tachycardia, headache, irritability, anxiety, postural hypotension, insomnia, moderate diaphoresis, hyperreflexic DTRs, disorientation. Usually the extent of mild withdrawal syndrome. Only approximately 10% of persons will progress to following symptoms of extreme autonomic excess; i.e., extreme sympathetic nervous system stimulation (see (b) below).
        - (b) Multiple generalized seizures; most common within the first 72 hours of withdrawal syndrome. More likely to progress to "status epilepticus" in barbiturate withdrawal.
        - (c) Myoclonic contractions.
        - (d) Hallucinosis, usually auditory as a third person voice, occurring while sensorium is clear and memory intact; patient may recognize as hallucinations.
        - (e) Withdrawal delirium (referred to as delirium tremens or DTs in ETOH withdrawal). Characterized by impaired recent and remote memory, disorientation, terrifying visual, auditory or tactile hallucinations.
        - (f) Extreme hypertension.
        - (g) Profuse diarrhea.
        - (h) Hyperpyrexia with profound diaphoresis.
        - (i) Vascular collapse and death.
    - (4) Common concomitant medical problems which complicate physiological state:
        - (a) Malnutrition.
        - (b) Opportunistic infections; i.e., pneumocystic carini pneumonia, cytomegaly virus.
        - (c) Liver disease.
        - (d) Trauma, burns.
        - (e) Aspiration pneumonia.
        - (f) Pressure necrosis, skin breakdown.

Module II.5

2. CNS stimulants (amphetamine, cocaine):
   a. Stimulants act at the neurotransmitter level to provide subjective feelings of euphoria, activation, disinhibition, well-being, and alertness. Withdrawal symptoms are subtle and not obviously manifested systemically; best documented and understood within the psychological realm.
   b. Onset of withdrawal symptoms varies with half-life of stimulant; i.e., cocaine 30–60 minutes, amphetamine 4–6 hours.
   c. Recently reported physiological sequelae of stimulant withdrawal theoretically relate to alterations in systemic neurotransmitter systems.
      (1) Myocardial ischemia noted up to four weeks post-cocaine abstinence, perhaps due to cocaine-medicated chronic dopamine depletion which increases risk for coronary artery vasospasm.
      (2) Acute dystonia reported during acute cocaine withdrawal, perhaps due to cocaine-medicated chronic dopamine and norepinephrine depletion which lowers the threshold for sytonia responses.
   d. Common concomitant medical problems which complicate physiological health state:
      (1) Malnutrition.
      (2) Opportunistic infections.
      (3) Trauma.
3. Narcotics:
   a. Narcotics bind to endogenous *mu opiate receptors* in the CNS and produce actions of euphoria, analgesia, and respiratory depression. Withdrawal is characterized by rebound excitability in those organs whose functions were previously depressed.
   b. Withdrawal syndrome results in moderate discomfort; never leads to life-threatening illness.
   c. Great individual variation noted in withdrawal syndrome intensity; depends upon chronicity of opiate use, tolerance, and rate at which drug is removed from receptors.
   d. Withdrawal syndrome onset varies with half-life of opiate; i.e., heroin and morphine 10–12 hours, methadone 24–36 hours.
   e. Physiological manifestations:
      (1) Stomach cramps, nausea and vomiting.
      (2) Diaphoresis.
      (3) Hypertension.
      (4) Backaches or muscle aches.
      (5) Lacrimation and rhinorrhea.
      (6) Gooseflesh.
      (7) Yawning.
      (8) Mydriasis.
      (9) Diarrhea.

Nursing Care in Withdrawal

- f. Common concomitant medical problems which complicate health status:
    - (1) HIV, hepatitis, TB.
    - (2) Opportunistic infections.
    - (3) Cellulitis.
    - (4) Bacterial endocarditis.
    - (5) Aspiration pneumonia.
    - (6) Pressure necrosis.

B. Psychological States Associated with Withdrawal

1. CNS depressants:
    a. In mild withdrawal, acute anxiety, irritability and nervousness are evident which may be manifested as demanding or annoying behavior. The client may complain of difficulty in concentrating. Insomnia and nightmares are also common.
    b. In more severe withdrawal, psychological responses related to disorientation and delirium are evident, including paranoia, violence, fear, and depersonalization.
    c. Protracted withdrawal syndrome lasting at least three weeks post-depressant abstinence evidenced by complaints of spontaneous anxiety, depressive episodes, transient psychotic reactions, impaired cognitive performance, increased irritability and impatience, fatigue, low stress tolerance, emotional lability, and distractibility.
2. CNS stimulants:
    a. Withdrawal syndrome accompanying stimulant abstinence believed to be related to central neurotransmitter derangements secondary to chronic stimulant use.
    b. Described as occurring in three temporally-related phases, best described with cocaine abstinence.
        (1) The "Crash" phase, usually occurring between 9 and 96 hours post-cocaine use, is manifested by early symptoms of depression, agitation, and high drug craving. Proceeds to feelings of increased depression, fatigue with desire for sleep, and an absence of drug craving. Depressant use is common during this phase. Late in the crash phase, client behaviors include hypersomnolence and hyperphagia.
        (2) The withdrawal phase, occurring for the next 8–10 weeks after cocaine abstinence (similar temporally to the protracted withdrawal syndrome described with depressant withdrawal), results in marked anhedonia, anenergia, anxiety, and high cocaine craving.
        (3) If relapse is not experienced during the withdrawal phase, the client enters an indefinite extinction phase, characterized by a return to normal moods and hedonic response with episodic craving.
3. Narcotics:
    a. Distinct psychologic sequelae of opiate withdrawal are not evident.

Module II.5

      b. Similar to mild depressant withdrawal; generalized anxiety, restlessness, and dysphoria common.

      c. Inconclusive evidence exists that a protracted withdrawal syndrome may also occur, with subtle disturbances of mood and sleep persisting for weeks to months.

III. NURSING INTERVENTION

A. Assessment for Impending or Actual Withdrawal Syndrome

1. Nursing history:
   a. Drug of choice or substance primarily used.
   b. Other types of drugs used and possible interactions.
   c. Frequency, amount, duration of drug use.
   d. Half-life of substance(s) ingested.
   e. Minutes/hours since last use of substance(s) and amount of substance(s) last taken.
   f. Past history of and response to withdrawal.
   g. Patient's acceptance/knowledge of dependence and desired outcome.

2. Nursing examination:
   a. Mental status including level of consciousness, orientation, memory, mood, affect, and reality testing.
   b. Presence of anxiety, restlessness, drug-seeking behaviors.
   c. Vital signs.
   d. Plasma or urine toxicology reports.
   e. Presenting symptoms.
   f. Hydration status.
   g. Nutritional status.
   h. Skin assessment and integrity.

B. Establish Nursing Diagnoses

1. ANA Addictions Nursing Diagnoses and NANDA Nursing Diagnoses common in nursing practice when caring for clients experiencing a substance withdrawal syndrome.
   a. CNS depressant withdrawal syndrome:
      (1) Sensory-perceptual alteration related to uncontrolled CNS excitation, as evidenced by fluctuation in level of consciousness, disorientation, visual, auditory or tactile hallucinations, inability to process information.
      (2) Potential for injury related to uncontrolled CNS excitation, as evidenced by seizure activity, altered level of consciousness, impaired judgment, disorientation, sensory-perceptual deficits.

Nursing Care in Withdrawal

- (3) Potential for fluid and electrolyte imbalance related to profound autonomic stimulation, as evidenced by profuse diaphoresis, hyperpyrexia, hyperventilation, diarrhea and vomiting, increased serum sodium, and serum osmolarity.
- (4) Hyperthermia related to increased metabolic rate as evidenced by sustained temperature >39° C, flushed, warm skin.
- (5) Severe anxiety, related to uncontrolled CNS excitation/loss of substance believed to be necessary to maintain psychological stability/personality structure preceding substance use, as evidenced by restlessness, drug-seeking behavior, impatience, nervousness, difficulty concentrating, confusion, irritability.
- (6) Potential for violence related to disorientation and sensory-perceptual disturbances, as evidenced by aggressive behavior, threats of anger, hostility and rage, perception of environment as hostile and threatening, suspicion, delusional patterns of thinking related to anger.

b. CNS stimulant withdrawal syndrome:
- (1) Hopelessness related to depression, as evidenced by anhedonia, verbalizations of depression, verbalization of suicidality, apathy, anenergia, lack of ambition, initiative and/or interest, unable to recognize sources of hope.
- (2) Ineffective individual coping related to feelings of depression and anhedonia, as evidenced by relapse, feelings of self-defeat, replacing one addiction with another.
- (3) Alteration in nutritional status related to chronic anorexia, as evidenced by weight 10%–20% below ideal body weight, presence of opportunistic infections, poor skin, hair and/or nail integrity, evidence of immunocompromise in WBC count.
- (4) Potential alteration in cardiac tissue perfusion related to coronary artery vasospasm, as evidenced by EKG changes, anginal pain upon exertion, activity intolerance.

c. Narcotic withdrawal syndrome:
- (1) Alteration in comfort related to unbound opiate receptors, as evidenced by stomach cramps, backache and muscle aches, diaphoresis, crying/moaning, tense body posture.
- (2) Sleep patterns disturbance related to insomnia, as evidenced by verbal complaints, interrupted sleep, restlessness during sleep, increased irritability, lethargy, mood alterations.
- (3) Knowledge deficit related to experience of protracted withdrawal symptoms, as evidenced by lack of awareness of protracted symptoms, attribution of protracted symptoms to alternate environmental/situational stressors, relapse, replacing one addiction for another.

C. Intervention

1. Address acute physiological state:
   a. Frequent vital signs.

b. Accurate intake and output and aggressive intravenous fluid replacement; watch for signs of fluid overload.

c. Monitor laboratory values.

d. Administer vitamin supplements as ordered.

e. Administer pharmacological treatments as ordered and evaluate response; watch for oversedation and respiratory depression.

f. Place patient on seizure precautions with suction available.

g. Provide comfort measures.

h. Maintain skin integrity.

i. Ensure adequate nutritional intake.

j. Promote pulmonary hygiene.

k. Monitor client responses and behaviors after guest visits.

2. Assess psychological state:

   a. Perform mental status examination (instrument such as Mini-Mental State Exam helpful).

      (1) Level of consciousness.

      (2) Affect and mood; assess for presence of anxiety, depression, and mood swings.

      (3) Suicidal or homicidal thoughts.

      (4) Memory.

      (5) Judgment.

      (6) Reality testing.

   b. Coping and defense mechanisms.

3. Communication:

   a. Establish a short-term trusting relationship:

      (1) Attempt to be nonjudgmental in interactions.

      (2) Examine personal opinions/feelings about substance use and personal pattern of substance use; appreciate how these affect interactions with substance-abusing client.

      (3) Be honest and clear in interactions.

      (4) Anticipate anger, denial and defensiveness from client; accept as part of disease.

      (5) Treat client with respect and in self-esteem enhancing ways.

   b. Gather data on drug history:

      (1) Keep in mind that while in acute withdrawal, obtaining complete drug history may be impossible. Focus on information important to determining withdrawal response.

4. Interventions for behavioral disturbance:

   a. Offer emotional and psychological support.

Nursing Care in Withdrawal

    b. Provide a safe, nonthreatening environment. A private, well-lit, quiet room is ideal. Avoid placing in ICU as possible.

    c. Provide frequent reorientation cues as appropriate. Avoid the use of physical restraints. Ambulate client with assistance as appropriate to decrease anxiety and allow environmental exploration.

    d. Provide client with short-term alternative ways to deal with anxiety and dysphoria.

    e. Administer pharmacological agents and antidotes as appropriate. Evaluate effects.

    f. Utilize interpersonal supports as indicated.

    g. Utilize methods for interpersonal security.

    h. Do not attempt to address and change substance use behavior while client is experiencing acute withdrawal.

5. Following crisis intervention, evaluate need and potential for referral:

    a. Assess client's readiness and desire to change substance use behavior.

    b. Discuss potential referrals with client.

    c. Obtain consultation as necessary.

    d. Become familiar with and refer client to institution and/or community agencies.

MODULE II.5
NURSING CARE
IN WITHDRAWAL

INSTRUCTOR'S GUIDE

Margaret Compton, MS, RN

Madeline A. Naegle, PhD, RN, FAAN
Project Director
Janet S. D'Arcangelo, MA, RN, C
Project Coordinator

Project SAEN
SUBSTANCE ABUSE
EDUCATION IN NURSING

CONTENTS

Component	Page
Module Description	424
Time Frame	424
Placement	424
Learner Objectives	425
Recommended Readings	426
Faculty Readings	426
Student Readings	427
Recommended Audiovisual and Other Resources	428
Overhead Masters	429
Handout Masters	449
Recommended Teaching Strategies and Sample Assignments	454
Test Questions and Answers	456
Bibliography	460

Module II.5

MODULE DESCRIPTION

This module assists the student in developing an understanding of the physiological and psychological responses manifested by persons withdrawing from states of alcohol and drug dependence. Nursing interventions in the acute phase of withdrawal will be presented and the implications for long-term care and rehabilitation will be reviewed.

TIME FRAME

3 hours

PLACEMENT

Adult Health, Adult Acute Illness, Psychiatric-Mental Health

Instructor's Guide

LEARNER OBJECTIVES

Upon successful completion of this module, the learner will:

1. Describe signs and symptoms of withdrawal from alcohol and other drugs.
2. List nursing diagnoses which correspond to human responses in withdrawal from alcohol and other drugs.
3. Identify nursing skills utilized in the care of the client withdrawing from dependence on alcohol and other drugs.
4. Formulate nursing interventions with the client withdrawing from alcohol and other drugs.
5. Evaluate nursing interventions with the client withdrawing from alcohol and other drugs.
6. Describe anticipated outcomes of nursing intervention with the client withdrawing from alcohol and other drugs.

Module II.5

RECOMMENDED READINGS

FACULTY READINGS

Alpert, M. A. (1990). Modern management of delirium tremens. *Hospital Medicine*, 111–136.

American Nurses' Association, & National Nurses Society on Addictions. (1988). *Standards of addiction nursing practice with selected diagnoses and criteria.* Kansas City, MO: ANA.

Bissell, L. (1971). *Guidelines to management of alcohol withdrawal.* New York: National Council on Alcoholism.

Busto, V., Sellers, E. M., Naranjo, C. A., Cappell, H., et al. (1986). Withdrawal reaction after long-term therapeutic use of benzodiazepines. *New England Journal of Medicine, 315,* 854–859.

Charney, D. S., Riordan, E. E., Kleber, H. D., et al. (1982). Clonidine and naltrexone: A safe, effective and rapid treatment of abrupt withdrawal from methadone therapy. *Archives of General Psychiatry, 39,* 1327–1332.

Gawin, F. H., & Kleber, H. D. (1986). Abstinence symptomatology and psychiatric diagnosis in cocaine abusers. *Archives of General Psychiatry, 43,* 107–113.

Giannini, A. J. (1982). *Handbook of overdose and detoxification emergencies.* New Hyde Park, NY: Medical Examination Publication.

Gottheil, E., McLellam, T., & Druley, K. (1981). *Matching patient needs and treatment methods in alcoholism and drug abuse.* Springfield, IL: Charles C. Thomas.

Greenblatt, D. J., & Shader, R. I. (1975). Treatment of the alcohol withdrawal syndrome. In R. I. Shader (Ed.), *Manual of psychiatric therapeutics: Practical psychopharmacology and psychiatry.* Boston: Little Brown.

Jaffe, J. H., & Kleber, H. D. (1989). Opioids: General issues and detoxification. In American Psychiatric Association, *Treatments of psychiatric disorders* (Vol. 2, pp. 1309–1331). Washington, DC: Author.

Khantzian, E. J., & McKenna, G. J. (1979). Acute toxic and withdrawal reactions associated with drug use and abuse. *Annals of Internal Medicine, 90,* 361–372.

Smith, D. E., Landry, M. J., & Wesson, D. R. (1989). Barbiturate, sedative, hypnotic agents. In American Psychiatric Association, *Treatments of psychiatric disorders* (Vol. 2, pp. 1294–1308). Washington, DC: Author.

Instructor's Guide

STUDENT READINGS

American Nurses' Association. (1982, December). The hospitalized alcoholic (programmed instruction). *American Journal of Nursing, 82*, 1861–1879.

Bluhm, J. (1981, February). When you face the alcoholic patient. *Nursing, 81*, 71–73.

Estes, N., & Heinemann, E. (1982). *Alcoholism, development, consequences, and intervention*. St. Louis, MO: C. V. Mosby.

Henningfield, J. (1984). Pharmacologic basis and treatment of cigarette smoking. *Journal of Clinical Psychiatry, 45*(12, pt. 2), 24–34.

Hoff, L. A. (1984). *People in crisis: Understanding and helping*. New York: Addison-Wesley.

Kelly, F. M. (1986). Caring for the patient in acute alcohol withdrawal. *Critical Care Quarterly, 8*(4), 11–19.

Module II.5

RECOMMENDED AUDIOVISUAL AND OTHER RESOURCES

1. **Conquering Cocaine . . . Early Stages of Recovery**

   The process of the early stages of withdrawal from cocaine is described by medical experts and recovering addicts. Among the millions of people who use cocaine excessively, a growing number are asking for and receiving help. Their experiences affirm the need for professional treatment to get well. Treatment, ranging from hospitalization to outside support groups such as Cocaine Anonymous, provides a necessary, supportive environment and psychological motivation for withdrawal. For recovery there must be recognition of a tremendous problem, a desire to get well, and complete abstinence from all drugs and alcohol. The processes of detoxification, withdrawal symptoms, and counseling are described. This 18-minute program emphasizes that recovery is a lifelong process and that being part of an aftercare or self-help group is the only way to stay sober. To help users determine if they are dependent on cocaine, the program presents them with a number of questions to ask themselves. At the powerful conclusion of this program, a recovering addict describes the conditions that led to treatment and subsequent recovery. **Available from AIMS Media, #8097, rental ($75) or purchase ($245).**

2. **Drug and Alcohol Rehabilitation**

   One in ten Americans has a drinking problem; one in five has at least dabbled with drugs. This program focuses on the treatments in use to overcome these chemical dependencies and on the four stages of treatment: detoxification, counseling, acceptance, and recovery. The program also covers two controversial therapies currently in use: aversion therapy for alcoholism and methadone treatment for drug addiction. Viewers learn what the addict must do to avoid relapse, including taking it "one day at a time"—a basic tenet of self-help groups like Alcoholics Anonymous. **Available from Films for the Humanities and Sciences. VHS #BD-1369, purchase ($149).**

OVERHEAD MASTERS

MODULE II.5   NURSING CARE IN WITHDRAWAL

1. General Facts about Withdrawal Relevant to All Classes of Drugs
2. Physiological Withdrawal from Classes of Drugs
3. Psychological Withdrawal from Classes of Drugs
4. Delirium Tremens—General Considerations
5. Delirium Tremens—Clinical Picture
6. Delirium Tremens—General Principles of Treatment
7. Nursing Assessment for Impending or Actual Withdrawal Syndrome—Nursing History
8. Nursing Assessment for Impending or Actual Withdrawal Syndrome—Nursing Examination
9. Scope of Nursing Interventions for Impending or Actual Withdrawal Syndrome

Module II.5—Overhead #1

GENERAL FACTS ABOUT WITHDRAWAL RELEVANT TO ALL CLASSES OF DRUGS

1. Severity of withdrawal is related to:
   a. Chronicity.
   b. Tolerance.
   c. Rate of Abstinence.
2. Syndrome onset varies with half-life of substance used. For example:
   a. ETOH: 6–8 hours
   b. Cocaine: 30–60 minutes
   c. Heroin: 10–12 hours
3. Typically, withdrawal symptoms are somewhat opposite in nature from the direct effects of the substance.
4. Withdrawals from all classes of drugs are similar in producing symptoms of acute anxiety and protracted depression.

Instructor's Guide

Module II.5—Overhead #2

PHYSIOLOGICAL WITHDRAWAL FROM CLASSES OF DRUGS

1. CNS Depressants.

    a. This is the *most dangerous* withdrawal syndrome. Abrupt withdrawal may be life-threatening.

    b. General manifestation is CNS hyperactivity manifested at levels of the cerebral cortex, limbic system, and brainstem, with potential for uncontrolled CNS stimulation.

2. CNS Stimulants.

    a. Symptoms may not be obvious systemically.

    b. General manifestation is at the neurotransmitter level.

    c. Symptoms commonly manifested in subjective feelings, psychological realm.

3. Narcotics.

    a. Least life-threatening withdrawal.

    b. Symptoms are dramatic, temporarily disabling, and painful.

    c. General manifestation is a rebound excitability in organs depressed by the drugs.

    d. Typical symptoms.

        (1) Stomach cramps.
        (2) GI upset.
        (3) Diaphoresis.
        (4) Lacrimation.
        (5) Rhinorrhea.
        (6) Diarrhea.
        (7) Mydriasis.
        (8) Gooseflesh.
        (9) Yawning.
        (10) Backache.
        (11) Muscle aches.

Module II.5—Overhead #3

PSYCHOLOGICAL WITHDRAWAL FROM CLASSES OF DRUGS

1. CNS Depressants.
       a. Feelings and manifestations of anxiety and irritability.
       b. Severe reactions include disorientation, delirium, paranoia, and violence.
       c. Protracted syndrome may occur, lasting at least three weeks, with a wide range of symptoms.
2. CNS Stimulants.
       a. Manifestations are due to neurotransmitter derangement.
       b. Three temporally related phases are described.
           (1) "Crash": 9–96 hours, with a range of manifestations.
               (a) Depression → Increased depression → Hypersomnolence.
               (b) Agitation → Fatigue.
               (c) High drug craving → Low drug craving → Hyperphagia.
           (2) Withdrawal: 8–10 weeks.
               (a) Anhedonia, anergia, and anxiety.
               (b) High cocaine craving.
           (3) Extinction: Indefinite.
               (a) Episodic craving.
               (b) Potential for relapse.
3. Narcotics.
       a. Similar to mild depressant withdrawal.
       b. May have protracted withdrawal syndrome and disturbances of mood and sleep for weeks to months (research evidence inconclusive).

Instructor's Guide

Module II.5—Overhead #4

DELIRIUM TREMENS—GENERAL CONSIDERATIONS

1. General Facts.
   a. Most extreme form of alcohol withdrawal syndrome.
   b. Acute, potentially fatal, and psychotic reaction.
   c. Onset, 3–5 days following cessation of drinking.
   d. Duration, 72 hours (80% of cases), followed by a deep sleep up to 24 hours.
   e. Early symptoms.
      (1) Tremulousness.
      (2) Hallucinosis (visual, auditory, tactile, or combined with clear sensorium).
      (3) Seizure.
      (4) Difficulty concentrating.
      (5) Restlessness.
      (6) Irritability.
2. Diagnostic Criteria.
   a. Delirium component.
      (1) Mental clouding.
      (2) Hallucinations.
      (3) Misperceptions.
      (4) Disorientation.
      (5) Fluctuating levels of awareness.
   b. Tremens component (at least two of the following):
      (1) Tachycardia (pulse rate >100/min).
      (2) Hypertension (>150/100 mm/Hg).
      (3) Tremors.
      (4) Diaphoresis.
      (5) Diarrhea.
      (6) Fever (>100°).

From: Cushman, P. (1987). Delirium tremens: Update on an old disorder. *Postgraduate Medicine, 82*(5), 117–122.

Instructor's Guide

Module II.5—Overhead #5

DELIRIUM TREMENS—CLINICAL PICTURE

The patient develops characteristic physiologic changes, which set this syndrome apart from the other alcohol withdrawal states and from other forms of delirium.

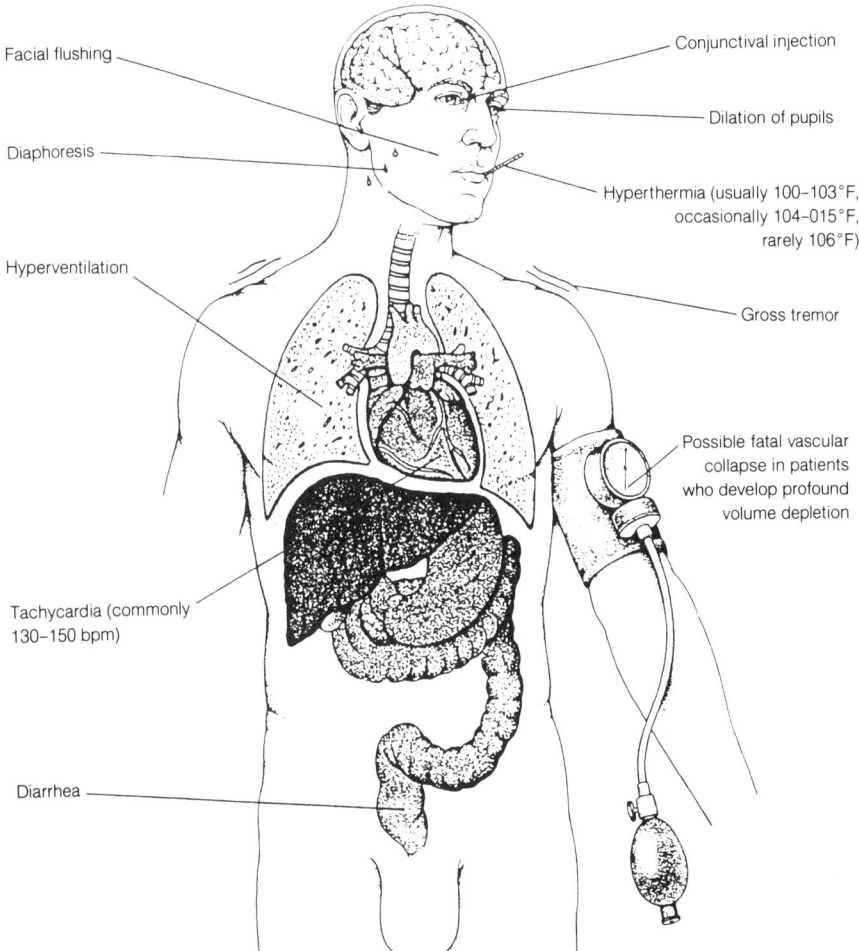

As the clinical manifestations of delirium tremens abate, the exhausted patient falls into a deep and prolonged sleep that may last up to 24 hours. If no complications supervene, the patient awakens from this sleep physically drained but otherwise sound.

From: Alpert, M. A. (1990). Modern management of delirium tremens. *Hospital Medicine,* 125. Copyright Cahners Publishing Company.

Instructor's Guide

Module II.5—Overhead #6

DELIRIUM TREMENS—GENERAL PRINCIPLES OF TREATMENT

1. Placement in private, well-lit room.
2. Minimize noises and diversions.
3. Thorough history and physical.
4. IV line inserted for fluid administration.
5. Thiamine (100 mg) administered intravenously for the first two days of hospitalization to prevent Wernicke's encephalopathy.
6. Multivitamins administered orally or intravenously.
7. Vital signs every half hour, temperature every hour since physiologic changes, including vascular collapse, may occur suddenly.
8. Baseline laboratory tests including:
   a. CBC.
   b. Prothrombin time.
   c. Serum electrolyte, including calcium and magnesium.
   d. Glucose levels.
   e. BUN.
   f. Liver function studies.
   g. Urinalysis.
   h. Stool occult blood assay.

From: Alpert, M.A. (1990). Modern management of delirium tremens. *Hospital Medicine,* 125.

Module II.5—Overhead #7

NURSING ASSESSMENT FOR IMPENDING OR ACTUAL WITHDRAWAL SYNDROME—NURSING HISTORY

1. Drug of choice or substance primarily used.
2. Other types of drugs used and possible interactions.
3. Frequency, amount, duration of drug use.
4. Half-life of substance(s) ingested.
5. Minutes/hours since last use of substance(s) and amount of substance(s) taken.
6. Past history of and response to withdrawal.
7. Patient's acceptance/knowledge of dependence and desired outcome.

Module II.5—Overhead #8

NURSING ASSESSMENT FOR IMPENDING OR ACTUAL WITHDRAWAL SYNDROME—NURSING EXAMINATION

1. Mental status, including level of consciousness, orientation, memory, mood, affect and reality testing.
2. Presence of anxiety, restlessness, drug-seeking behaviors.
3. Vital signs.
4. Plasma or urine toxicology reports.
5. Presenting symptoms.
6. Hydration status.
7. Nutritional status.
8. Skin assessment and integrity.

Module II.5—Overhead #9

SCOPE OF NURSING INTERVENTIONS FOR IMPENDING OR ACTUAL WITHDRAWAL SYNDROME

1. Address acute physiological state.
2. Assess psychological state.
3. Communicate effectively.
4. Intervene for behavioral disturbances.
5. Following crisis intervention, evaluate need and potential for referral.

Instructor's Guide

HANDOUT MASTERS

MODULE II.5   NURSING CARE IN WITHDRAWAL

1. Symptoms of Opiate Withdrawal/Overdose
2. Abstinence Symptom Rating Scales: Subscale 1
3. Abstinence Symptom Rating Scales: Subscale 2
4. Nursing Assessment for Impending or Actual Withdrawal Syndrome

Module II.5

Module II.5—Handout #1

SYMPTOMS OF OPIATE WITHDRAWAL/OVERDOSE

Symptoms of Opiate Withdrawal	Symptoms of Opiate Overdose
Increased temperature	Decreased temperature
Tachycardia	Bradycardia
Hypertension	Hypotension
Increase in rate and depth of respirations	Decrease in rate and depth of respirations
Piloerection	Pruritis
Perspiration	Flushing
Restlessness	Lethargy
Mydriasis	Miosis

From: Schloemer, N. F., & Skidmore, J. W. (1983). Opiate withdrawal with clonidine. *Journal of Psychosocial Nursing and Mental Health Services, 21*(10), 8–14.

Instructor's Guide

Module II.5—Handout #2

ABSTINENCE SYMPTOM RATING SCALES

SUBSCALE I

	Symptoms			
	None	Mild	Moderate	Severe
1. Loss of appetite				
2. Stomach cramps				
3. Nausea				
4. Diarrhea				
5. Sweating				
6. Chills				
7. Goose flesh				
8. Runny nose				
9. Tearing				
10. Yawning				
11. Joint pains				
12. Muscle pains				
13. Craving				
14. Insomnia				
15. Drowsiness				
16. Low energy				
17. Feeling blah				
18. Nervousness				
19. Irritability				
20. Mydriasis				
21. Spontaneous orgasm				

R.N.'s Signature _____ Date: _____

Time: _____

From: Schloemer, N. F., & Skidmore, J. W. (1983). Opiate withdrawal with clonidine. *Journal of Psychosocial Nursing and Mental Health Services, 21*(10), 8–14.

Module II.5—Handout #3

ABSTINENCE SYMPTOM RATING SCALES

SUBSCALE II

How Are You Feeling Right Now?

	None	Mild	Moderate	Severe
I feel calm.				
I feel secure.				
I am tense.				
I am regretful.				
I feel at ease.				
I feel upset.				
I am presently worried about possible misfortunes.				

From: Schloemer, N. F., & Skidmore, J. W. (1983). Opiate withdrawal with clonidine. *Journal of Psychosocial Nursing and Mental Health Services, 21*(10), 8–14.

Instructor's Guide

Module II.5—Handout #4

NURSING ASSESSMENT FOR IMPENDING OR ACTUAL WITHDRAWAL SYNDROME

A. Nursing History:
   1. Drug of choice or substance primarily used.
   2. Other types of drugs used and possible interactions.
   3. Frequency, amount, duration of drug use.
   4. Half-life of substance(s) ingested.
   5. Minutes/hours since last use of substance(s) and amount of substance(s) taken.
   6. Past history and response to withdrawal.
   7. Patient's acceptance/knowledge of dependence and desired outcome.

B. Nursing Examination:
   1. Mental status, including level of consciousness, orientation, memory, mood, affect, and reality testing.
   2. Presence of anxiety, restlessness, drug-seeking behaviors.
   3. Vital signs.
   4. Plasma or urine toxicology reports.
   5. Presenting symptoms.
   6. Hydration status.
   7. Nutritional status.
   8. Skin assessment and integrity.

Module II.5

RECOMMENDED TEACHING STRATEGIES AND SAMPLE ASSIGNMENTS

RECOMMENDED TEACHING STRATEGIES

- Lecture
- Clinical placement
- Case study and role play

CASE VIGNETTE

Peter Lindenson

Peter Lindenson is a 35-year-old middle manager at a large computing corporation. He was about to complete his MBA degree when his wife became seriously ill with breast cancer. She did not respond to several forms of therapy and died three months ago, leaving Peter to raise their two children. Throughout her illness, Peter kept putting off attending to his own physical health problem with low back pain. In order to keep up with the demands of caring for a terminally ill wife, seeing that the children were cared for and their home maintained, Peter began using a combination of valium, marijuana, and alcohol. He realized his drug use was out of control when he experienced withdrawal symptoms when hospitalized for acute low back syndrome recently. He completed detox while receiving extensive physical therapy. His physicians have been unable to diagnose any physical cause for his back pain and they have recommended that he seek counseling as well as remaining abstinent. Peter is withdrawn and sullen on approach by the nurse in a mental health out-patient clinic.

SAMPLE ASSIGNMENT

Role-Play Teaching Format

As the nurse in the mental health clinic:

1. Explore Peter's understanding of the addiction process.
2. Clarify the clinical data needed to support the appropriate nursing diagnoses relative to his withdrawal from alcohol and drugs, his physical pain, and his bereavement.

Instructor's Guide

3. Demonstrate the nursing skill of affective exploration in caring for this client.
4. Intervene with Peter; for example, by:
   a. Teaching alternative pain management measures, such as relaxation techniques and guided imagery.
   b. Assisting him in the identification of actual and potential losses.
   c. Encouraging him to keep a journal when unable to sleep and attend to his dream patterns when he does sleep.
   d. Providing rich emotional support.

Module II.5

TEST QUESTIONS AND ANSWERS

TEST QUESTIONS

1. Mr. Dan Drake, 25 years old, has a history of stealing money to buy barbiturates to sustain his drug habit. He is admitted to a psychiatric unit for treatment of his current withdrawal symptoms. In addition to finding out as far as possible how much of the addictive drug he has been taking, which of the following additional information would be basic to developing his treatment plan?

    a. The type of barbiturate he customarily uses.

    b. Where he gets his drug supply.

    c. If he has ever undergone treatment before.

    d. In what setting he usually takes the drug.

2. Mr. Drake is to be maintained on a stable dosage of phenobarbital for two days. Which of these symptoms would indicate a too-rapid withdrawal that could result in a serious complication?

    a. Tremulousness and insomnia.

    b. Rhinitis and goose flesh.

    c. Bradycardia and halitosis.

    d. Nystagmus and slurred speech.

3. Barbiturate withdrawal is best accomplished by which of the following treatment approaches?

    a. Abrupt cessation of the drug.

    b. Gradual cessation of the drug with the support of other former users.

    c. Substituting methadone for the barbiturate.

    d. Detoxification in a well-supervised medical setting.

4. Which of the following symptoms should a nurse expect to encounter in clients who are experiencing alcohol withdrawal?

    a. Slurred speech, ataxia.

    b. Coarse tremors of the hand, general malaise, anxiety.

    c. Hallucinations and seizures.

    d. Cirrhosis of the liver.

Instructor's Guide

5. During acute withdrawal after prolonged use of alcohol, a client cries out to the nurse that she sees ants swarming all over her. The nurse should:

   a. Apply restraints immediately to prevent the client from harming herself.

   b. Tell the client that visual and tactile disturbances are part of the withdrawal from alcohol.

   c. Ask the client to say some more about this upsetting experience.

   d. Ask the client if she has recently been using drugs other than alcohol.

6. For clients with alcoholism, the primary rehabilitator is the:

   a. Nurse.

   b. Physician.

   c. Entire health team.

   d. Client.

7. Symptoms of alcohol withdrawal syndrome include which of the following:

   a. Bizarre tongue movements and tremors.

   b. Thirst and bradycardia.

   c. Lethargy and anorexia.

   d. Hallucinations and convulsions.

8. Which behavioral problem of the alcoholic client requires the most exacting limit-setting?

   a. Manipulation

   b. Impulsiveness.

   c. Avoidance.

   d. Grandiosity.

9. David, 28-years-old, was recently admitted to the drug abuse unit. His history includes an alcoholic father, problems with the law as a teenager, and a broken marriage. He is a truck driver by trade. To establish a therapeutic relationship you would do everything *except*:

   a. Give vivid examples that point out the futility of drug use.

   b. Attempt to see his point of view.

   c. Examine your own prejudices and face them squarely.

   d. Avoid drug stereotypes.

10. James has been living with three other people in a run-down apartment in a deteriorating neighborhood. James knows most of the drug users in the neighborhood and participates in heavy use of LSD and alcohol. He supports himself with welfare, shoplifting, and drug peddling. James would be *least* likely to have:

    a. Flashbacks of bad trips.

    b. Psychological dependence on drugs.

c. A strong relationship with his family.

d. AIDS and a police record.

11. A client on a drug rehabilitation unit says to you that his friends in his former neighborhood are now into bluebells. You have never heard the term before and the client senses this. He shouts: "What are you doing working in this place if you don't know anything about drugs?" Your best response is:

    a. "I'm not familiar with those. What kind of drug is it?"

    b. "I don't have time to talk now. There is a staff meeting."

    c. "How am I supposed to know every street drug these days?"

    d. "It offends me when you shout at me."

12. Steve McFadden is a 48-year-old chronic alcoholic who looks 60. He has been on the alcohol rehabilitation unit for three weeks and says to the nurse, "My feet have been burning and tingling for three months now and no one has done a damn thing." Mr. McFadden may be suffering from:

    a. Korsakoff's syndrome.

    b. Pancreatitis.

    c. Inadequate circulation to his extremities.

    d. Peripheral polyneuropathy.

13. Tim, age 31, is to be discharged soon after successfully withdrawing from drugs. He found a part-time job as a dispatcher and has been accepted into a half-way house. He has made good progress on the unit, changed a lot of his old patterns, and has been supportive of his peers. He reports to the nursing station at midnight saying, "I'm having a really bad flashback." Your most therapeutic response would be:

    a. "Tim, I'll be right with you as soon as report is over."

    b. "I'll get you a _____ (antipsychotic) and a sleeping pill."

    c. "Feel free to pace the halls, Tim. It will pass."

    d. "What are you experiencing, Tim?"

14. Sarah Simmons, age 18, has just been admitted to your unit. She has been on high doses of nembutal, a barbiturate, for the last 20 days. She has had none since yesterday morning. The most appropriate nursing intervention would be:

    a. Administer barbiturates as ordered.

    b. Take her into the day room and introduce her to others.

    c. Monitor her knowledge of drug abuse.

    d. Suggest sleep.

Instructor's Guide

ANSWER KEY

1. c
2. a
3. d
4. b
5. b
6. d
7. d
8. a
9. a
10. c
11. a
12. d
13. d
14. a

Module II.5

BIBLIOGRAPHY

MODULE II.5 NURSING CARE IN WITHDRAWAL

Alpert, M. A. (1990). Modern management of delirium tremens. *Hospital Medicine*, 111–136.

American Nurses' Association, & National Nurses Society on Addictions. (1988). *Standards of addiction nursing practice with selected diagnoses and criteria.* Kansas City, MO: ANA.

American Nurses' Association. (1982, December). The hospitalized alcoholic (programmed instruction). *American Journal of Nursing, 82,* 1861–1879.

American Psychiatric Association. (1987). *DSM-IIIR.* Washington, DC: Author.

Bissell, L. (1971). *Guidelines to management of alcohol withdrawal.* New York: National Council on Alcoholism.

Bluhm, J. (1981, February). When you face the alcoholic patient. *Nursing, 81,* 71–73.

Brower, K. J., & Paredes, A. (1987). Cocaine withdrawal. *Archives of General Psychiatry, 44,* 297–298.

Busby, H. C., & Sieffort, W. (1982). Acute gastrointestinal bleeding. In C. M. Hudak, B. Gallo, & J. Benz (Eds.), *Critical care nursing* (3rd ed.). Philadelphia: J. B. Lippincott.

Busto, V., Sellers, E. M., Naranjo, C. A., Cappell, H., et al. (1986). Withdrawal reaction after long-term therapeutic use of benzodiazepines. *New England Journal of Medicine, 315,* 854–859.

Charney, D. S., Riordan, E. E., Kleber, H. D., et al. (1982). Clonidine and naltrexone: A safe, effective and rapid treatment of abrupt withdrawal from methadone therapy. *Archives of General Psychiatry, 39,* 1327–1332.

Choy-Kwong, M., & Lipton, R. B. (1989). Dystonia related to cocaine withdrawal. *Neurology, 39,* 996–997.

Cushman, P. (1987). Delirium tremens: Update on an old disorder. *Postgraduate Medicine, 82*(5), 117–122.

Daghestani, A. N. (1987). Alcohol withdrawal: A comprehensive approach to treatment. *Postgraduate Medicine, 81*(6), 111–118.

Estes, N., & Heinemann, E. (1982). *Alcoholism, development, consequences, and intervention.* St. Louis, MO: C. V. Mosby.

Gallant, D. M. (1989). Treatment of organic mental disorders. In American Psychiatric Association, *Treatments of psychiatric disorders, Volume 2* (pp. 1076–1093). Washington, DC: Author.

Gawin, F. H., & Ellinwood, E. H. (1989). Stimulants. In American Psychiatric Association, *Treatments of psychiatric disorders, Volume 2* (pp. 1218–1240). Washington, DC: Author.

Gawin, F. H., & Kleber, H. D. (1986). Abstinence symptomatology and psychiatric diagnosis in cocaine abusers. *Archives of General Psychiatry, 43*, 107–113.

Giannini, A. J. (1982). *Handbook of overdose and detoxification emergencies.* New Hyde Park, NY: Medical Examination Publication.

Gottheil, E., McLellam, T., & Druley, K. (1981). *Matching patient needs and treatment methods in alcoholism and drug abuse.* Springfield, IL: Charles C. Thomas.

Greenblatt, D. J., & Shader, R. I. (1975). Treatment of the alcohol withdrawal syndrome. In R. I. Shader (Ed.), *Manual of psychiatric therapeutics: Practical psychopharmacology and psychiatry.* Boston: Little Brown.

Henningfield, J. (1984). Pharmacologic basis and treatment of cigarette smoking. *Journal of Clinical Psychiatry, 45*(12, pt. 2), 24–34.

Hoff, L. A. (1984). *People in crisis: Understanding and helping.* New York: Addison-Wesley.

Jaffe, J. H., & Kleber, H. D. (1989). Opioids: General issues and detoxification. In American Psychiatric Association, *Treatments of psychiatric disorders, Volume 2* (pp. 1309–1331). Washington, DC: Author.

Kelly, F. M. (1986). Caring for the patient in acute alcohol withdrawal. *Critical Care Quarterly, 8*(4), 11–19.

Khantzian, E. J., & McKenna, G. J. (1979). Acute toxic and withdrawal reactions associated with drug use and abuse. *Annals of Internal Medicine, 90*, 361–372.

McManus, M. E., & Moisan, D. (1982). Drug and poison overdose. In C. M. Hudak, B. Gallo, & J. Benz (Eds.), *Critical care nursing* (3rd ed.). Philadelphia: J. B. Lippincott.

Nademanee, K., et al. (1989). Myocardial ischemia during cocaine withdrawal. *Annals of Internal Medicine, 111*, 876–880.

National Nurses' Society on Addictions. (1989). *Nursing care planning with the addicted client, Volume I.* Skokie, IL: Author.

O'Brien, R., & Cohen, S. (Eds.). (1984). *The encyclopedia of drug abuse.* New York: Facts on File, Inc.

Pike, R. F. (1989). Cocaine withdrawal. *Postgraduate Medicine, 85*(4), 115–121.

Rounsaville, B. J. (1989). Clinical assessment of drug abusers. In American Psychiatric Association, *Treatments of psychiatric disorders, Volume 2* (pp. 1183–1191). Washington, DC: Author.

Roy-Byrne, P. P., & Hommer, D. (1988). Benzodiazepine withdrawal: Overview and implications for the treatment of anxiety. *American Journal of Medicine, 84*, 1041–1052.

Schenck, E. (1987). Substance abuse. In W. Phipps, B. Long, & N. Woods (Eds.), *Medical-Surgical nursing: Concepts and practices.* St. Louis, MO: C. V. Mosby.

Schloemer, N. F., & Skidmore, J. W. (1983). Opiate withdrawal with clonidine. *Journal of Psychosocial Nursing and Mental Health Services, 21*(10), 8–14.

Module II.5

Sheehy, S. B., & Sheehy, B. J. (1986). *Emergency nursing: Principles and practice.* St. Louis, MO: C. V. Mosby.

Smith, D. E., Landry, M. J., & Wesson, D. R. (1989). Barbiturate, sedative, hypnotic agents. In American Psychiatric Association, *Treatments of psychiatric disorders, Volume 2* (pp. 1294–1308). Washington, DC: Author.

Stuart, G. W., & Sundeen, S. J. (Eds.). (1987). *Principles and practice of psychiatric nursing* (pp. 616–648). St. Louis, MO: C. V. Mosby.

MODULE II.6
DRUG MISUSE AND DEPENDENCE IN THE ELDERLY

Gean Mathwig, PhD, RN
Janet S. D'Arcangelo, MA, RN, C

Madeline A. Naegle, PhD, RN, FAAN
Project Director
Janet S. D'Arcangelo, MA, RN, C
Project Coordinator

Project SAEN
SUBSTANCE ABUSE
EDUCATION IN NURSING

CONTENT OUTLINE

I. Drug and Alcohol Use in Elderly Populations
    A. Commonly Held Attitudes among Elderly (65+) Clients Regarding Medication, Alcohol, and Other Drug Use
    B. Attitudes of Health Care Providers about Elders' Drug Use/Abuse
    C. Health Care Practices in Prescribing and Drug Administration Which Influence Drug Use in Elderly Clients
    D. Patterns of Drug Use, Misuse, and Dependence in Elderly Clients
        1. Definitions
        2. Differentiating patterns of use, abuse, misuse, and dependence
            a. Over-the-counter medication
            b. Prescription drugs
            c. Alcohol
            d. Other drugs
            e. Drug interactions
        3. Epidemiology
        4. Other patterns characteristic of drug use among the elderly

II. Patterns of Aging Which Influence Drug Effects
    A. Psychological Patterns
    B. Physiological Patterns

III. The Impact of Drug and Alcohol Use on the Health of the Elderly Client
    A. Behavioral Signs and Symptoms Secondary to Drug Abuse
    B. Health Problems Associated with Alcohol and Drug Misuse and Dependence

IV. Nursing Interventions to Address Alcohol and Drug Use Patterns
    A. Rapport
    B. Self-Assessment of Attitude and Values about the Elderly

Module II.6

C. Client Assessment
D. Develop an Individualized Plan of Care
E. Interventions Targeted at Specific Levels of Alcohol/Drug Use
   1. Active alcoholism
   2. Acute alterations in physical states, thought processes, or functional abilities
   3. Risk control among the elderly
   4. Health teaching of clients as primary prevention of alcohol and drug problems
   5. Health teaching of health care providers as primary prevention
F. Intervention with Family System
G. Intervention with Community System

Drug Misuse and Dependence in the Elderly

CONTENTS

I. DRUG AND ALCOHOL USE IN ELDERLY POPULATIONS

A. Commonly Held Attitudes Among Elderly (65+) Clients Regarding Medication, Alcohol, and Other Drug Use

1. Attitudes and personal feelings of the patient/client about medication will influence the individual's use.
2. There may be preferences for specific remedies on the part of the elderly.
3. Some clients believe that there is a drug to cure or control every ailment.
4. Fear of dependency: Some clients resist the loss of control that they perceive a medical regimen imposes on them.

B. Attitudes of Health Care Providers about Elders' Drug Use/Abuse

1. General lack of interest in health care for the elderly; consequently, problems are neither studied nor addressed in clinical settings.
2. Attitudes on the parts of physicians and nurses that the elderly have only a limited time left may support prescribing practices.
3. Negative public and health professional attitudes toward the elderly alcoholic compromise access to services.
4. General biases regarding the elderly.
5. Caregivers who are accustomed to the acute illness model may foster the notion of cure or attempt to achieve an unrealistic relief from the normal aging process.
6. Adopting standards of care dictated by reimbursement sources. For example, drugs may be a "covered" expense but not other therapies which provide non-medicated symptom control, such as psychotherapy, physical therapy, or nutritional counseling.

C. Health Care Practices in Prescribing and Drug Administration Which Influence Drug Use in Elderly Clients

1. Use of two or more pharmacies and medication prescriptions by two or more physicians are significantly associated with drug misuse (Raffoul, Cooper, & Love, 1981).
2. Behavioral problems associated with cognitive declines may evoke efforts to over-medicate the elderly in an attempt to control behavior.
3. Economic factors, including the ability to purchase medication, may be important determinants of medication use.
4. Miscommunication between the caregiver and the patient can result in misuse. For example, an error or misunderstanding in history-taking could result in treating side effects of one drug with a second drug. Side effects often mimic a disease process.

5. Patterns of socialization may aggravate tendencies to consume alcohol or support medication misuse in the elder client; e.g., sharing or trading medications with friends.

D. Patterns of Drug Use, Misuse, and Dependence in Elderly Clients

1. Definitions.
   a. Psychoactive drug abuse: A maladaptive pattern of alcohol or other drug abuse indicated by continued use, despite knowledge of persistent or recurrent social, occupational, psychological, or physical problems caused or exacerbated by use of the substance, and/or symptoms persisting for at least one month.
   b. Psychoactive substance dependence:
      (1) Use of a substance in increasing amounts or over a longer period than intended.
      (2) A persistent desire for one or more unsuccessful attempts to cut down on or control substance use.
      (3) A great deal of time spent using the substance.
      (4) Frequent intoxication or withdrawal symptoms.
      (5) Reduction or giving up of activities.
      (6) Continued use despite knowledge of recurrent, associated problems.
      (7) A marked tolerance for the substance.
      (8) Characteristic withdrawal symptoms and use of the substance to relieve or avoid withdrawal symptoms (modified from APA, 1987).
   c. Abuse/Misuse patterns of drugs can also be categorized in these three ways (Ellor & Kurz, 1982):
      (1) Overuse (intentional or accidental) resulting in an overdosage or too high levels of medication.
      (2) Underuse as a result of forgetfulness or by choice.
      (3) Erratic use, which incorporates elements of the other two; i.e., omitting one dose, compensating by taking two.
2. Differentiating patterns of use, abuse, misuse, and dependence.
   a. Over-the-Counter (OTC) medications:
      (1) This category of drugs is used more frequently by the elderly than by any other age group, both on a regular and a p.r.n. basis.
      (2) The most common OTC medications are analgesics, antidiarrheal/laxatives, vitamins/minerals/iron, antacids, cough/cold formulas, emetics/anti-emetics, hemorrhoidal, and ophthalmic/otic preparations.
      (3) These drugs may have significant alcohol, sodium, and sugar content.
   b. Prescription drugs:
      (1) Multiple chronic pathologies result in polypharmacy. Polypharmacy increases risk of adverse reactions; errors or drug patient confusion are increased.

(2) Evaluation for renewal or discontinuation of use may lack coordination due to multiple caregivers.

(3) The elderly use three times as many prescription drugs as all other groups combined (Hanan, 1978).

c. Alcohol:

(1) Variations and longevity in lifestyle affect definition of pattern of use as abusive.

(2) Proper use is characterized by controlled consumption in therapeutic, social, or recreational settings according to learned habits of moderation and safety, which results in minimal or no adverse medical or social consequences (Staab & Lyles, 1989).

d. Other drugs:

(1) Illicit drugs are not commonly used by older persons. Opioids are the most frequently used by people who manage to survive through addictions established early in life. Much of this population is among criminals. The percentage of clients over 60 in methadone programs is increasing.

(2) Caffeine is used daily by a majority of elderly people.

(3) Nicotine ingestion through cigarette smoking decreases with age.

e. Drug interactions:

(1) Physiological age changes and multiple chronic conditions contribute to polypharmacy.

(2) Complete and updated medication history should be done more frequently in this age group.

(3) Patterns of alcohol and dietary intake are usually well-established, and the ability to engage in new learning may be diminished. These factors must be considered in planning the nature of education and monitoring schedules.

(4) Interdisciplinary collaboration facilitates consistency of observations and reinforcement of new routines.

(5) There is a similarity between drug interaction symptoms and symptoms of old age; e.g., forgetfulness, weakness, anxiety.

3. Epidemiology.

a. The prevalence of alcohol abuse dependence or misuse peaks between ages 35–50 but affects 2.2% of individuals between ages 65–74, and 1.2% of those over 75 (Mezey, 1985).

b. In specific situations, alcoholism affects the elderly at higher rates.

(1) Prevalence among elderly on medical wards is 10%.

(2) Prevalence among elderly in nursing homes is 20%.

(3) Prevalence among elderly in psychiatric hospitals is 28–50%.

c. Factors affecting determination of prevalence rates:

(1) Lack of consensus among agencies/institutions about criteria for diagnosis of alcoholism.

(2) Variable inclusion of inactive cases with those demonstrating current alcohol problems (Lawson, 1989).

 d. Elderly alcoholics fall into two categories:

  (1) Those who developed alcoholism before age 40 but, despite reduced intake, present with residual complications.

  (2) Individuals with light to moderate intake early in life who develop severe alcohol problems after age 50.

 e. Non-prescription or over-the-counter preparations most frequently used and misused are analgesics, antacids, laxatives, and sedatives.

 f. Elderly clients abuse and misuse psychotherapeutic drugs, including anxiolytics, sedatives, hypnotics, and analgesics.

 g. The narcotic to which the older client most frequently becomes addicted is Dilaudid.

4. Other patterns characteristic of drug use among the elderly.

 a. Alcoholism in the elderly can also be categorized according to onset:

  (1) Reactive alcoholics, for example, are individuals who had no history of excessive drinking and then drift into drinking in response to the experience of aging.

  (2) Chronic alcoholics, on the other hand, are individuals who have always been heavy drinkers who then continue to drink, or decrease their drinking, before old age (Rosin & Glatt, 1971).

 b. Elderly individuals are more likely to misuse drugs and be "at risk" for drug misuse than any other group. The high percentage of drugs prescribed for them, characteristics of aging, and cultural and social patterns interact to influence drug-taking.

 c. Manifestations of alcoholism in the elderly include more daily drinking, shorter time periods of consumption, symptoms apparent at a lower dose, and a decreased predictability between the volume and frequency of alcohol consumption and alcohol dependence.

II. PATTERNS OF AGING WHICH INFLUENCE DRUG EFFECTS

A. Psychological Patterns

1. The losses associated with aging require adjustment. These include loss of friends and spouse to death, retirement, relocation to new communities, loss of a lifestyle as a function of economic constraints, and loss of health.

2. Maladaptive drug-using patterns may emerge in attempts to cope with perceived life stresses.

3. Responses to changes in the older person's life are often feelings of sadness, depression, and anxiety.

4. Social stigma associated with aging, estrangement from family members, and economic stress create psychological burdens for many elderly people.

Drug Misuse and Dependence in the Elderly

5. Declines in intellectual and problem-solving difficulties impact on self-concept as well as on overall function.
6. Role changes create the need for adaptation and increase the potential for role strain.

B. Physiological Patterns

The physiology of aging results in changes which influence the response by older persons to drugs and their impact on health.

1. The central nervous system of the older individual is increasingly sensitive to the depressant effects of alcohol.
2. Higher peak levels of alcohol occur in the older person although intake of an amount of the drug is the same as in a younger person.
3. Decreased food intake characteristic of the elderly individual, in combination with alcohol, is more likely to result in malnutrition.
4. The adverse effects of the interaction of alcohol with other drugs are increased in the aged.
5. Ethanol may accelerate or inhibit the metabolism of other drugs.
6. When taken with alcohol, sedative hypnotic drugs, minor tranquilizers, and central nervous system depressants have additive and/or synergistic effects to which the aged person is particularly sensitive.
7. Decreased activity due to sight and hearing loss, altered fine and gross motor coordination, existing and drug-induced memory impairment, and pre-existing chronic pathology contribute to changes in drug effects.
8. Impaired drug absorption may occur due to altered gastric PH, decreased intestinal motility, reduced blood circulation, and declining metabolic and excretion rates.
9. Diminishing changes in the functional neuronal tissue of the brain, as well as age-related changes in receptor sites, contribute to increased CNS sensitivity.
10. Overall decrease in levels of physiological reserve in response to stresses of illness.

III. THE IMPACT OF DRUG AND ALCOHOL USE ON THE HEALTH OF THE ELDERLY CLIENT

A. Behavioral Signs and Symptoms Secondary to Drug Abuse

1. The interaction of physiological, psychological, and drug effects results in behavioral patterns particular to the elder individual. These include both acute and chronic responses to drug intake.
2. Drug-induced memory deficits may precipitate drug misuse.
3. Social problems and legal entanglements secondary to intoxication may occur.
4. Financial problems can result due to impaired judgment.

5. Confusion, disorientation and memory loss are direct effects of alcohol abuse, drug misuse, and normal aging; overlapping causes are problematic.

6. Disturbed motor functions result from drug interactions.

7. Isolation and withdrawal from usual activities may occur.

B. Health Problems Associated with Alcohol and Drug Misuse and Dependence

1. Osteoporosis results when calcium absorption is impaired by alcohol intake and malnutrition.

2. Alcohol interacting with other medications may lead to the following negative effects:

   a. Interaction with anticoagulants.

   b. Hypotension when taken with antihypertensives.

   c. GI bleeding when taken with aspirin.

   d. Hypotension when taken with antidiabetics, including insulin.

   e. Hypertensive response with monoamine oxidase inhibiting antidepressants.

   f. Interaction with nitroglycerine to cause hypotension.

   g. Potentiates CNS depressant effects when taken with sedatives, barbiturates, and minor tranquilizers.

3. Short-term effects of alcohol use include slowed wound healing, erectile dysfunction, gastrointestinal bleeding, insomnia, fluid and electrolyte imbalance, and myopathy.

4. Long-term alcohol dependence is associated with congestive heart failure, pneumonia, feminization syndrome in men, pancreatitis, peripheral neuropathy, hepatitis, cirrhosis, Wernicke's encephalopathy, and Korsakoff's syndrome.

5. Drug misuse, even in the absence of alcoholism, affects the established predictability of pharmacokinetic parameters for the elderly. Absorption, distribution metabolism, and excretion are altered by interactions and improper use.

6. Vitamin deficiencies are sometimes directly or indirectly caused by prescription medications and OTC drugs. For example, Digotrim induces thiamin deficiency; Estrogen induces deficiencies in folic acid, riboflavin, thiamin, and vitamins B_6, B_{12}, and C. Ingestion of mineral oil produces a physical barrier to all fat soluble vitamins (Ebersole & Hess, 1990).

IV. NURSING INTERVENTIONS TO ADDRESS ALCOHOL AND DRUG USE PATTERNS

A. Rapport

1. Develop a nurse-patient relationship characterized by trust, advocacy behaviors on the part of the nurse, and when possible, continuity of the same caregivers over time.

Drug Misuse and Dependence in the Elderly

B. **Self-Assessment of Attitudes and Values about the Elderly**

   1. Understanding the characteristics and limitations of the elderly, and a belief that the elderly are valuable and able to change, are important components which the nurse brings to the interaction.

C. **Client Assessment**

   1. Evaluate the medical history with special attention to drug use.
   2. Obtain a detailed history of past and present drug use, including alcohol, coffee, tea, vitamins, tobacco.
   3. Obtain a history of past and present experiences of loss.
   4. Identify patterns of adaptation and coping.
   5. Include an account of a typical day in the life of the older person.
   6. Identify collateral services (family, friends) in reference to drug and alcohol use by the older person.
   7. Identify sources of social support for the elderly.
      a. Involvement with clubs and religious groups.
      b. Networks of family and friends.
      c. Attitudes toward religion.
      d. Involvement with community agencies.

D. **Develop an Individualized Plan of Care**
E. **Interventions Targeted at Specific Levels of Alcohol/Drug Use**

   1. Active alcoholism.
      a. Recognize alcoholism as a separate chronic illness.
      b. Treat elderly in places that they already are frequenting, such as senior centers.
      c. Use therapies that have been helpful with the elderly: socialization, group work with age-related peers (Lawson, 1989).
      d. Incorporate treatment that considers alleviating some of the environmental stress to which the elderly react with alcohol or other drug abuse. Survival needs of food and shelter must be adequately met first.
      e. Make home visits for the advantage of getting direct assessment data.
   2. Acute alterations in physical states, thought processes, or functional abilities.
      a. A problem with medications must be considered as a possible etiology in the assessment of any disturbances. If not, it is possible that the administration of additional medication and/or the stress of a hospitalization will complicate the existing condition.
      b. Medication intake history up to two weeks prior to presenting symptoms should be taken, including reasons for discontinuing, since excretion time varies.

Module II.6

    c. When memory is affected, obtain from the individual or other person any prescribed and OTC medications that appear to be currently in use by the patient. A paper bag of these items can yield much relevant data (Ebersole & Hess, 1990).

3. Risk control among the elderly.
   a. Frequent, thorough review of medical regimens and monitoring of medication schedules to reduce risks of over-medication, drug interaction, and drug misuse.
   b. Personal rather than telephone contact with client.
   c. Direct communication among providers: doctor, nurse, pharmacist, and personal/family caregivers.
   d. Regular monitoring of changes in patterns and activities of daily living in order to mitigate stress reactions.

4. Health teaching of clients as primary prevention of alcohol and drug problems.
   a. General principles of patient education relevant to drug and alcohol use (Staab & Lyles, 1989):
      (1) Explain expected effects, possible side effects, and storage requirements of prescribed and OTC medications.
      (2) Ask patients to relate to you what they know about the drugs they are taking, both prescription and non-prescription.
      (3) Be certain that patients understand the treatment program, including the importance of non-drug therapy.
      (4) Choose a suitable memory aid and explain its use to the patient. Color coding or use of an egg carton may be needed for illiterate patients or the visually impaired.
      (5) Suggest that the patient use only one pharmacy. Many pharmacies now maintain computer medication profiles on their customers and may provide helpful information on drug interactions.
      (6) Discourage self-medication.
      (7) Advise patients not to drink alcohol if and when they use drugs.
   b. Principles of consumer advocacy to foster self-management of health care and prevent drug misuse.
      (1) Teach patient consumer rights.
      (2) Assist patient in identifying, remembering, and communicating concerns. A list of questions, a daily log, or notations on a drug calendar are common aids to bring to provider visits.

5. Health teaching of health care providers as primary prevention:
   a. Regarding the disease concept of dependency.
   b. In order to decrease the stigma associated with alcoholism in the elderly client.
   c. In more prudent prescribing practice and case management for monitoring of drug treatment.

Drug Misuse and Dependence in the Elderly

   d. On the need to adequately evaluate emergency states and episodes of illness in relation to toxic or adverse effects, and especially with signs of dementia and confusion.

   e. On the risk for development of dependence, danger of extended use, scope of side effects, and dangers of prescribing drugs in combination.

F. Intervention with Family System: Work with Client and Family to:

1. Develop a system to remind the individual about what drugs should be taken and when.
2. Engage family members in the provision of information, monitoring, and assistance.
3. Identify attitudes and values about medication and drug use.
4. Inform family members of available support systems and treatment modalities.

G. Intervention with Community System: Develop Community Resources to:

1. Educate health care professionals employed in all varieties of health care agencies.
2. Organize and implement information and education on drugs and the elderly.
3. Encourage agencies to utilize interviewing and assessment for screening elderly populations for problems.
4. Establish telephone hot lines as sources for referral and information.
5. Organize media and community campaigns promoting drug-free living.

MODULE II.6
DRUG MISUSE AND DEPENDENCE IN THE ELDERLY

INSTRUCTOR'S GUIDE

Gean Mathwig, PhD, RN
Janet S. D'Arcangelo, MA, RN, C

Madeline A. Naegle, PhD, RN, FAAN
Project Director
Janet S. D'Arcangelo, MA, RN, C
Project Coordinator

Project SAEN
SUBSTANCE ABUSE
EDUCATION IN NURSING

CONTENTS

Component	Page
Module Description	480
Time Frame	480
Placement	480
Learner Objectives	481
Recommended Readings	482
Faculty Readings	482
Student Readings	482
Recommended Audiovisual and Other Resources	483
Overhead Masters	485
Handout Masters	513
Recommended Teaching Strategies and Sample Assignments	521
Test Questions and Answers	523
Bibliography	527

Module II.6

MODULE DESCRIPTION

This module assists the student in identifying common drug-using patterns of elderly clients. Patterns of misuse of prescription drugs, over-the-counter drugs, and alcohol will be described. Attitudes and behaviors specific to the older client will be emphasized, as well as physiological characteristics which potentiate drug effects. The influence of life patterns common to the older client will be discussed, and the formulation of nursing interventions described.

TIME FRAME

2 hours

PLACEMENT

Adult Health, Community Health, Psychiatric-Mental Health Nursing, Gerontological Nursing

Instructor's Guide

LEARNER OBJECTIVES

Upon successful completion of this module, the learner will:

1. Describe attitudes and factors which influence drug use in the elderly.
2. Describe patterns of drinking, drug misuse, and drug abuse common to older clients.
3. Describe problems of over-reliance on medication observed in institutionalized and community-based elderly clients.
4. Identify physiological and psychological patterns of aging which differentiate therapeutic outcomes from dysfunctional drug use.
5. List behavioral effects observed in elderly clients who are alcohol- or drug-dependent.
6. Identify health problems of the elderly associated with drug and alcohol use.
7. Formulate nursing interventions related to drug and alcohol use in groups of the elderly.

Module II.6

RECOMMENDED READINGS

FACULTY READINGS

Brogatta, E. F., Montgomery, R. J. V., & Brogatta, M. L. (1982). Alcohol use and abuse: Life crisis events and the elderly. *Research in Aging, 4,* 378–408.

Lasker, M. N. (1986). Aging alcoholics need nursing help. *Journal of Gerontological Nursing, 12*(1), 16–19.

Norwark, C. A. (1985). Life events and drinking behavior in later years. In E. Gottheil, K. A. Druley, T. E. Skoida, & H. M. Waxman (Eds.), *The combined problems of alcoholism, drug addiction and aging* (pp. 37–50). Springfield, IL: Charles Thomas.

Stall, R. (1987). Research issues concerning alcohol consumption among aging populations. *Drug and Alcohol Dependence, 19*(3), 195–213.

STUDENT READINGS

Caroselli-Karinja, M. (1985). Drug abuse and the elderly. *Journal of Psychosocial Nursing and Mental Health Services, 23*(6), 25–30.

Ellor, J. K., & Kurz, D. J. (1982). Misuse and abuse of prescription drugs by the elderly. *Nursing Clinics of North America, 17,* 319–330.

Felker, M. P. (1988). A recovery group for elderly alcoholics. *Geriatric Nursing, 9*(2), 110–113.

Goodwin, J. S., Sanchez, C. J., Thomas, P., Hunt, C., Garry, P. J., & Goodwin, J. M. (1987). Alcohol intake in a healthy elderly population. *American Journal of Public Health, 77*(2), 173–177.

Gulino, C., & Kadin, M. (1986). Aging and reactive alcoholism. *Geriatric Nursing, 7*(3), 148–151.

RECOMMENDED AUDIOVISUAL AND OTHER RESOURCES

AUDIOVISUAL RESOURCES

Drug Issues

1. **Aging: The Losses**

   Covers losses of family and friends, changed lifestyles, and economic and role adjustments. 30 minutes. **Available from the American Journal of Nursing Company, Educational Services Division, 555 West 57th Street, New York, New York 10019-2961. Phone: 1-800-223-2282 or (212) 582-8820.** #4063, film rental ($60) or purchase ($350); Videocassette rental ($60) or purchase ($250).

2. **Medicating the Elderly**

   Problems specific to drug use and misuse in the elderly; includes physiological aspects of aging and its therapeutic implications. 28 minutes. **Available from the American Journal of Nursing Company, Educational Services Division, 555 West 57th Street, New York, New York 10019-2961. Phone: 1-800-223-2282 or (212) 582-8820.** #7508, videocassette rental ($60) or purchase ($275).

3. **Medications: A Prescription for Health**

   Dramatizes how two elderly patients work with their pharmacist and physician to manage the multiple medications they take and avoid medication-related problems. This videotape will help educate elderly patients about the following: how to prepare for visits to the health care provider, the potential problems associated with multiple drug use, and how to make it easier to comply with drug therapy. 13 minutes. **Available from Health Sciences Consortium, 201 Silver Cedar Court, Chapel Hill, North Carolina 27514. Phone: (919) 942-8731.** VHS #R851-VI-069, purchase ($195).

4. **The Medicated Generation**

   Reviewed in *The Gerontologist,* 25(1), 1985. 28 minutes. **Available from Video Services (distributor), University of Maryland, Department of Physical Therapy, 32 South Green Street, Baltimore, Maryland 21201, (301) 528-7720.** ½″ VHS, rental ($75), sale ($300).

Module II.6

Alcoholism Issues

1. **Alcohol, Drugs, and Seniors: Tarnished Dreams**

   Dramatic case history vignettes illustrate that nowhere is the abuse and misuse of alcohol and drugs more cruelly felt than among older adults. The film shows how alcohol and drugs make it difficult for seniors to deal effectively with the everyday stresses and strains of life. It teaches that the risk of accident and illness is increased, and life expectancy is shortened by as much as fifteen years. The several major warning signs of addiction are shown, and suggestions are given that will help seniors obtain professional assistance. 23 minutes. **Available from AIMS Media, Inc., 6901 Woodley Avenue, Van Nuys, California 91406-4878. Phone: 1-800-267-2467 or (818) 785-4111. #9864, rental ($75) or purchase ($395).**

2. **Seniors and Alcohol Abuse**

   An examination of the subtleties and complexities in the lives of those who are no longer in the work force and are therefore frequently isolated from society. This video graphically portrays the pain of aging coupled with addiction. 23 minutes. **Available from FMS Productions, P.O. Box 4428, 520 East Montecito Street, Suite F, Santa Barbara, California 93140. Rental ($50) or purchase ($450). Also available from the New York State Council on Alcoholism, Film Library, 155 Washington Avenue, Albany, New York 12210. Phone: (518) 432-8281 or 1-800-252-2557.**

3. **Senior Adults, Traffic Safety and Alcohol**

   This video is part of the AAA series. It is an imaginative, animated film designed for presentation to senior adult groups to help them put alcohol in perspective— to assess the genuine good times that can go along with drinking against the consequences of drinking too much to drive or walk safely home in traffic. 11 minutes. **Available from the New York State Council on Alcoholism, Film Library, 155 Washington Avenue, Albany, New York 12210. Phone: (518) 432-8281 or 1-800-252-2557.**

4. **The Older Adult Alcoholic—Feelings Shared**

   Seniors tell their stories of how and when their use of alcohol began, the effect that their use of alcohol had on them and on others, and how they turned their lives around through treatment and self-help groups. **Available from the New York State Council on Alcoholism, Film Library, 155 Washington Avenue, Albany, New York 12210. Phone: (518) 432-8281 or 1-800-252-2557.**

Instructor's Guide

OVERHEAD MASTERS

MODULE II.6   DRUG MISUSE AND DEPENDENCE IN THE ELDERLY

1. Who Becomes a Problem Drinker?
2. Prevalence of Alcohol Abuse, Dependence or Misuse
3. Psychological Patterns of Aging Which Influence Substance Use, Misuse and Dependence
4. Metabolic and Physiological Changes that Affect Drug Use in the Elderly
5. Common Medication Errors among the Elderly and Reported Problems with Taking Medications
6. Misuse of Prescription Drugs
7. Strategies to Improve Compliance with Prescribed Medication Schedules
8. Guidelines for Providers: General Prescribing Case Management Principles
9. Drugs and the Elderly: Practitioner Responsibility
10. Guidelines for Patients: General Principles of Patient Education Relevant to Drug and Alcohol Use
11. Guidelines for Patients: Sample Questions About Medicines
12. Consumer Rights Relative to Medications
13. Community Resources to Address Drug Misuse in the Elderly

Instructor's Guide

Module II.6—Overhead #1

WHO BECOMES A PROBLEM DRINKER?

In old age, problem drinkers seem to be of two types.

1. The first are chronic abusers, those who have used alcohol heavily throughout life. Although most chronic abusers die by middle age, some survive into old age. Approximately two-thirds of older alcoholics are in this group.

2. The second type begins excessive drinking late in life, often in response to "situational" factors—retirement, lowered income, declining health, and the deaths of friends and loved ones. In these cases, alcohol is first used for temporary relief but later becomes a problem.

From: National Institute on Aging. (1983, November). *Age page: Aging and alcohol abuse* (Public Health Service Publication No. 1983-418-427). Washington, DC: U.S. Government Printing Office.

Module II.6—Overhead #2

PREVALENCE OF ALCOHOL ABUSE, DEPENDENCE OR MISUSE (MEZEY, 1985)

1. Peaks between ages 35–50.
2. Affects 2.2% of individuals 65–74 years of age.
3. Affects 1.2% of those over 75.

SELECTED INSTITUTIONAL PREVALENCE OF ALCOHOL ABUSE, DEPENDENCE, AND MISUSE

1. Prevalence among elderly on medical wards is 10%.
2. Prevalence among elderly in nursing homes is 20%.
3. Prevalence among elderly in psychiatric hospitals is 28–50%.

FACTORS AFFECTING PREVALENCE RATES IN INSTITUTIONS (LAWSON, 1989)

1. Lack of consensus among agencies/institutions about criteria for diagnosis of alcoholism.
2. Variable inclusion of inactive cases with those demonstrating current alcohol problems.

Module II.6—Overhead #3

PSYCHOLOGICAL PATTERNS OF AGING WHICH INFLUENCE SUBSTANCE USE, MISUSE, AND DEPENDENCE

1. Losses in multiple dimensions of life.
2. Reduction of available coping strategies to deal with stresses.
3. Characteristic responses of sadness, depression, and anxiety regarding life changes.
4. Social stigma of aging process, family estrangement, and declining financial resources.
5. Decreased self-esteem and direct overall function due to cognitive declines.
6. Shifting of roles, role strains.

The psychological patterns described above may affect selection of alcohol and other substances for symptoms relief. They may also affect motivation and abilities to manage self-care.

Module II.6—Overhead #4

METABOLIC AND PHYSIOLOGICAL CHANGES THAT AFFECT DRUG USE IN THE ELDERLY

1. Deterioration of organs and enzyme systems.
2. Presence of multiple diseases.
3. Undernutrition.
4. Changes in GI tract.
5. Less body water and lean body mass.
6. Less efficient renal excretion.
7. Diminished capacity to metabolize drugs.
8. Decreased liver function and hepatic blood flow.
9. Increased sensitivity of central nervous system.
10. Drug sensitivity altered by disease.
11. Impaired homeostatic mechanisms.

The metabolic and physiological changes described above determine expected effects of drugs but also cause unexpected effects when combined with alcohol or when monitored improperly.

From: Commonwealth of Pennsylvania, Department of Aging. (1986). *Drug use and the elderly: A training program* (Document #T-19). Erie, PA: Keystone University Research Corporation.

Module II.6—Overhead #5

COMMON MEDICATION ERRORS AMONG THE ELDERLY AND REPORTED PROBLEMS WITH TAKING MEDICATIONS

A. Medication Errors.
   1. Errors in omission.
   2. Inappropriate self-medication.
   3. Incorrect dosage.
   4. Improper timing.
   5. Incorrect knowledge of purpose of drugs and lack of knowledge about side effects.

B. Problems with Taking Medications.

Trouble taking at nighttime	8.0%
Trouble remembering	22.9%
Trouble opening bottle	36.5%
Trouble separating or breaking tabs	4.6%
Trouble mixing or preparing medication	1.1%
Trouble keeping adequate supply	6.2%
Trouble reading label	9.0%
Taking more or less than label says	4.3%
Medications look alike	1.1%
Other	2.3%

From: National Institute on Drug Abuse. (1982). *Drug-taking among the elderly.* Washington, DC: Author.

Instructor's Guide

Module II.6—Overhead #6

MISUSE OF PRESCRIPTION DRUGS

A person is considered to be misusing medicine when he or she:

1. Does not know its name or why it was prescribed.
2. Does not know how or when to take it to make it most effective.
3. Forgets to take it.
4. Forgets to take it one time and doubles the dosage the next time.
5. Takes doses at improper time.
6. Does not recognize side effects.
7. Discontinues it without notifying the physician.
8. Stretches it to make it last longer than intended.
9. Seeks a refill long after the rational need for it has disappeared.
10. Saves old medicine for self-treatment at a later time.
11. Borrows or lends medicine.
12. Takes too much, thinking that if one dose is helpful, two would be even better.
13. Takes too much by taking duplicate medicines prescribed by two different physicians.
14. Mixes alcohol with such drugs as tranquilizers, barbiturates, and antihistamines.

From: Commonwealth of Pennsylvania, Department of Aging. (1986). *Drug use and the elderly: A training program* (Document #T-19). Erie, PA: Keystone University Research Corporation.

Module II.6—Overhead #7

STRATEGIES TO IMPROVE COMPLIANCE WITH PRESCRIBED MEDICATION SCHEDULES

1. Make drug regimens as simple as possible.
2. Instruct relatives and caregivers on the drug regimen.
3. Enlist others (e.g., home health aides, pharmacists) to help ensure compliance.
4. Make sure the elderly patient can get to a pharmacist (or vice versa), can afford the prescriptions, and can open the container.
5. Use aids (such as special pill boxes and drug calendars) whenever appropriate.
6. Keep updated medication records.
7. Review knowledge of, and compliance with, drug regimens regularly.

From: Kane, R., Ouslander, J., & Abrass, I. (1986). *Essentials of clinical geriatrics.* New York: McGraw Hill.

Module II.6—Overhead #8

GUIDELINES FOR PROVIDERS: GENERAL PRESCRIBING/CASE MANAGEMENT PRINCIPLES

1. Obtaining a complete medication history is critical. It must include all medications, including OTCs. Ask about allergies and intolerances.

2. Determine use of alcohol: history, frequencies.

3. Avoid using medications to treat non-specific complaints.

4. When treating a chronic disease, try to select drugs that will not diminish the quality of life. The effect of treatment must be clearly better than no treatment.

5. Chronic diseases can impair and exaggerate drug response. (For example, demented patients are disposed to exaggerated CNS side effects of drugs.) Alcoholism is considered a chronic condition.

6. Multiple pathology is the rule, so a priority order regarding treatment is essential.

7. The number of drugs administered concurrently must be kept to a minimum.

8. Stopping a drug may be more beneficial than starting one.

9. Know the pharmacology of each drug prescribed.

10. When dosing a drug, start low and go slow.

11. Use of serum drug levels is helpful in determining the appropriate dose of some medications.

12. Don't prescribe a drug without some consideration of the patient's social and economic resources and alternate treatment modalities.

13. Implement a regular mechanism for monitoring drug effects and changes in life events.

From: Staab, A., & Lyles, M. (1989). *Manual of geriatric nursing* (pp. 119–121). Glenview, IL: Scott, Foresman, & Company.

Module II.6—Overhead #9

DRUGS AND THE ELDERLY: PRACTITIONER RESPONSIBILITY

1. Help client obtain accurate drug information.
2. Encourage client to participate in treatment decisions.
3. Verify doctor appointments and drug regimen.
4. Assess client health practices and drug usage.
5. Coordinate drug treatment activities.
6. Provide drug education programs for clients, their families, and other practitioners.
7. Advocate better geriatric pharmacology.

From: Commonwealth of Pennsylvania, Department of Aging. (1986). *Drug use and the elderly: A training program* (Document #T-19). Erie, PA: Keystone University Research Corporation.

Module II.6—Overhead #10

GUIDELINES FOR PATIENTS: GENERAL PRINCIPLES OF PATIENT EDUCATION RELEVANT TO DRUG AND ALCOHOL USE

1. Explain expected effects, possible side effects, and storage requirements of prescribed and OTC medication.

2. Ask patients to relate to you what they know about the drugs they are taking, both prescription and non-prescription.

3. Be certain that patients understand the treatment program, including the importance of non-drug therapy.

4. Choose a suitable memory aid and explain its use to the patient. Color coding or use of an egg carton may be needed for illiterate patients or the visually impaired.

5. Suggest that the patient use only one pharmacy. Many pharmacies now maintain computer medication profiles on their customers and may provide helpful information on drug interactions, and so on.

6. Discourage self-medication.

7. Advise patients not to use drugs if they drink alcohol.

From: Staab, A., & Lyles, M. (1989). *Manual of geriatric nursing* (p. 119). Glenview, IL: Scott, Foresman, & Company.

Module II.6—Overhead #11

GUIDELINES FOR PATIENTS: SAMPLE QUESTIONS ABOUT MEDICINES

To be asked periodically about entire medication regimen and also whenever a medication is changed or a new one prescribed.

1. Is the drug needed? Are there any alternative non-drug treatments available?
2. What are the name and purpose of the drug?
3. How and when should it be taken?
4. How long should it be taken?
5. Can it be stopped when the symptoms disappear?
6. What should be done if a dose is missed?
7. Can it be taken with other drugs, including over-the-counter drugs and/or alcohol?
8. What possible effects or reactions are there?
9. Are there any side effects that should be reported immediately?
10. Are there any special precautions to be taken?
11. Can the prescription be refilled?
12. Is there a less expensive substitute which is as effective?

Instructor's Guide

Module II.6—Overhead #12

CONSUMER RIGHTS RELATIVE TO MEDICATIONS

1. **Right to Safety:**

   FDA is the government agency charged with enforcing laws about safety. Discuss risks, benefits, and alternatives.

2. **Right to Be Informed:**

   Discuss labelling, clarity of information, and limits of effectiveness uncontaminated by commercial motives.

3. **Right to Choose:**

   Clarify differences between brand names and generic, as well as comparable or competitive prices. Identify "active ingredients" as critical factors in decision making.

4. **Right to Be Heard:**

   All individual drug reactions are valid and should be reported. The Adverse Drug Reporting System is a mechanism of the FDA which collects data on drug effects.

Module II.6—Overhead #13

COMMUNITY RESOURCES TO ADDRESS DRUG MISUSE IN THE ELDERLY

1. Education of health professionals employed in ambulatory care, in-patient and mental health centers.

2. Information and education programs on drug misuse and abuse in the aged.

3. Community agency screening using interviewing and assessment to identify problems.

4. Utilization of churches and synagogues in "drug awareness" programming.

5. Central telephone hot lines as sources of referral and information.

6. Media and community campaigns promoting drug-free living.

Instructor's Guide

HANDOUT MASTERS

MODULE II.6   DRUG MISUSE AND DEPENDENCE IN THE ELDERLY

1. Misuse of Prescription Drugs
2. Guidelines for Providers: General Prescribing/Case Management Principles
3. Drugs and the Elderly: Practitioner Responsibility
4. Guidelines for Patients: General Principles of Patient Education Relevant to Drug and Alcohol Use
5. Guidelines for Patients: Sample Questions About Medicines
6. Consumer Rights Relative to Medications
7. Patient-Care Provider Expectations

Module II.6

Module II.6—Handout #1

MISUSE OF PRESCRIPTION DRUGS

A person is considered to be misusing medicine when he or she:

- Does not know its name or why it was prescribed.
- Does not know how or when to take it to make it most effective.
- Forgets to take it.
- Forgets to take it one time and doubles the dosage the next time.
- Takes doses at improper time.
- Does not recognize side effects.
- Discontinues it without notifying the physician.
- Stretches it to make it last longer than intended.
- Seeks a refill long after the rational need for it has disappeared.
- Saves old medicine for self-treatment at a later time.
- Borrows or lends medicine.
- Takes too much, thinking that if one dose is helpful, two would be even better.
- Takes too much by taking duplicate medicines prescribed by two different physicians.
- Mixes alcohol with such drugs as tranquilizers, barbiturates, and antihistamines.

From: Commonwealth of Pennsylvania, Department of Aging. (1986). *Drug use and the elderly: A training program* (Document #T-19). Erie, PA: Keystone University Research Corporation.

Instructor's Guide

Module II.6—Handout #2

GUIDELINES FOR PROVIDERS: GENERAL PRESCRIBING/CASE MANAGEMENT PRINCIPLES

1. Obtaining a complete medication history is critical. It must include all medications, including OTCs. Ask about allergies and intolerances.
2. Determine use of alcohol: history, frequencies.
3. Avoid using medications to treat non-specific complaints.
4. When treating a chronic disease, try to select drugs that will not diminish the quality of life. The effect of treatment must be clearly better than no treatment.
5. Chronic diseases can impair and exaggerate drug response. (For example, demented patients are disposed to exaggerated CHS side effects of drugs.) Alcoholism is considered a chronic condition.
6. Multiple pathology is the rule, so a priority order regarding treatment is essential.
7. The number of drugs administered concurrently must be kept to a minimum.
8. Stopping a drug may be more beneficial than starting one.
9. Know the pharmacology of each drug prescribed.
10. When dosing a drug, start low and go slow.
11. Use of serum drug levels is helpful in determining the appropriate dose of some medications.
12. Don't prescribe a drug without some consideration of the patient's social and economic resources and alternate treatment modalities.
13. Implement a regular mechanism for monitoring drug effects and changes in life events.

From: Staab, A., & Lyles, M. (1989). *Manual of geriatric nursing* (pp. 119–121). Glenview, IL: Scott, Foresman, & Company.

Module II.6—Handout #3

DRUGS AND THE ELDERLY: PRACTITIONER RESPONSIBILITY

1. Help client obtain accurate drug information.
2. Encourage client to participate in treatment decisions.
3. Verify doctor appointments and drug regimen.
4. Assess client health practices and drug usage.
5. Coordinate drug treatment activities.
6. Provide drug education programs for clients, their families, and other practitioners.
7. Advocate better geriatric pharmacology.

From: Commonwealth of Pennsylvania, Department of Aging. (1986). *Drug use and the elderly: A training program* (Document #T-19). Erie, PA: Keystone University Research Corporation.

Instructor's Guide

Module II.6—Handout #4

GUIDELINES FOR PATIENTS: GENERAL PRINCIPLES OF PATIENT EDUCATION RELEVANT TO DRUG AND ALCOHOL USE

1. Explain expected effects, possible side effects, and storage requirements of prescribed and OTC medication.

2. Ask patients to relate to you what they know about the drugs they are taking, both prescription and non-prescription.

3. Be certain that patients understand the treatment program, including the importance of non-drug therapy.

4. Choose a suitable memory aid and explain its use to the patient. Color coding or use of an egg carton may be needed for illiterate patients or the visually impaired.

5. Suggest that the patient use only one pharmacy. Many pharmacies now maintain computer medication profiles on their customers and may provide helpful information on drug interactions, and so on.

6. Discourage self-medication.

7. Advise patients not to use drugs if they drink alcohol.

From: Staab, A., & Lyles, M. (1989). *Manual of geriatric nursing* (p. 119). Glenview, IL: Scott, Foresman, & Company.

Module II.6—Handout #5

GUIDELINES FOR PATIENTS: SAMPLE QUESTIONS ABOUT MEDICINES

To be asked periodically about entire medication regimen and also whenever a medication is changed or a new one prescribed.

1. Is the drug needed? Are there any alternative non-drug treatments available?
2. What are the name and purpose of the drug?
3. How and when should it be taken?
4. How long should it be taken?
5. Can it be stopped when the symptoms disappear?
6. What should be done if a dose is missed?
7. Can it be taken with other drugs, including over-the-counter drugs and/or alcohol?
8. What possible effects or reactions are there?
9. Are there any side effects that should be reported immediately?
10. Are there any special precautions to be taken?
11. Can the prescription be refilled?
12. Is there a less expensive substitute which is as effective?

Instructor's Guide

Module II.6—Handout #6

CONSUMER RIGHTS RELATIVE TO MEDICATIONS

1. Right to Safety:

    FDA is the government agency charged with enforcing laws about safety. Discuss risks, benefits, and alternatives.

2. Right to Be Informed:

    Discuss labelling, clarity of information, and limits of effectiveness uncontaminated by commercial motives.

3. Right to Choose:

    Clarify differences between brand names and generic, as well as comparable or competitive prices. Identify "active ingredients" as critical factors in decision making.

4. Right to Be Heard:

    All individual drug reactions are valid and should be reported. The Adverse Drug Reporting System is a mechanism of the FDA which collects data on drug effects.

Module II.6

Module II.6—Handout #7

PATIENT-CARE PROVIDER EXPECTATIONS

1. Care-provider should be willing to listen, explain, and discuss health care.
2. Care-provider should facilitate communication by willingness to talk on the phone, and arrange appointments easily.
3. Waiting time should be reasonable.
4. Office and billing policies should be clear.
5. Emergency procedures should be stated.
6. Exchange of expectations about decision making and compliance should occur.
7. A mechanism to facilitate communication, such as a "Questions to Ask" list (below), should be encouraged.

QUESTIONS TO ASK

QUESTION	ASKED
1. _____	_____
2. _____	_____
3. _____	_____
4. _____	_____
5. _____	_____
6. _____	_____
7. _____	_____
8. _____	_____
9. _____	_____
10. _____	_____
11. _____	_____
12. _____	_____
13. _____	_____
14. _____	_____
15. _____	_____

Instructor's Guide

RECOMMENDED TEACHING STRATEGIES AND SAMPLE ASSIGNMENTS

RECOMMENDED TEACHING STRATEGIES

- Lecture
- Audiovisual and media resources
- Home visits
- Clinical placements in community agencies, nursing homes
- Case studies

SAMPLE ASSIGNMENTS

CASE STUDY #1

Mr. Jones (Aged 72)

Mr. Jones, aged 72, lives alone in rent controlled housing for the elderly. At the request of a social worker, a registered nurse has scheduled a home visit to assess Mr. Jones' ability and safety to continue to live alone.

During the course of the interview, the registered nurse learns that Mr. Jones is a retired dock worker. He has no close relatives and no close friends in the housing complex. His income is limited to his Social Security and pension benefits. The registered nurse obtains the following additional observations:

1. Mr. Jones is a slender, although not thin, male slightly unsteady in his ambulation. He says that he has been especially healthy, has no current health problems, and doesn't go to a physician on a regular basis.

2. His speech and thought processes are coherent and in the context of the nurse-client interview.

3. Mr. Jones has several bruises on his left arm and left leg. Mr. Jones says he fell when he got up to go to the bathroom one night. In discussing the incident, Mr. Jones says he fell because he didn't turn on the lights and he stumbled in the dark.

4. Every time the registered nurse makes her home visit, Mr. Jones always has a water glass half-filled with whiskey sitting on the table by his chair. Mr. Jones says that he has always drunk only whiskey, and that this is his "daily cocktail."

Module II.6

When reporting back to the social worker, the registered nurse's opinion is that, at present, Mr. Jones is able to carry out the activities of daily living and to live alone. However, a risk of further falls and injury due to his alcohol abuse is present.

Mr. Jones denies an alcohol abuse problem and the registered nurse and social worker are continuing to consider the management of Mr. Jones' related housing/health/alcohol abuse problem.

CASE STUDY #2

Mrs. Smith (Aged 65)

Mrs. Smith, aged 65, has been admitted to an alcohol treatment center. Her husband, who has accompanied Mrs. Smith to the treatment center, tells the admitting nurse that Mrs. Smith has been drinking "a bottle" of gin every day for the past five years. Mrs. Smith is mumbling incoherently and is unable to stand erect at the time of admission.

Mr. Smith further tells the admitting nurse that he has tried to help Mrs. Smith but everything that he has tried to do for her just seems to make Mrs. Smith's drinking pattern worse. Mr. Smith goes on to say that neither he nor Mrs. Smith belong to any alcohol abuse treatment or support groups. Mr. Smith states that he has convinced Mrs. Smith to come to this treatment center, as he "just can't deal with the home situation any longer."

After the admission process has been completed, the admitting nurse meets with the unit staff to prepare the following short- and long-term nursing care plan for Mr. and Mrs. Smith.

OTHER SAMPLE ASSIGNMENTS

1. Discuss current self-treatment practices among the elderly. Develop a client education plan that could be used in a care setting for the elderly.

2. Have students discuss their views on use of medications for the elderly with respect to:

    a. Altering behavior.

    b. Pain control.

    c. Use of placebos.

From: McKenry, L., & Salerno, E. (1989). *Mosby's pharmacology in nursing* (17th ed.). St. Louis, MO: C.V. Mosby.

Instructor's Guide

TEST QUESTIONS AND ANSWERS

TEST QUESTIONS

Mr. Jones, aged 60, has been admitted to an alcohol treatment center. Mr. Jones has been drinking up to the time he was admitted. His wife, who has accompanied Mr. Jones, states that her husband drinks a quart or more of whiskey a day.

1. The nurse admitting Mr. Jones would anticipate that which of the following would most likely be included in Mr. Jones' admission orders?
    a. High fat diet, vitamins B and E, thiamin.
    b. High protein diet, vitamins B complex and C, Librium.
    c. Liquid diet, vitamins A and E, Demerol.
    d. Liquid diet, vitamins B complex and C, Dilantin.
2. Prolonged use of alcohol may result in central nervous system damage. This may be manifested as Korsakoff's syndrome. The physiological basis for this condition is:
    a. Convulsions during withdrawal.
    b. Dystonic reactions.
    c. Encephalomalacia.
    d. Marked vitamin B deficiency.
3. The nurse observes Mr. Jones for signs of Korsakoff's psychosis which would include:
    a. Amnesia and confabulation.
    b. Delusions and fear.
    c. Nihilistic ideas and tearfulness.
    d. Sullenness and suspiciousness.
4. Which of the following environmental factors should the nurse anticipate would be the most disturbing to Mr. Jones if he should develop delirium tremens?
    a. Medical odors.
    b. Shadows.
    c. Strangers.
    d. Unfamiliar procedures.
5. On the evening of his admission, Mr. Jones begins to manifest alcohol withdrawal. The first symptoms are:
    a. Diaphoresis, nervousness, and tremors.

Module II.6

    b. Fever, dehydration, and convulsions.

    c. Hypotension and bradycardia.

    d. Vomiting, diarrhea, and incontinence.

6. Mrs. Jones tells the nurse she would like to help her husband stop drinking but that everything that she does just seems to make Mr. Jones drink more. The primary goal of the nurse's response should be:

    a. Encourage Mrs. Jones to join Al-Anon.

    b. Help Mrs. Jones understand that alcohol abuse is a problem only Mr. Jones can solve.

    c. Help Mrs. Jones clarify the problem as she sees it.

    d. Tell Mrs. Jones that she has done all she can do to help her husband.

7. Mr. Jones tells the nurse he has never been able to face life without alcohol. The most appropriate response for the nurse should be:

    a. "But now you know where to go for help."

    b. "I know how you feel, Mr. Jones. We all have difficulty in dealing with our problems."

    c. "Perhaps you can if you join Alcoholics Anonymous."

    d. "That has been the way you have dealt with your problems, Mr. Jones."

8. Mr. Jones is taking antabuse and will continue to do so after he is discharged. Which medications should he be instructed not to take?

    a. Antacids and laxatives.

    b. Aspirin and Tylenol.

    c. Elixir terpin hydrate.

    d. Heart and blood pressure medication.

9. Mrs. Jones asks the nurse about Al-Anon. After explaining that Al-Anon is a support group for families of alcoholics, the nurse's best response would be:

    a. "Do you feel that you need this?"

    b. "Everyone who has a spouse who abuses alcohol should join."

    c. "How do you feel about joining?"

10. Mr. Jones attends Alcoholics Anonymous prior to being discharged home. Which statement about Alcoholics Anonymous is most correct?

    a. It is a self-help group led by professionals who have achieved sobriety.

    b. It is a self-help group where members acknowledge their illness and share experiences concerning abuse and control of alcohol intake.

    c. It is a therapy group in which membership is recommended after discharge from a substance-abuse program.

    d. It is a therapy group that discourages relationships outside the organization.

11. Mrs. Smith, aged 68, has been admitted to your unit for a diagnostic work-up, including alcohol abuse. You correctly identify which of the following two manifestations as characteristics of alcohol abuse in the elderly?

Instructor's Guide

   a. History of alcohol abuse: Heavy, severe drinking.
   b. History of alcohol abuse: Mildly severe drinking.
   c. More prone to binge drink.
   d. More prone to drink on a daily basis.
12. Alcohol consumption for the patient taking medications frequently results in increased drug interaction. Two interactions that could occur include which two of the following?
   a. Alcohol and Antihypertensives may result in: hypertension.
   b. Alcohol and Antihypertensives may result in: hypotension.
   c. Alcohol and Nitroglycerine may result in: hypertension.
   d. Alcohol and Nitroglycerine may result in: hypotension.

Module II.6

ANSWER KEY

1. a
2. d
3. a
4. b
5. a
6. c
7. d
8. c
9. c
10. b
11. b,d
12. b,d

Instructor's Guide

BIBLIOGRAPHY

MODULE II.6 DRUG MISUSE AND DEPENDENCE IN THE ELDERLY

Abrams, R. C., & Alexopoulos, G. S. (1987). Substance abuse in the elderly: Alcohol and prescription drugs. *Hospital and Community Psychiatry, 38*(12), 1285–1287.

American Nurses' Association, Drug and Alcohol Nurses' Association, & National Nurses' Society on Addictions. (1987). *The care of clients with addictions: Dimensions of nursing practice.* Kansas City, MO: Author.

American Nurses' Association, & National Nurses' Society on Addictions. (1988). *Standards of addictions nursing practice with selected diagnoses and criteria.* Kansas City, MO: Author.

American Psychiatric Association. (1987). *DSM-IIIR.* Washington, DC: Author.

Atkinson, R. M. (1984). Substance use and abuse in late life. In R. M. Atkinson (Ed.), *Alcohol and drug abuse in old age* (pp. 1–21). Washington, DC: American Psychiatric Press.

Basen, M. (1977). The elderly and drug problems: Overview and programs strategy. *Public Health Reports, 92*(1), 43–48.

Beatie, B. L., & Sellers, E. M. (1979). Psychoactive drug use in the elderly: The pharmacokinetics. *Psychosomatics, 20,* 474–479.

Brody, J. A. (1982, February). Aging and alcohol abuse. *Journal of the American Geriatrics Society, 30*(2), 123–126.

Brogatta, E. F., Montgomery, R. J. V., & Brogatta, M. L. (1982). Alcohol use and abuse, life crisis events and the elderly. *Research in Aging, 4,* 378–408.

Brown, B., & Chiang, C. P. (1983–1984). Drug and alcohol abuse among the elderly: Is being alone key? *International Journal of Aging and Human Development, 18,* 1–12.

Caroselli-Karinja, M. (1985). Drug abuse and the elderly. *Journal of Psychosocial Nursing and Mental Health Services, 23*(6), 25–30.

Chien, C. P., Townsend, E. J., & Ross-Townsend, A. (1978). Substance use and abuse among the community elderly: The medical aspect. *Addiction Diseases, 3,* 357–372.

Commonwealth of Pennsylvania, Department of Aging. (1986). *Drug use and the elderly: A training program* (Document #T-19). Erie, PA: Keystone University Research Corporation.

Cotton, P. G., Beno-Kociemba, A., & Kelly, C. E. (1978). A community program for elderly hospital patients. *Journal of Geriatric Psychiatry, 11,* 217–230.

Module II.6

Crandall, R. C. (1980). Aged alcohol abuser. *Catalyst, 1*(3), 56–63.

Ebersole, P., & Hess, P. (1990). *Toward healthy aging: Human needs and nursing response* (3rd ed.). (pp. 234–268, 501–503, 631–632). St. Louis, MO: C. V. Mosby.

Eliopoulos, C. (1989). *Caring for the elderly in diverse care settings.* New York: Lippincott.

Ellor, J. K., & Kurz, D. J. (1982). Misuse and abuse of prescription drugs by the elderly. *Nursing Clinics of North America, 17,* 319–330.

Etemad, B. (1980). Alcoholism and aging. In J. H. Masserman (Ed.), *Current psychiatric therapies* (pp. 111–114). New York: Grune & Stratton.

Felker, M. P. (1988). A recovery group for elderly alcoholics. *Geriatric Nursing, 9*(2), 110–113.

Finlayson, R. E. (1984). Prescription drug abuse in older persons. In R. M. Atkinson (Ed.), *Alcohol and drug abuse in old age* (pp. 61–70). Washington, DC: American Psychiatric Press.

Gerbino, P. P. (1982). Complications of alcohol use combined with drug therapy in the elderly. *Journal of American Geriatric Society, 30*(11), 88–93.

Giannini, A. J. (1988). Drug abuse and depression: Possible models for geriatric anorexia. *Neurobiology of Aging, 9*(1), 26–27.

Giordano, J. A., & Beckham, K. (1985). Alcohol use and abuse in old age: An examination of type II alcoholism. *Journal of Gerontological Social Work, 9*(1), 65–83.

Goodwin, J. S., Sanchez, C. J., Thomas, P., Hunt, C., Garry, P. J., & Goodwin, J. M. (1987). Alcohol intake in a healthy elderly population. *American Journal of Public Health, 77*(2), 173–177.

Greenblatt, D. J., Sellers, E. M., & Shader, R. I. (1982). Drug therapy: Drug disposition in old age. *New England Journal of Medicine, 306,* 1081–1088.

Gulino, C., & Kadin, M. (1986). Aging and reactive alcoholism. *Geriatric Nursing, 7*(3), 148–151.

Hunan, Z. I. (1978, January). Geriatric medications: How the aged are hurt by drugs meant to help. *RN,* 57–59.

Huntington, D. D. (1990). Home care of the elderly alcoholic. *Home Health Care Nurse, 8*(5), 26–32.

Kane, R., Ouslander, J., & Abrass, I. (1986). *Essentials of clinical geriatrics.* New York: McGraw Hill.

Kofoed, L. L. (1984). Abuse and misuse of over-the-counter drugs by the elderly. In R. M. Atkinson (Ed.), *Alcohol and drug abuse in old age* (pp. 49–59). Washington, DC: American Psychiatric Press.

Lamy, P. P. (1980). Misuse and abuse of drugs by the elderly. In R. Faulternberry (Ed.), *Drug problems of the '70's, solutions for the '80's* (pp. 161–166). Lafayette, LA: Endac Enterprises.

LaSage, J. (1982). Drug therapy in long-term facilities. *Nursing Clinics of North America, 17,* 331–340.

Lasker, M. N. (1986). Aging alcoholics need nursing help. *Journal of Gerontological Nursing, 12*(1), 16–19.

Lawson, A. W. (1989). Substance abuse problems of the elderly: Consideration for treatment and prevention. In G. Lawson & A. Lawson (Eds.), *Alcoholism and substance abuse in special populations.* Rockville, MD: Aspen.

Lesnoff-Caravaglia, G. (Ed.). (1980). *Health care of the elderly: Strategies for prevention and intervention.* New York: Human Sciences.

Lundin, D. V. (1978). Medication-taking behavior of the elderly: A pilot study. *Drug Intelligence Clinical Pharmacology, 11,* 518–522.

McKenry, L., & Salerno, E. (1989). *Mosby's pharmacology in nursing* (17th ed.). St. Louis, MO: C. V. Mosby Co.

McPherson, M. (1989). Medicating the elderly in home health care. *Journal of Home Health Care Practice, 2*(1), 16–28.

Meyers, A., Hingston, R., Mucatel, M., & Goldman, E. (1982). Social and psychological correlates of problem drinking in old age. *Journal of the American Geriatrics Society, 30,* 452–456.

Mezey, E. (1985). Alcohol. In R. Andres, E. L. Bierman, & W. R. Hazzard (Eds.), *Principles of geriatric medicine* (pp. 507–511). New York: McGraw Hill.

Morrant, J. C. A. (1989). Use and abuse of psychoactive drugs in the elderly. *Canada Medical Association Journal, 129,* 245–248.

National Institute on Aging. (1983, November). *Age page: Aging and alcohol abuse* (Public Health Service Publication No. 1983-418-427). Washington, DC: U. S. Government Printing Office.

National Institute on Drug Abuse. (1982). *Drug-taking among the elderly.* Washington, DC: Author.

Norwark, C. A. (1985). Life events and drinking behavior in later years. In E. Gottheil, K. A. Druley, T. E. Skoioda, & H. M. Waxman (Eds.), *The combined problems of alcoholism, drug addiction and aging* (pp. 37–50). Springfield, IL: Charles Thomas.

Nelson, R. A. (1982). Use and misuse of vitamins in the elderly. *Geriatrics, 37,* 138–140.

Pettee, J. (1982). Uncovering the "hidden alcoholic." *Geriatrics, 37,* 145–146.

Peterson, D. M. (1978). Introduction: Drug use among the aged. *Addiction Disease, 3,* 305–309.

Raffoul, P. R., Cooper, J. K., & Love, D. W. (1981). Drug misuse in older people. *Gerontologist, 21,* 146–150.

Richelson, E. (1984). Psychotropics and the elderly: Interactions to watch for. *Geriatrics, 39*(12), 30–36, 39–42.

Rosin, A. J., & Glatt, N. M. (1971). Alcohol excess in the elderly. *Quarterly Journal of Studies on Alcohol, 32,* 53–59.

Sanberg, P., & Krena, R. M. T. (1986). *Over the counter drugs.* New York: Chelsea House.

Module II.6

Schrock, M. M. (1980). *Holistic assessment of the healthy aged.* New York: John Wiley & Sons.

Schuckit, M. A. (1982). A clinical review of alcohol, alcoholism and the elderly patients. *Journal of Clinical Psychiatry, 43,* 396–399.

Schuckit, M. A., & Moore, M. (1979). Drug problems in the elderly. In O. Kaplan (Ed.), *Psychopathology of aging* (pp. 53–59). New York: Academic Press.

Schuckit, M. A., Atkinson, J. H., Miller, P. L., & Berman, J. (1980). A three-year follow-up of elderly alcoholics. *Journal of Clinical Psychiatry, 41,* 412–416.

Sellers, E. M., Frecker, R. C., & Romach, M. K. (1983). Drug metabolism in the elderly: Confounding of age, smoking and ethanol effects. *Drug Metabolism Review, 14,* 225–250.

Shoemaker, D. M. (1980). Use and abuse of OTC medications by the elderly. *Journal of Gerontological Nursing, 6,* 21–24.

Simon, A. (1989). The neuroses, personality disorders, alcoholism, drug use and misuse, and crime in the aged. In J. Birren & R. B. Sloan (Eds.), *Handbook of mental health and aging* (pp. 653–670). Englewood Cliffs, NJ: Prentice-Hall.

Staab, A. S., & Lyles, M. F. (1989). *Manual of geriatric nursing.* Glenview, IL: Scott, Foresman, & Company.

Stall, R. (1987). Research issues concerning alcohol consumption among aging populations. *Drug and Alcohol Dependence, 19*(3), 195–213.

Ward, R. A. (1981–1982). Aging, the use of time and social change. *The International Journal of Aging and Human Development, 14,* 177–185.

Watts, J. P. (1984). Alcohol problems in the elderly. *Journal of the American Geriatrics Society, 45,* 417–428.

MODULE II.7
DRUG AND ALCOHOL PROBLEMS IN SPECIAL POPULATIONS

Aileen H. Clucas, MSN, RN, CCDN
Vivian P. J. Clarke, EdD, CHES
Consultant

Madeline A. Naegle, PhD, RN, FAAN
Project Director
Janet S. D'Arcangelo, MA, RN, C
Project Coordinator

Project SAEN
SUBSTANCE ABUSE
EDUCATION IN NURSING

CONTENT OUTLINE

I. Drug and Alcohol Use in Groups at Risk—Ethnic Minorities
   A. Prevalence of Alcohol and Drug Abuse and Dependence in Racial and Ethnic Minorities
      1. Statistics of limited value
      2. African-Americans
      3. Hispanics
      4. Native Americans
      5. Homeless
   B. Patterns of Drug and Alcohol Use in Special Populations
      1. Drugs commonly used
      2. Age as a factor in drug use
   C. Cultural Factors and Traditions Which Influence Drug Use Patterns
   D. Social and Economic Factors Which Shape Alcohol/Drug Use
   E. Many Health Problems Are Secondary to Alcohol and Drug Dependence
   F. Access to Institutional and Community-Based Treatment
II. Intravenous Drug Users
   A. Prevalence of Intravenous Drug Use
   B. Patterns of Intravenous Drug Use and Other Drug Use
   C. Social and Community Factors Which Influence the Prevalence of Intravenous Drug Use
   D. Social Responses in the Community and Health Care Delivery System to IV Drug Abusers
   E. Health Risks and Health Deviations Associated with Intravenous Drug Use
III. Women
   A. Prevalence of Alcohol and Drug Use and Dependence in Women

Module II.7

- B. Patterns of Women's Drug and Alcohol Use and Dependence
    1. Gender-related differences
    2. Drug use patterns among women
    3. Onset of dependence for women
- C. Factors Which Influence Drug Using Patterns and Social Responses to Women with Drug and Alcohol Problems
- D. Institutional and Community Resources
- E. Treatment Considerations

IV. Glossary

Drug and Alcohol Problems in Special Populations

CONTENTS

I. DRUG AND ALCOHOL USE IN GROUPS AT RISK—ETHNIC MINORITIES

A. Prevalence of Alcohol and Drug Abuse and Dependence in Racial and Ethnic Minorities

1. Available statistics are limited in value because:
   a. Minorities are not homogeneous populations; i.e., groups include African-Americans, African blacks and Caribbean blacks.
   b. Regional differences can be significant as intervening variables.
   c. Major household surveys for national drug use do not include the undomiciled, persons without fixed residences, prison inmates, college dormitory students, or emancipated youth.
   d. Patterns of use and the drug of choice may fluctuate over time as a function of trends, accessibility, geographic region, and socioeconomic class.
2. African-Americans.
   a. Largest racial minority: twelve percent (12%) of the United States population is African-American or composed of blacks with other ethnic heritages.
   b. There is a prevailing stereotype of the drug user as an African-American or Hispanic male. However, white males have the highest lifetime use of cigarettes, alcohol, stimulants, and hallucinogens (NIDA, 1989).
   c. More African-American men and women abstain from alcohol than white men and women (NIDA, 1989).
   d. The overall rate of alcohol consumption is consistent among all racial groups.
   e. Rates of "ever used" illicit drugs for African-Americans over age 12 is about the same as for white Americans (NIDA, 1989).
   f. Rates of "current use" of illicit drugs are greater among African-Americans than for either whites or Hispanics in *all* age groups, except for those ages 12–17 (NIDA, 1989).
   g. In 1988, data from the Drug Abuse Warning Network (DAWN) indicated:
      (1) Fifty-seven percent (57%) of all cocaine-related emergency room episodes involved African-American men.
      (2) Sixty-eight percent (68%) of cocaine or cocaine and other drug-related deaths involved African-American men.
      (3) African-Americans accounted for 48% of heroin-related emergency room episodes.
      (4) A higher population of drug dependent African-American clients seek drug treatment than Hispanics or whites.
   h. African-Americans and Hispanics are over-represented in data obtained from drug use surveys (NIDA, 1988).

Module II.7

3. Hispanics.
   a. Represent the fastest growing ethnic minority. Currently Hispanics are 7% of the United States population.
   b. Three major Hispanic cultural groups are observed in America:
      (1) Mexican American.
      (2) Puerto Rican.
      (3) Cuban.
   c. Nationally, drug and alcohol use among Hispanics are no more than that of other groups. However, differences are found when one looks at usage patterns and prevalence in specific subgroups related to regions, economic class, and degree of acculturation, etc.
      (1) The Puerto Rican single male, aged 18–24 years, whose first language is English, has the highest rate of illegal drug use. In contrast, the married Cuban female, over age 35, whose first language is Spanish, is the least likely to have used illegal drugs (NIDA, 1988).
      (2) Gender differences are more pronounced among Hispanics than among other groups.
         (a) Seventy percent (70%) of Hispanic women drink less than one drink per month or not at all.
         (b) Seventy percent (70%) of Hispanic men drink; the more acculturated the man is, the more he tends to drink (U.S. Department of Health and Human Services, 1990).
      (3) Of the three subcultures listed above, Mexican Americans drink the most (Institute of Medicine, 1990).
4. Native Americans.
   a. Constitute 1% of the U.S. population. Three hundred (300) tribes inhabit the continental U.S. and Alaska.
   b. Significant intertribal differences exist in alcohol/drug consumption and usage patterns.
   c. Alcohol-related mortality is highest for Native Americans; 1.35% of all Native American deaths are alcohol-related. Five of the ten most frequent causes of death among Native Americans are alcohol-related. However, there are also high rates of abstinence.
   d. Clinical alcoholism among Native Americans is 5.4–5.5% greater than in the general U.S. population (Institute of Medicine, 1990).
   e. Motor vehicular accidental deaths among Native Americans are 2.5–5.5 times greater than in the general population. Alcohol-related arrests among Native Americans are 12 times greater than those for the general population.
   f. Seventy-five percent (75%) of traumatic deaths and suicides among Native Americans are alcohol-related.
   g. Fetal alcohol syndrome statistics are significantly higher among Native Americans than those for the general population (NIDA, 1988).

Drug and Alcohol Problems in Special Populations

5. Homeless.
   a. There are approximately 250,000 homeless men, women, and children in the United States (DHHS, 1990a).
   b. Few epidemiological studies have been done on the homeless; those available address the homeless "alcoholic" rather than crack/cocaine and poly-substance abusers.
   c. Twenty to forty-five percent (20–45%) of homeless people are estimated to have alcohol problems (Seventh Special Report to Congress, 1990).
   d. Twenty to sixty percent (20–60%) of participants in a study reported that alcoholism was the cause of their homeless status (Fischer & Breakey, 1987).
   e. Rates of multiple psychiatric illness among homeless alcoholics are high. Twenty-five percent (25%) male homeless alcoholics and 50% female homeless alcoholics are estimated to also have a major psychiatric diagnosis (Seventh Special Report to Congress, 1990).

B. Patterns of Drug and Alcohol Use in Special Populations

1. Drugs commonly used include alcohol, cocaine and crack, heroin, inhalants, PCP, and marijuana.
   a. African-Americans and Hispanics.
      (1) A general trend suggests a greater preference for intravenous drug use, and for more use of drugs which are potentially more lethal.
      (2) From 1984 to 1987 cocaine-related deaths tripled for African-Americans and Hispanics, and doubled for whites.
      (3) Mortality rates for African-Americans and Hispanics from narcotics are disproportionate to their representation in the population.
      (4) Heroin use is very prevalent in certain African-American and Hispanic groups in specific geographic regions of the United States, particularly in the Northeast and Southwest.
      (5) When lifetime "ever used" drugs are estimated, use is actually lower for Hispanics than for either African-Americans or whites.
      (6) Generally speaking, Hispanic people living above the poverty line are more likely to use marijuana and cocaine than those living in poverty (NIDA, 1989).
      (7) Use of inhalants and sedatives are less common among Hispanics than in the general population.
   b. Native Americans.
      (1) Binge drinking is a common pattern.
      (2) Use of inhalants is more common than in the general population.
      (3) Alcoholism rates for Native American males are twice those of white males.

c. Homeless.
   (1) Little research is available on patterns of use.
   (2) Twenty percent (20%) of the homeless male population uses drugs other than alcohol. For the homeless female population, this figure rises to 25%.
   (3) The use of all drugs by the homeless fluctuates with changes in income; i.e., drug use increases when public assistance checks arrive.
2. Age as a factor in drug use.
   a. African-American.
      (1) African-American men increase alcohol consumption after age 30; the lower their income, the greater their usage of alcohol. Among white males, consumption decreases with age; additionally, there is a higher prevalence of usage as level of income rises.
      (2) African-American men are at lowest risk for alcohol problems between ages 18–29; white males are at highest risk in this age group (DHHS, 1990a).
   b. Hispanics.
      (1) Older, more tradition-bound Hispanics are less likely to drink alcohol or use drugs (Glick & Moore, 1990).
      (2) Some specific cohorts of Hispanic women under the age of 35 are more likely to use drugs (Glick & Moore, 1990).
   c. Native Americans.
      (1) Native American high school seniors have higher lifetime prevalence rates for illicit drug and alcohol use than other cohort groups (DHHS, 1990a).
      (2) Alaskan Natives and other Native Americans living in Alaska have the highest rate of alcohol and other drug use (DHHS, 1990a).
      (3) Native American adolescents begin alcohol/drug use at a younger age than cohorts in other populations (DHHS, 1990a).
      (4) Alcoholism is most prevalent among Native American men aged 25–44 years.
   d. Homeless.
      (1) Middle-aged (45–64 years old) homeless individuals appear to use alcohol more than younger or older peers.
      (2) According to a 1984 study, the homeless alcoholic is more likely to be male, older (41+ years), divorced, have past criminal activity, experience homelessness for longer periods, have physical and emotional problems, and a past history of psychiatric hospitalization (as cited in Fischer & Breakey, 1987).

C. Cultural Factors and Traditions Which Influence Drug Use Patterns

1. All aspects of alcohol and/or drug abuse, first use, choice of drugs, patterns of abuse, perception of treatment, and relapse are influenced by cultural factors and ethnic traditions.

2. Acculturation, the degree to which the dominant cultural values and behaviors are accepted, influences use of alcohol and other drugs.
3. The more a group retains original cultural values, the less prevalent is the use of alcohol and drugs.
4. Some stressors appear to be culture-specific; e.g., among immigrants without documentation (illegal alien status) and barriers to employment based on language.
5. Family cohesiveness and values of the extended family appear to influence and reduce alcohol/drug abuse patterns in Hispanic populations.
6. Church attendance is a positive influence and a source of support and strength in the African-American and Hispanic communities.
7. There is a wide range of alcohol/drug use and abuse prevalence among Native American tribes.
   a. In Oklahoma, alcohol-related deaths vary 1%–24% among tribes. These variations appear to be related to tribal traditions and socioeconomic factors.
   b. Native Americans caught between two completely different cultural systems experience cultural role strain, which influences alcohol/drug use.

D. Social and Economic Factors as Influences Which Shape Alcohol/Drug Use

1. Many factors interact to contribute to drug using patterns:
   a. Poverty.
   b. Illiteracy.
   c. Limited job opportunities.
   d. Discrimination.
   e. Availability of drugs/alcohol.
   f. Stresses of urban life.
   g. Money and peer status associated with drug dealing in a sub-culture.
2. African-Americans and Hispanics.
   a. Thirty-four percent (34%) of African-Americans live below poverty level (National Black Alcoholism Council, NIDA, 1987).
   b. White Americans are more likely to be admitted into hospitals for alcohol and drug abuse; African-Americans and Hispanics are more often treated and released (NIDA, 1987).
   c. Ethnic minorities appear more frequently in populations of addicts in the criminal justice system than in treatment facilities (NIDA, 1987).
   d. African-Americans are over-represented in inner city populations.
      (1) The interface of social and economic factors appears to influence drug/alcohol seeking behaviors.
      (2) Central Harlem has the highest mortality rate in New York City; it is twice that for whites in the city's general population and 50% greater

than for African-Americans living elsewhere. Causes for this high mortality rate in Harlem include cardiovascular disease, cirrhosis, and homicide (McCord & Freeman, 1990).

e. Hispanics have lower high school completion rates than any other ethnic group (NIDA, 1987). With the exception of Cuban Americans, Hispanics are more likely to be poor than other Americans, and the poverty rate in Hispanic communities is increasing.

(1) In 1987, 30% of Mexican-Americans lived below the poverty line.

(2) In 1987, the Puerto Rican mean income was 47% that of Caucasians (Glick & Moore, 1990).

f. Native Americans.

(1) Some reservations are very isolated and provide few opportunities for employment, while supporting large numbers of welfare recipients.

(2) The interface of social and economic oppression, combined with the loss of valued cultural traditions, may influence a fatalistic acceptance of tribal alcohol/drug use.

g. Homeless.

(1) Social and economic factors may be overwhelming and lead to hopelessness, helplessness, despair, and multiplicity of needs which are unmet.

(2) Homelessness and alcoholism are seen as interrelated.

(3) Alcohol and drugs are potent anesthetics which can dull emotional pain.

(4) Priorities for homeless individuals are primary survival needs such as housing and income—not alcoholism and drug abuse treatment.

(5) There are fewer social supports for sobriety available to the homeless population.

E. Many Health Problems Are Secondary to Alcohol and Drug Dependence

1. Alcoholism is considered to be the # 1 health problem for both African-Americans and Native Americans.

   a. Although overall alcohol consumption is similar for both African-Americans and whites, African-Americans suffer greater health consequences.

   (1) Rates of cirrhosis, alcoholic fatty liver, and hepatitis are higher among African-Americans than among Caucasians.

   (2) Esophageal cancer in certain African-American age groups is ten times higher than among Caucasians.

   b. Native Americans have rates of cirrhosis of the liver which are 2.6–3.5 times higher than those of the general population (Institute of Medicine, 1990).

   c. Fetal alcoholism syndrome and fetal effects occur disproportionally higher among Native Americans than in any other female population in the U.S.

Drug and Alcohol Problems in Special Populations

    2. Homeless.

        a. The interactions of many factors contribute to health problems in this population:

          (1) Exposure.

          (2) Dietary problems of undernutrition and malnutrition.

          (3) Lack of sleep.

          (4) Environmental, social, and economic stresses as well as the stress of maintaining "hypervigilance" for personal safety.

          (5) Alcohol/drug use further stresses the immune system.

          (6) Homeless individuals experience a greater prevalence of:

              (a) Trauma.

              (b) Thermoregulatory disorders; e.g., frostbite.

              (c) Peripheral vascular disorders; e.g., edema, cellulitis, ulcers.

              (d) Infestations.

              (e) Incidence of tuberculosis among the homeless is 100–200 times greater than in the general population. In addition, the disease is difficult to treat; isoniazid administration for tuberculosis is contraindicated for the alcohol abusing individual.

          (7) Compliance with therapeutic recommendations is hard to achieve in the context of a multiplicity of needs, few sober supports, and social discrimination.

F. Access to Institutional and Community-Based Treatment

1. There is a limited research based on effectiveness of culturally sensitive treatment approaches.

2. Lack of availability of bilingual health workers is a barrier for many clients seeking treatment.

3. Requirements for extensive documentation compromise accessibility of services.

4. Many alcohol and drug rehabilitation centers do not accept medicaid clients.

5. Therapeutic community drug treatment centers have long waiting lists (six months or longer).

6. Alcohol/drug abusing patients in general hospital care are often not diagnosed and not referred for treatment.

7. Treatment resources for minorities are often unavailable in geographic areas of need.

8. Aftercare social supports and services are limited and hard to access; e.g., alcohol-free housing for the homeless.

Module II.7

II. INTRAVENOUS DRUG USERS

A. Prevalence of Intravenous Drug Use

1. Approximately 1.1–1.3 million individuals are estimated to be intravenous drug abusers (NIDA, 1986).
2. An estimated 500,000 people regularly inject heroin, cocaine, and/or methamphetamines alone and in combinations (NIDA, 1986).
3. African-Americans and Hispanics are over-represented in AIDS surveillance data (New York City AIDS Surveillance Report, 1990).
   a. They constitute 41% of AIDS cases, but only 19% of the U.S. population.
   b. Of heterosexual IV substance abusers who also have AIDS, 81% are minority group members.

B. Patterns of Intravenous Drug Use and Other Drug Use

1. Research limitations relate to problems of self-report and problems accessing illicit users.
2. Use may be experimental or casual.
3. Use may be intravenous or subcutaneous ("skin popping").
4. Cocaine is more frequently associated with higher prevalence of daily use and/or binge use. The AIDS study funded by the National Institute on Drug Abuse (NIDA, 1986) suggests:
   a. Nineteen percent (19%) of cocaine IV users inject daily—some 10 times per day.
   b. Six percent (6%) use heroin as drug of choice.
5. Numbers of heroin abusers have remained stable over time. However, some evidence suggests that cocaine is replacing heroin as the drug of choice.
6. Greater numbers of IV substance abusers (50%) than previously are now using combinations of drugs; e.g., "speedballing" (injecting heroin and cocaine).
7. Intravenous drug use is often associated with communal use ("shooting galleries") and sharing of works.

C. Social and Community Factors Which Influence the Prevalence of Intravenous Drug Use

1. Poverty, lack of employment.
2. Availability; all drugs now have widespread distribution.
3. Family disintegration related to social and economic factors.
4. Lack of community support to sustain abstinence.

D. Social Responses in the Community and Health Care Delivery System to IV Drug Abusers

1. Some communities demonstrate great resistance to implementation of locally-based treatment centers related to stigma of IV substance abusers.

2. Health care institutions, e.g., hospital emergency departments and/or medical wards, often do not even intervene on addictions *per se;* they just treat emergency or medical conditions secondary to substance abuse.
3. Health care providers.
    a. Experience denial.
    b. Stigmatize the IV substance abuser as hopeless.
    c. Are overwhelmed and/or discouraged by the numbers of abusers; their multiplicity of problems; and the users' own denial, returns for multiple ER/hospital visits, and histories of manipulative behavior.
4. Grass roots, lay, and professional organizations provide outreach and offer referrals and/or treatment, including
    a. Needle exchange programs.
    b. Outreach to shooting galleries with literature and supplies for cleaning works.
    c. Efforts that are often specific and culturally sensitive.
5. Therapeutic communities.
    a. Waiting lists are generally very long.
    b. Treatment commitments required are often one and one-half years.
    c. Rehabilitation must extend over several years.
6. Church-based local organizations.
7. Self-help programs based on Twelve-Step models; e.g., Narcotics Anonymous, Cocaine Anonymous.

E. **Health Risks and Health Deviations Associated with Intravenous Drug Use**

1. AIDS transmission.
    a. To the intravenous substance abuser (needle sharing, contaminated works).
    b. To sexual partners (sex without condoms, fluid transmission).
    c. In children born to seropositive mothers.
2. Hepatitis.
3. Bacterial endocarditis.
4. Septic conditions.
5. Cellulitis, abscesses.
6. Ventricular arrhythmias related to cocaine use.
7. Pulmonary congestion and edema with heroin use.
8. Pulmonary fibrosis and granulomas associated with adulterants mixed in solution with injectable cocaine/heroin.
9. Seizures related to overdosing.
10. Sleep deprivation and/or abnormal REM sleep associated with habitual use.
11. Nutritional deficits.

12. Compromised immune system functioning related to:
    a. Stress.
    b. Nutritional status.
    c. Poor sleep patterns.
    d. Direct toxic effects of alcohol and other drugs on immune system.
13. Concomitant alcohol and/or multiple drug use damaging to health.
14. Intravenous substance abuse and sexual behavior.
    a. As many as 50% of IV substance abusers had two or more sexual partners; 70% did not use condoms. Most did not sterilize works, increasing risk of HIV transmission.
    b. High rates of compulsive sexual activity associated with cocaine abuse, leading to high rates of possible HIV transmission and other sexually transmitted diseases (STDs).
    c. Prostitution.
    d. Engaging in high risk sexual practices.
15. Trauma and physical abuse secondary to IV substance abuse.
    a. Dangerous situations related to drug culture and drug trafficking (gunshot wounds, stabbing).
    b. Accidents and overdose; suicide.
    c. Physical and sexual abuse from partner.
16. Reproductive system trauma.
    a. Decreased fertility in men secondary to alcoholism.
    b. Frequent reproductive incompetence in alcohol and drug addicted women.
    c. Gynecological problems; e.g., amenorrhea.

III. WOMEN

A. Prevalence of Alcohol and Drug Use and Dependence in Women

1. Sixty percent (60%) of women over age 18 drink; 5% drink heavily (in excess of 2–3 drinks daily).
2. At risk women are: single, working, aged 18–35; also those divorced, separated, aged 35–50 years old.
3. Male alcoholics outnumber female alcoholics 2:1.
4. More men are in treatment for alcoholism than women by a ratio of 4:1.
5. Thirty-four percent (34%) of the people attending Alcoholics Anonymous are women (Institute of Medicine, 1990).
6. Of African-American women who drink, drinkers consume more than white women, and report more health problems than their African-American male peers.
7. There are few female Hispanic alcoholics, nearly none who are over 60 years old. Hispanic women drink less and use fewer drugs than women in white and African-American groups.

Drug and Alcohol Problems in Special Populations

8. Native American women ages 15–34 develop cirrhosis at a rate 36 times higher than that of white women.

B. **Patterns of Women's Drug and Alcohol Use and Dependence**

1. Gender-related differences.
   a. Women may experience an increased physiological bio-availability of alcohol, increasing physiological vulnerability to end organ effects.
      (1) Women experience more serious liver disease at lower rates of consumption (Penniman & Agnew, 1988).
      (2) Women experience earlier onset of alcoholic cirrhosis (Penniman & Agnew, 1988).
      (3) Women demonstrate earlier alcohol-related CAT scan changes (Jacobsen, 1986).
      (4) Women die from alcoholism at an earlier age than men (Penniman & Agnew, 1988).
   b. Women experience greater prevalence of primary affective disorders in self and female relatives (Institute of Medicine, 1990).
   c. Women report greater marital instability with higher divorce rates.
   d. Women are less likely than men to be supported by their families in treatment attempts.
   e. Women report incest, sexual, and physical abuse at rates higher than those reported by men. They also more frequently report sexual dysfunction as a predictor of subsequent substance abuse.
   f. Women are prescribed sedatives and tranquilizers more often than men.
   g. Women are less likely to be arrested for drunken driving than men; often women are remanded to treatment.
2. Drug use patterns among women.
   a. Women use prescription drugs, particularly sedatives and tranquilizers, in greater amounts than men.
   b. Women take over-the-counter drugs more frequently.
   c. Women use prescription drugs and alcohol in combination to self-medicate.
   d. Crack/cocaine use by African-American women is highest among all groups.
   e. Women attending Alcoholics Anonymous report combination alcohol/drug use, including prescription drugs/illicit drugs in increasing numbers.
3. Onset of dependence for women.
   a. At a later age than for men.
   b. Has more effects, and damage is "telescoped"; i.e., end organ damage occurs more quickly.
   c. More often reported to be associated with life transitions.
   d. Occurs at earlier ages; more high school age females are drinking than previously.

Module II.7

C. Factors Which Influence Drug Using Patterns and Social Responses to Women with Drug and Alcohol Problems

1. Women are more frequently prescribed sedatives and hypnotics.
2. Women are more prone to use CNS stimulants to maintain weight control, leading to eventual abuse.
3. Females in certain groups report using drugs to maintain significant relationships.
4. Women who are alcoholic or who abuse drugs are stigmatized.
5. Alcoholism and drug abuse may be regarded as less serious in women.
6. Misdiagnosis is more common than in men.

D. Institutional and Community Resources

1. Women experience greater barriers to accessing treatment.
    a. Few drug treatment programs admit pregnant substance abusers.
    b. Few programs provide child care during hospitalizations.
    c. Women are reluctant to enter treatment for fear of foster placement of their children.
    d. Women are ambivalent about suspending caretaking roles to enter inpatient treatment.
    e. Women have fewer financial resources and less insurance coverage.
    f. Stigma and shame which women experience may interfere with attempts to seek treatment.
2. Homeless women and homeless women with children have the fewest resources for treatment.

E. Treatment Considerations

1. Child care provision.
2. Gender-specific assessment.
    a. Differential diagnosis; e.g., alcohol-related depression vs. post menopausal depression vs. pituitary tumor.
3. Assessment of history of incest, sexual abuse, physical abuse, and treatment and/or referral.
4. Psychiatric assessment and treatment when indicated.
5. Personal growth and efforts to increase self-esteem are especially important.
6. Assertiveness training.
7. Vocational training and/or referral to educational and vocational preparation.

IV. GLOSSARY

African-American—Americans of African heritage.

Drug Abuse—Maladaptive patterns of alcohol or other drug use which occur despite recurrent social, occupational, or physical problems.

Drug Addiction/Dependence—Maladaptive patterns of alcohol or other drug use with recurrent social, occupational, psychological, or physical problems, and the existence of tolerance to the drug as well as withdrawal symptoms on abstinence.

Ethnic Minorities—Groups with particular cultural backgrounds as indicated by nationality.

MODULE II.7
DRUG AND ALCOHOL PROBLEMS IN SPECIAL POPULATIONS

INSTRUCTOR'S GUIDE

Aileen H. Clucas, MSN, RN, CCDN
Vivian P. J. Clarke, EdD, CHES
Consultant

Madeline A. Naegle, PhD, RN, FAAN
Project Director
Janet S. D'Arcangelo, MA, RN, C
Project Coordinator

Project SAEN
SUBSTANCE ABUSE
EDUCATION IN NURSING

CONTENTS

Component	Page
Module Description	552
Time Frame	552
Placement	552
Learner Objectives	553
Recommended Readings	554
Faculty Readings	554
Student Readings	554
Recommended Audiovisual and Other Resources	555
Overhead Masters	557
Handout Masters	575
Recommended Teaching Strategies and Sample Assignments	589
Test Questions and Answers	594
Bibliography	597

Module II.7

MODULE DESCRIPTION

This module is designed to promote student recognition and understanding of drug and alcohol use patterns in selected populations at high risk and/or manifesting a high prevalence and atypical needs. Identification of special population groups residing in institutions and the community and their characteristics are emphasized.

TIME FRAME

3 hours

PLACEMENT

Community Health Nursing, Nursing Care of the Adolescent, Psychiatric-Mental Health Nursing, Adult Health

Instructor's Guide

LEARNER OBJECTIVES

Upon successful completion of this module, the learner will:

1. Describe the prevalence of drug and alcohol dependence and related health deviations in special population groups, including ethnic minorities, intravenous drug users, and women.

2. Describe patterns of drug and alcohol use in relation to social and cultural traditions as well as lifestyle factors.

3. Develop an awareness of the impact of health policy on drug and alcohol problems in special populations.

4. Identify trends in society which impact on drug- and alcohol-related problems in special populations.

5. Describe multiple factors which interact to result in health deviations secondary to dependence on drugs and alcohol.

6. List factors which influence the accessibility of resources to special population groups.

Module II.7

RECOMMENDED READINGS

FACULTY READINGS

Brunswick, A., & Messeri, P. (1984). Causal factors in onset of adolescents' cigarette smoking: A prospective study of urban black youth. *Advances in Alcohol and Substance Abuse, 3*(1–2), 35–52.

Johnson, E. M. (1987). Women's health: Issues in mental health, alcoholism and substance abuse. *Public Health Reports, 7–8,* 42–48.

Stall, R. (1988). Prevention of HIV infection associated with drug and alcohol abuse. *Advances in Alcohol and Abuse, 7*(2), 73–81.

Wright, R., & Watts, T. D. (1988). Alcohol and minority youth. *Journal of Drug Issues, 18*(1), 1–7.

STUDENT READINGS

May, P. A. (1986). Alcohol and drug misuse prevention programs for American Indians: Needs and opportunities. *Journal of Studies on Alcohol, 47*(3), 187–195.

Moore, M. H., & Gernstein, D. K. (Eds.). (1981). *Alcohol and public policy: Beyond the shadow of prohibition.* Washington, DC: National Academy Press.

Naegle, M. A. (1988). Substance abuse among women: Prevalence patterns and treatment issues. *Issues in Mental Health Nursing, 9*(2).

Rynerson, B. C. (1989). Cops and counselors: Counseling issues with prison inmate substance abusers. *Journal of Psychosocial Nursing and Mental Health Services, 27*(2), 12–17.

Vener, A. M., Kreyoka, L. R., & Climo, J. J. (1980). Drug use and health characteristics in non-institutionalized Mexican-American elderly. *Journal of Drug Education, 10,* 343–353.

Instructor's Guide

RECOMMENDED AUDIOVISUAL AND OTHER RESOURCES

AUDIOVISUAL RESOURCES

1. **Beyond Black and White**

    This video, dramatizing the psychological and sociological origins of prejudice against minorities and women, reveals that for some of its victims, prejudice frequently results in alcohol or drug abuse, and for some, criminal behavior. Dramatic vignettes present positive, believable behavior models, and encourage the utilization of programs designed to provide career opportunities for young adult minorities and women. **Available from the New York State Council on Alcoholism, Film Library, 155 Washington Avenue, Albany, New York 12210. Telephone: (518) 432-8281 or 1-800-252-2557.**

2. **The Bottom Line: Women and Alcohol**

    Women alcoholics, social drinkers, treatment people, and a researcher candidly describe on camera the problems faced by women in an era of increased opportunity and motivation. This video explores some difficulties and survival techniques developed by modern women with respect to alcohol use and abuse. It is for general audiences. 20 minutes. **Available from Addiction Research Foundation, 33 Russell Street, Toronto, Canada M5S2S1. Telephone: (416) 595-6059. Purchase ($160).**

3. **Female Alcoholism**

    Alcoholism among women is a growing problem. This program examines the changing stereotype of the female alcoholic, as well as analyzing some case histories of recovered alcoholic women. It explains the dangers of drinking during pregnancy, the effect of the fetal alcohol syndrome on newborns and the emotional effect on children of being raised by an alcoholic mother. The program also explains why women are reluctant to seek help—and suggests ways to overcome this reluctance. 19 minutes. **Available from Films for the Humanities and Sciences, P.O. Box 2053, Princeton, New Jersey. Telephone: 1-800-257-5126. # BD-1366, purchase ($199).**

4. **The Honour of All**

    This three-part docu-drama captures the amazing, real-life story of the Alkali Indian Band's heroic struggle to overcome its widespread alcoholism. The people who lived it tell the story in their own words and portray themselves in these videos that recreate the Band's gradual slide into alcoholism, beginning in 1940. The deterioration of this community from British Columbia is shown and how, in 1971, tribal member Phyllis Chelsea's recovery helped inspire the Band to attain a 95% sobriety rate within 14 years. These videos offer Native Americans an inspiring example of how their peers could and did recover from the alcoholism that was destroying their community and their culture.

Part One recreates the story of the Band's struggle to overcome and conquer its alcoholism. It dramatically portrays the painfully slow, often lonely, but ultimately rewarding road back to sobriety. 56 minutes.

Part Two outlines the community development process that occurred at Alkali Lake, British Columbia, as the Band moved from alcoholism to sobriety. Various members of the Band discuss what it was like, what happened, and what it's like now. 43 minutes.

Part Three expands on the general theme of community development and personal growth begun in Parts One and Two. 26 minutes.

Available from Hazelden Educational Materials, Pleasant Valley Road, Box 176, Center City, Minnesota 55012-0176. Telephone: 1-800-328-3000. Purchase: Part One ($150), Part Two ($100), Part Three ($100).

5. **Junkie**

   Explores the many faces of women's addiction, detailing not only the belief systems which sustain addictions but also the support systems which can free addicts to live healthy lives. Created out of the life experiences of company members of At the Foot of the Mountain Theater, all of whom are recovering addicts, the film explores addiction to alcohol, food, speed, work, sex, violence, marijuana, and romantic love. Each woman is forced to confront her own loneliness and fear as her personal story is dramatized and examined. Unable to sustain their denial, the women urge one another to let go of the controlling behavior and delusions which keep them trapped and find a spiritual path of healing. 60 minutes. **Available from Hazelden Educational Materials, Pleasant Valley Road, Box 176, Center City, Minnesota 55012-0176. Telephone: 1-800-328-3000.** 16mm film only. Rental ($100) or purchase ($850).

6. **The Last to Know**

   A thirty-minute dramatization of women's experience of addiction. **Available from the New York State Council on Alcoholism, Film Library, 155 Washington Avenue, Albany, New York 12210. Telephone: (518) 432-8281 or 1-800-252-2557.**

7. **Women and Their Use of Mood-Altering Drugs: The Immigrant Experience**

   This tape presents some of the stresses that immigrants, particularly women, may have to face in adjusting to a new society. The program shows some of the short- and long-term effects of using minor tranquilizers as a way of coping. A consumer's approach to medical care is presented, stressing the importance of informed consent. 16 minutes. **Available from Addiction Research Foundation, 33 Russell Street, Toronto, Canada M5S2S1. Telephone: (416) 595-6059.** Purchase ($150).

Instructor's Guide

OVERHEAD MASTERS

MODULE II.7   DRUGS AND ALCOHOL PROBLEMS IN SPECIAL POPULATIONS

1. African-Americans
2. Hispanic Americans
3. Native Americans
4. Women
5. Homeless
6. Sample Nursing Diagnosis: Impaired Communication—Psychosocial
7. Sample Nursing Diagnosis: Hopelessness—Spiritual Distress
8. Structure of the Rehabilitation Network for the Single, Homeless, and Problem Drinkers

Instructor's Guide

Module II.7—Overhead #1

AFRICAN-AMERICANS

- **Patterns of AOD use are roughly similar for blacks and whites.**
    - **Black and white men have similar patterns of use.**
    - **More black women than white women completely abstain from alcohol.**
- **Blacks experience more significant consequences of AOD use.**
- **Blacks (particularly youth) are over-represented in:**
    - **Arrest records.**
    - **Treatment admissions.**
    - **Emergency room visits.**
- **High HIV infection rate.**
- **Positive cultural factors can facilitate prevention and intervention.**
    - **Strong kinship ties.**
    - **Role of church.**

Module II.7—Overhead #2

HISPANIC AMERICANS

- Second largest ethnic group in United States.
- Highly heterogeneous, many subgroups.
  - Cubans.
  - Mexican-Americans.
  - Puerto Ricans.
  - Central Americans.
  - Caribbean Islanders.
  - South Americans.
  - Spanish.
- Several factors relevant to patient assessment and counseling are consistent.
  - Concept of Machismo.
  - Concept of Barrio.
  - Extended family.
  - Use of Spanish language.
- Changes with acculturation.

Module II.7—Overhead #3

NATIVE AMERICANS

- **Highly heterogeneous population.**
  - **500 tribes and Alaskan villages.**
  - **Distinct language, customs, ceremonies, and socioeconomic status.**
- **Tribe's members live in urban and rural settings.**
- **Alcohol is most often drug of choice.**
- **Culturally determined behavior needs to be respected in dealing with Native Americans.**
  - **Reticence about self-disclosure.**
  - **Avoidance of direct eye contact.**

Instructor's Guide

Module II.7—Overhead #4

WOMEN

- Alcohol more toxic to women than to men.
- Women suffer more medical complications than men.
- Women likely to characterize AOD use as solution to some other problem.
- Women likely to be in relationships with addicted men.
- Treatment services should:
  - Be sensitive to issues of low self-esteem, depression, anxiety, and feelings of isolation.
  - Build on women's expressive and relationship skills.
  - Include child care.
  - Be able to deal with related issues of incest and family violence.

Module II.7—Overhead #5

HOMELESS

- **Portrait of the Homeless (from National Coalition for the Homeless, 1990).**
  - Over one-third are families with children.
  - One-half are single men.
  - 14% are single women.
  - 20–30% are employed.
  - 30% are veterans.
- **Patterns of AOD among the Homeless.**
  - Most epidemiological studies address the homeless "alcoholic" rather than users of crack/cocaine and poly-substance abuse.
    — 20–45% of the homeless have alcohol problems.
    — 20–60% report that alcoholism was the cause of their homeless status.
  - Relative to other drug use among the homeless.
    — 20–25% of the homeless use drugs other than alcohol.
  - Co-occurrence of alcohol abuse with drug abuse and mental illness (DHHS, 1990a):
    — 25% among homeless males.
    — 50% among homeless females.
- **The homeless alcoholic is more likely to be male, older (41+ years), divorced, have past criminal activity, be homeless for longer periods, with physical and emotional problems, and a past history of psychiatric hospitalization (Fisher & Breakey, 1987).**
- **Social and economic factors (deprivation of social support, housing, and income) may be overwhelming, leading to hopelessness, helplessness, and despair.**
- **Alcohol and drugs are potent anesthetics which can dull emotional pain.**

Module II.7—Overhead #6

SAMPLE NURSING DIAGNOSIS: IMPAIRED COMMUNICATION—PSYCHOSOCIAL

Defining Characteristics.

- Inability to express feelings.
- Lack of assertive behaviors reflected in messages.
- Lack of knowledge of English language.

Process Criteria.

- The nurse encourages the healthy expression of feelings.
- The nurse teaches methods of assertiveness and effective communication.
- The nurse enlists the assistance of translators.
- The nurse provides frequent contact with the individual.

Outcome Criteria.

- The individual states awareness of his or her needs.
- The individual demonstrates assertive behaviors.
- The individual demonstrates effective verbal and nonverbal communication skills in keeping with his or her capacity.

Module II.7—Overhead #7

SAMPLE NURSING DIAGNOSIS: HOPELESSNESS—SPIRITUAL DISTRESS

Defining Characteristics.

- Passivity.
- Feelings of hopelessness related to addiction and the outcome of treatment.
- Frequent crying spells.

Process Criteria.

- The nurse possesses a reality-oriented focus on the addiction process and recovery.
- The nurse helps the individual distinguish between attributes resulting from addictive behavior and positive qualities.
- The nurse helps the individual identify areas he or she can control.
- The nurse assists the individual in setting realistic goals for himself or herself.

Outcome Criteria.

- The individual demonstrates an increased energy level, showing more interest in self-care activities and less dependent behavior.
- The individual demonstrates ability to set a daily schedule that can realistically be met.

Instructor's Guide

Module II.7—Overhead #8

THE STRUCTURE OF THE REHABILITATION NETWORK FOR SINGLE, HOMELESS, AND PROBLEM DRINKERS

The lines indicate the frequency with which channels are used.

Problem Drinkers and Drug Takers

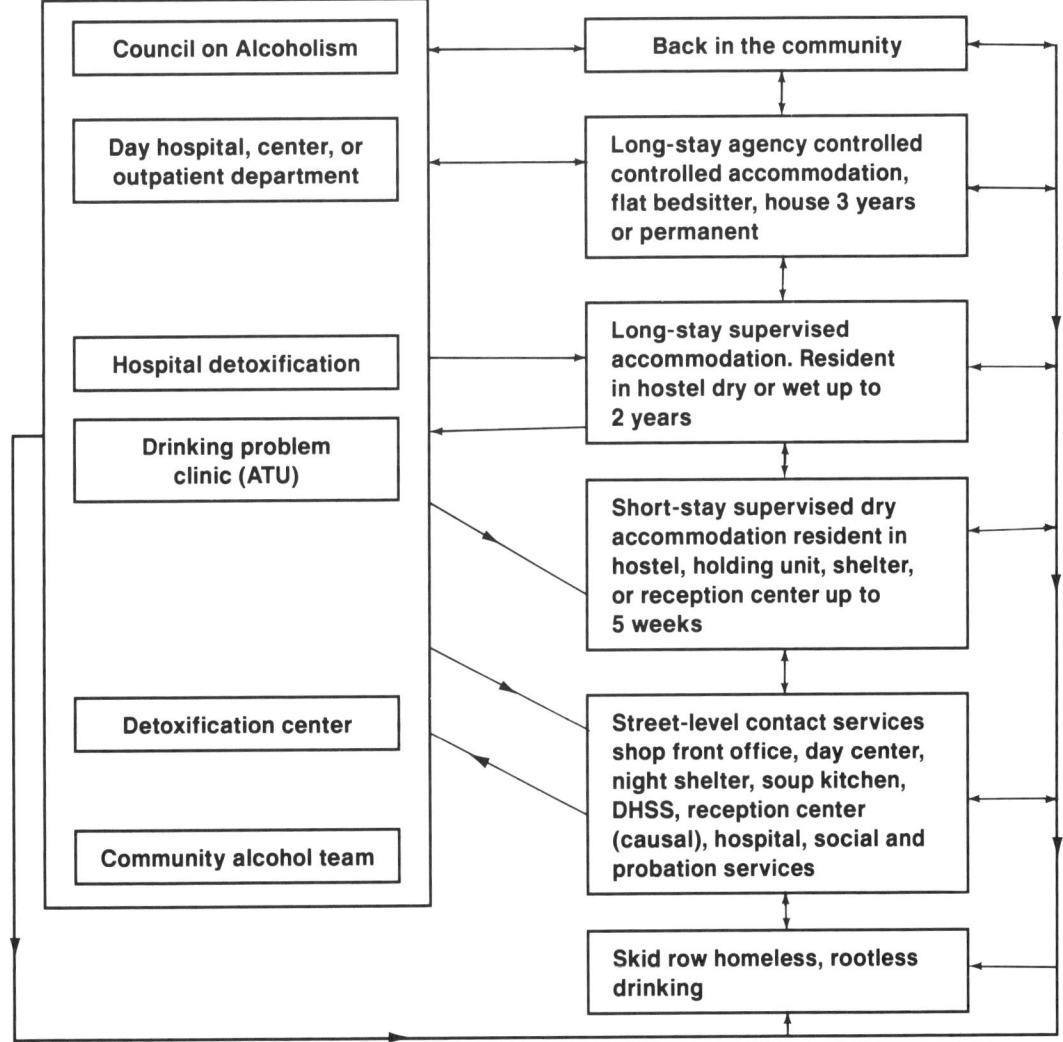

From: Thorley, A. (1983). Problem drinkers and drug takers. In F. N. Watts & D. H. Bennett, *Theory and practice of psychiatric rehabilitation* (p. 99). New York: John Wiley & Sons.

Instructor's Guide

HANDOUT MASTERS

MODULE II.7   DRUGS AND ALCOHOL PROBLEMS IN SPECIAL POPULATIONS

1. Substance Abuse among blacks in the U.S.
2. Substance Abuse among Hispanic Americans
3. Abuse de Drogas entre Hispanoamericanos (in Spanish)
4. Alcohol and Other Drug Problems Are a Major Concern in Native American Communities
5. National Institute on Drug Abuse: Major Drug Abuse Surveys with Data on Minority Populations
6. Resources for Data on the Homeless

Module II.7

Module II.7—Handout #1

SUBSTANCE ABUSE AMONG BLACKS IN THE U.S.

- Almost 8 million (36%) blacks have used marijuana, cocaine, or other illicit drugs at least once in their lifetimes; 3 million blacks used an illicit drug in the past year and 1.7 million blacks used an illicit drug in the past month (NIDA Household Survey, 1988).

- Among the population age 35 and older, blacks were more likely than whites or Hispanics to be using an illicit drug currently (past month). Current use of cocaine among blacks decreased from 3% in 1985 to 2% in 1988 (NIDA Household Survey, 1988).

- Black women are more likely than women in any other racial/ethnic group to have used crack/cocaine. Less than 1% of white women, 1.3% of Hispanic women and 1.5% of black women have used crack/cocaine (NIDA Household Survey, 1988).

- Black patients accounted for 39% (63,002) of the 160,170 drug-related emergency room (ER) cases reported to the Drug Abuse Warning Network (DAWN) in 1988. Of the ER cases involving black patients, 62% were male and 40% were 20–29 years old (NIDA DAWN, 1988).

- Cocaine was the most frequently mentioned drug in DAWN emergency room (ER) episodes. Almost 57% of cocaine ER cases involved black patients (NIDA DAWN, 1988).

- Black decedents accounted for 30% (1,999) of the 6,756 drug-related deaths reported by medical examiners (ME) to DAWN in 1988. Over 74% of black decedents were males and 46% were 30–39 years old (NIDA DAWN, 1988).

- Cocaine was the most frequently mentioned drug in DAWN ME cases, followed by heroin/morphine. Blacks accounted for 41% of cocaine-related deaths and for 31% of heroin/morphine deaths (NIDA DAWN, 1988).

- AIDS is a severe problem among blacks due to intravenous (IV) drug use. Of those living in households, blacks are twice as likely as whites to have used drugs intravenously. Although African-Americans represent 12% of the population in the U.S., they account for 27% of all people with AIDS. Of these cases, 44% (12,609) reported injection of an illicit substance prior to diagnosis with AIDS (CDC, 1989).

- The impact of AIDS associated with IV drug abuse on blacks is also reflected in cases of AIDS among the heterosexual partners of IV drug abusers. Blacks accounting for more than half of the AIDS cases were heterosexual partners of IV drug abusers (CDC, 1989).

Module II.7—Handout #1 *(continued)*

- Blacks account for 53% (939) of pediatric AIDS cases. Over 60% of the black pediatric cases are infected because their mothers were IV drug users or had sex with an IV drug user. (CDC, 1989).

- Data on drug abuse clients in treatment show that blacks represented about one-fourth of the drug abuse clients. The proportion of black clients was highest in the District of Columbia, Georgia, Illinois, and Maryland (NIDA NDATUS, 1987).

- Over one-third of 18–19-year-old blacks have dropped out of school. Drug use is generally higher among dropouts than among those who complete school. Black students who stay in school are less likely than white students to use illicit drugs. White seniors are twice as likely to report ever using cocaine than black seniors (13% vs. 6%), and more likely to ever use marijuana (50% vs. 37%). (U.S. Department of Education/NIDA High School Senior Survey, 1988).

Centers for Disease Control. (1989, September). *HIV/AIDS surveillance report.* Atlanta, GA: Author.

National Institute on Drug Abuse. (1987). *National drug and alcoholism treatment unit survey (NDATUS).* Rockville, MD: Author.

National Institute on Drug Abuse. (1988). *Drug abuse warning network (DAWN).* Rockville, MD: Author.

National Institute on Drug Abuse. (1988). *National household survey on drug abuse.* Rockville, MD: Author.

U.S. Department of Education and National Institute on Drug Abuse. (1988). *High school senior survey: Monitoring the future study.* Washington, DC: U.S. Government Printing Office.

Module II.7

Module II.7—Handout #2

SUBSTANCE ABUSE AMONG HISPANIC AMERICANS

- Between 1985 and 1988, the number of Hispanic Americans aged 12 and over who had ever used illicit drugs rose from 3.7 million to more than 4.8 million. The percentage of Hispanics who had ever used cocaine rose from 7.3% in 1985 to 11% in 1988. The percentage of Hispanics who used illicit drugs at least once in the past year, however, dropped from 16.7% to 14.7%, and the percentage of Hispanics who used illicit drugs at least once in the past month dropped from 10.7% in 1985 to 8.2% in 1988 (NIDA National Household Survey, 1988).

- As of December 1989, more than 18,200 Hispanic Americans had developed AIDS—at least 50% of these cases involved intravenous drug abuse. Also, more than 80% of those Hispanics who had developed AIDS through heterosexual contact had acquired the HIV infection through sex with an intravenous drug abuser (CDC, 1990).

- Of the 491 Hispanic children under the age of 13 who had developed AIDS by December 1989, more than 70% were born to mothers whose risk for contracting the HIV infection had been associated with their own intravenous drug abuse or sex with an intravenous drug abuser (CDC, 1990).

- Of the Hispanics using drugs intravenously, 29% of males and 29% of females inject heroin, cocaine, or a mixture of the two ("speedball") on a daily basis. Of those Hispanics who do not always use a new needle, 27% never use bleach or alcohol to clean their equipment before injecting, placing them at serious risk for contracting, as well as spreading the HIV infection (NIDA AIDS Demonstration Research, 1989).

- Although Hispanics accounted for less than 10% of all 1988 emergency room mentions in 21 metropolitan areas, they showed comparatively high rates of mention for certain drugs: for heroin—14.6%; inhalants—15.4%; methadone—18.7%. Nearly 18% of the 1988 emergency room episodes for Hispanics involved heroin and/or morphine. This is a higher percentage than for any other ethnic group. Nearly 13% of the 1988 deaths due to drugs in 27 metropolitan areas occurred among Hispanics (NIDA DAWN, 1988).

- Hispanics represented about one-sixth of the nearly 254,000 Americans who were in drug treatment in 1987. Relatively high proportions of Hispanic clients were reported in Arizona, California, New Mexico, New York, and Texas. Of Hispanics who use drugs intravenously, however, about 41% have never been in treatment (NIDA, 1987; NIDA, 1989).

- NIDA's toll-free Hispanic Hotline number for drug abuse treatment referral is 1-800-66-AYUDA.

Centers for Disease Control. (1990, January). *HIV/AIDS surveillance report*. Atlanta, GA: Author.

National Institute on Drug Abuse. (1987). *National drug and alcoholism treatment survey: Final report*. Rockville, MD: Author.

National Institute on Drug Abuse. (1988). *Data from the drug abuse warning network* (Series I, No. 8). Rockville, MD: Author.

National Institute on Drug Abuse. (1988). *National household survey on drug abuse*. Rockville, MD: Author.

National Institute on Drug Abuse. (1989, November). *NIDA AIDS demonstration research demonstration national database*. Rockville, MD: Author.

Instructor's Guide

Module II.7—Handout #3

ABUSO DE DROGAS ENTRE HISPANOAMERICANOS

- Entre 1985 y 1988, el número de Hispanoamericanos desde los 12 años de edad en adelante que nunca había usado drogas ilícitas acrecentó en más de 3.7 millones a más de 4.8 millones. El porcentaje de Hispanos que nunca habían usado cocaína se acrecentó de 7.3% en 1985 a 11% en 1988. Sin embargo, el porcentaje de Hispanos que usaron drogas por lo menos una vez en el año pasado, disminuyo de 16.7%, a 14% y el mes pasado el uso de drogas decreció de 10.7% en 1985 a 8.2% en 1988.

- A partir de diciembre de 1989, más de 18,200 Hispanoamericanos han contraido el SIDA. Por lo menos un 50% de estos casos incluían el uso intravenoso de drogas. También, más de un 80% de aquellos Hispanos que han contraido el SIDA por medio de contacto heterosexual habían adquirido la infección del Virus de Inmuno-Deficiencia Humanapor (VIH) por medio de contacto sexual con una persona que usa drogas por via intravenosa.

- De los 491 niños menores de 13 años de edad que han contraido el SIDA hasta 1989, más de 70% son hijos de madres cuyo riesgo de contraer la infección del VIH fue causado por el abuso de drogas intravenosas o por haber tenido relaciones sexuales con personas que usan drogas intravenosas. (Uno de cada tres Hispanos reportan haber contraido una enfermedad transmitida sexualmente.)

- Entre los Hispanos que usan drogas endovenosas, 23% del sexo masculino y 20% del sexo femenino, se inyectan a diario heroína, cocaína, o una mezcla de las dos ("speedball"). Entre aquello Hispanos que pocas veces usan una aguja nueva, 27% nunca usan blanqueo o alcohol para limpiar sus equipos antes de inyectarse, lo cual los pone a riesgo de contraer y a la vez de infectar a otros con las infección del VIH.

- A pesar de que el total de Hispanos es menos de un 10% de todos los casos reportados en las salas de emergencias entre 21 areas metropolitanas, los Hispanos tienen comparativamente un porcentaje más alto en el uso de ciertas drogas: heroína—14.6%; inhalables—15.4%; metadona—18.7%. Casi un 18% del total de Hispanos admitidos en salas de emergencias durante 1988 incluyeron heroína y/o morfina—lo que constituye el porcentaje más alto que ningun otro grupo étnico. Cerca de un 13% de las muertes ocasionadas por drogas en 27 areas metropolitanas ocurrieron entre Hispanos.

- Los Hispanos representan una sexta parte de los 254,000 Americanos que estaban en tratamiento por uso de drogas durante 1987. El porcentaje de pacientes Hispanos fue el más alto reportado en Arizona, California, Nuevo México, Nueva York y Texas. Sin embargo, entre aquellos Hispanos que usan drogas intravenosas, 41% nunca ha estado en tratamiento.

Para información sobre referencias a programas de tratamiento del abuso de drogas favor de llamar gratuitamente al telefono 1-800-66-**AYUDA** del NIDA.

Module II.7—Handout #4

ALCOHOL AND OTHER DRUG PROBLEMS ARE A MAJOR CONCERN IN NATIVE AMERICAN COMMUNITIES

In the United States, there are approximately 1.4 million Native Americans who belong to many tribes and Alaska Native groups. Over 500 tribes are recognized by the Bureau of Indian Affairs (*Federal Register*, 1986). Native Americans are one of the fastest growing population groups in this country.

There are vast cultural differences among Native American groups. In fact, differences between some Native American groups (such as Alaska Natives and Cherokee Indians) are as great as the differences between Native Americans and the dominant American culture. (As a matter of policy, the Office for Substance Abuse Prevention refers to these groups consistently as Native Americans.) In addition, although Native Americans originally resided in less populated areas, today they live in large cities and on reservations (or other rural areas) in about equal numbers.

Among Native Americans, alcohol and other drug abuse results in large numbers of preventable deaths, injuries, and illnesses, especially among adolescents and young adults. Most tribes consider alcohol and other drug problems as their most important health issue.

This fact sheet answers questions and provides resources for volunteers and professionals, such as teachers and prevention program planners, working with or preparing to work in Native American communities.

What type of drug is most commonly used among Native American young people?

Inhalants are among the drugs most frequently used by the Native American youth who use drugs.

Although there is variation among tribes, more Native American youth are observed to have tried inhalants than non-Native American youth. And more Native American than non-Native American youth continue to use inhalants on a regular basis.

Between 22 and 44% of different samples of Native American youth report having used inhalants. That compares with approximately 9.2% of a national sample of all youth ages 12–17 who report ever having used inhalants. In the past, boys abused inhalants more than girls, but recent data show that, at the 8th grade level, boys and girls are using inhalants at nearly the same rate. In fact, the level for girls may be slightly higher. Reports also suggest that young adolescents are likely to continue using inhalants while adding other drugs.

Another commonly used drug is smokeless tobacco (snuff). In a Washington State survey of 1,180 6th, 9th, and 11th graders, it was found that 34% of male Native Americans, 24% of female Native Americans, 20% of male non-Native Americans, and 4% of female non-Native Americans are current users of smokeless tobacco products.

What are the dangers of inhalant use?

Inhalant use can lead to irreversible brain damage, coma, and death. Even single time users run the risk of sudden or accidental death. Other serious effects include depression,

Module II.7—Handout #4 (continued)

leukemia, anemia, liver damage, and immune system damage. Violent outbursts can accompany heavy chronic inhalant use. Many youths who continue to use inhalants over a long period become antisocial and withdrawn—warning signs that differ from those of the youthful alcohol users, who tend to drink in groups.

Why do they do it? How old are the users?

Inhalants are probably the easiest mind-altering drugs to obtain. In addition, they are cheap and they reportedly offer a "high" of short duration, so users may experience several "highs" in a short time period. Although few Native American children as young as six years old report using inhalants, the usual age to start using appears to be about 10 years old. While many users stop using inhalants in their teens, often shifting to use of other drugs, there are many other users who have continued into their thirties.

What can be done about the use of inhalants and other drugs by Native American youth?

There are no easy answers. On an individual basis, Native American youth often feel hopeless and helpless and see no alternatives to alcohol and other drug use. To discourage use, parents, teachers, counselors, and others working with youth should keep glue, paints, aerosols, and gasoline locked up. They must also be aware of the signs of inhalant use; in all areas and groups, the best indicator of whether an adolescent is or will become a user is the use pattern of friends.

Since inhalants, snuff, and marijuana are often the gateway drugs for Native American youth, sometimes even preceding the first drink, it is important to begin prevention programs at young ages. Prevention programs need to be soundly planned, maintained over time, evaluated, and accompanied by economic and social improvement in realms other than health.

What other drugs are commonly used by young Native Americans?

Marijuana, stimulants, tranquilizers, hallucinogens, and cocaine are used by some young Native Americans. Marijuana, in particular, is used frequently. Native American youth are more likely than white youth to use marijuana and to begin using it at young ages. In fact, Indian youth have higher rates of drug use than non-Indian youth for nearly all drugs.

According to national survey data, approximately 24% of all American youth ages 12–17 report having used marijuana at least once. In comparison, 46% of Native American youth in grades 7–12 report having tried marijuana at least once, according to data collected from several major reservations across the United States. About half of these youth had tried it by age 13. In a study of 7th–12th graders between 1975 and 1983, it as found that 53% of Native American youth could be classified as "at risk" in their drug involvement, compared with 35% of non-Native American youth. Indian Health Service records over a three-year period indicate that almost two-thirds of all alcohol program clients also used marijuana.

Module II.7—Handout #4 (continued)

Does this mean that few young Native Americans drink alcohol?

Unfortunately, no. Drinking is prevalent among adolescent and even younger Native American children. In a recent survey, 82% of Native American 7th–12th graders living on several major reservations across the United States reported that they had used alcohol at least once.

This compares with 66% of non-Native American youth sampled at the same time. Also alcohol use appears to be heavy among Native American youth; reports of blacking out or being extremely intoxicated are common.

Is it true that most Native American people have trouble with alcohol? Are Native Americans more prone to alcoholism?

Native Americans and Native American tribes vary greatly with regard to alcohol use. Overall, a higher percentage of Native American adults never drink, compared to non-Native Americans. However, among Native American people who do drink, a large percentage drink heavily. And Native Americans have the highest prevalence of alcohol problems among all U.S. population groups. It appears that those Native Americans run twice the risk of becoming alcoholic. But it is important to remember that many Native Americans drink very little, and many others have made the safe and healthy choice not to drink at all.

Do Native Americans suffer from poorer health or die from alcohol- and other drug-related problems at rates higher than the general U.S. population?

Yes, current information indicates that Native Americans have poorer health and are dying at far higher rates than the U.S. population. It has long been thought that alcohol abuse plays a role in the poorer health of Native Americans, but few studies offer uncontested evidence. The Indian Health Service reports that hospital discharge rates during 1981 for Native Americans with alcohol-related diagnoses were three times higher than for people in the United States as a whole.

A 1987 survey of 49 hospitals revealed that one out of four Native American inpatients was hospitalized for an alcohol-related cause. The Indian Health Service began collecting other drug-related health information in 1988, and reports on those relationships are forthcoming.

Although the age-adjusted alcoholism death rate for Native Americans has decreased in the last 10 years, the rate in 1985 was still 4.2 times the rate for the United States. The age-adjusted cirrhosis mortality rate for Native Americans in 1986 was 26.4 as compared to 9.2 for the general population. In addition, motor vehicle crashes and other accidents are among the leading causes of death for Native American people. Native American death rates for both are over two times the U.S. rates. Causes include death from drowning, fire and smoke, excessive cold, and firearms. While alcohol abuse is thought to be a major factor in motor vehicle crashes and other accidents, there has been little research into the extent of alcohol involvement.

Instructor's Guide

Module II.7—Handout #4 (continued)

Are suicide rates high for Native Americans? Are these deaths related to alcohol and other drug use?

Suicide rates for Native Americans are higher than for other U.S. population groups, and current information indicates that alcohol and other drug use is an important factor. Over 80% of suicides among Native Americans appear to involve alcohol, according to several regional and tribal studies. This compares to other studies that show that 20–37% of suicides in general involve alcohol; however, research has not been reported for directly comparable population groups residing in the same part of the country.

The highest suicide rates among Native Americans are among young men ages 15–34, whereas among all American men, the highest rates are among men older than 34. Among Native Americans as in the dominant society, more men complete their suicide. Methods cited include firearms, hanging, and overdoses. The motive in most cases appeared to be "to change an important relationship or deal with an unacceptable interpersonal relationship." Violent death, suicide, homicide, accident, and alcoholism rates for Alaska Natives are higher than for Alaska non-Natives, Native Americans, and the U.S. population as a whole. It is important to note that there are significant differences in tribal rates, and there may be a tendency for suicide to be over-reported on reservations and under-reported elsewhere in the United States.

Is the difference in rates of problem drinking and alcoholism due to a genetic difference?

Some studies report that Native Americans metabolize alcohol more rapidly than whites and therefore may be especially susceptible to alcoholism due to genetic or biological factors.

However, little is known about the biological aspects of alcoholism in Native Americans. And, based on what we know, differences in rates of alcoholism cannot be tied to genetic or biological factors. Although many people believe biological factors play a role, the nature of that role is not known.

However, we do know that there appears to be a certain sensitivity to alcohol that is shared by Asians/Asian Americans and Native Americans of both North and South America.

This sensitivity is shown in a rapid rushing of blood to the face when drinking alcohol. Called "facial flushing," this physical response is related to a genetic difference in the key enzyme involved in the oxidation (that is, breakdown) of acetaldehyde, which is the primary metabolic product when alcohol breaks down in the human body. It continues to puzzle researchers, then, that alcoholism is relatively uncommon among Asians but more common in Native Americans.

Adding to the puzzle, comparisons of metabolism of alcohol between white Americans and Native Americans frequently show no significant differences. The data are so inconsistent that no firm hypothesis has been offered. A recent review points out that, in general, much greater genetic variation is found within ethnic groups than among racial groups. And, in fact, Native Americans vary greatly among themselves in regard to alcohol sensitivity.

Module II.7

Module II.7—Handout #4 *(continued)*

Are Indian people more prone to difficulties with alcohol because of social and cultural factors?

Some day researchers will probably discover that it is a complex mix of genetic, social, and cultural factors that leads to alcoholism in all peoples, not just Native American people. Nowhere are the answers to questions like this more uncertain than in the case of alcoholism. However, more researchers argue that sociocultural factors, rather than biological or psychological factors, underlie some Native Americans' abuse of alcohol.

Theories that attempt to explain the role of environmental factors include:

1. *Stock-in-Society Theory*—that people with a stake in the dominant society, such as steady employment, will be less likely to become alcoholic.

2. *Defiance-Rebel Theory*—that alcohol gives many Native Americans a feeling of power, which they so often lack when dealing with modern society. Drinking has been viewed as defiance against white authority and against prohibition on the reservations.

3. *Invasion Reaction Theory*—that alcohol abuse among Native Americans is a reaction to the loss of tradition and culture. Native Americans abuse alcohol in mourning the loss of historical tradition and in reaction to the demands to integrate with mainstream culture.

4. *Social Learning Theory*—that the group drinking style (including drinking until supplies are depleted) that characterizes much Native American drinking actually was learned from the frontiersmen settling the West.

5. *Bicultural Theory*—that Native American children who are "bicultural" show the lowest use of alcohol and other drugs among Native American youth. Bicultural means identifying with both the traditional Native American culture and with the non-Native American world. It does not mean a blend of these cultures so much as it means an ability to adapt to each, depending on the circumstance.

6. *Chemical Warfare Theory*—that alcohol was used against Native American people as one of the first "chemical warfare" weapons deployed in the New World. It was used to cloud judgment and to cheat people in trade relations, particularly in the fur trade and land negotiations. Because of its addicting nature, Native American people continued to use and abuse it for the release that it provided.

7. *Socioeconomic Theory*—that poverty and the adversity of Native American life contribute to stress and provide an environment where alcohol and other drug use can thrive. These background circumstances include social and economic disorganization resulting from the rapid, forced changes in culture experienced by Native Americans. This, in turn, has resulted in economic dependency on the government, as well as emotional depression in individuals.

Some experts warn that one must be careful with "cultural" interpretations of susceptibility to alcohol and other drug use and abuse. There is no evidence that there is anything inherent in Native American culture that leads to alcohol and other drug abuse. In fact, strong identification with one's culture may be a protective factor.

Instructor's Guide

Module II.7—Handout #4 (continued)

The "bottom line," of course, is that excessive drinking is destructive, no matter what the reasons for it. Some people, both Native American and white, who view themselves as being in a high-risk group for addiction problems choose to leave both alcohol and other drugs alone. Many Native American elders view abstinence as essential in the task of restoring tribal cultural values and traditions. Because times and cultures change, the reasons for excessive drinking may also be changing.

What about Native American women? Do they have trouble with alcohol and other drugs?

In general, more men than women drink in all population groups. And more Native American males than Native American females drink. Still, Native American women have high rates of alcoholism and alcohol-related health problems.

For instance, one indicator of the rate of alcoholism in a population is the liver cirrhosis death rate. Native American women are dying of cirrhosis at high rates and frequently at young ages. The 1975 national cirrhosis death rate per 100,000 Native American women was more than six times the rate of white women. The 1975 national cirrhosis death rate for Native American women ages 15–34 was 36 times the white rate. Cirrhosis mortality within the State of Minnesota was examined for the time period 1970 through 1981, and it was found that Native American women had the highest death rates of all groups (whites, blacks, Native Americans), and they had the lowest average age at death (44.5 years).

Also Native American women who use drugs begin using them at a young age, often at 10 or 11 years. Marijuana, stimulants, and inhalants are as popular with many young women as with young men.

Do many Native American women give birth to infants with fetal alcohol defects?

Virtually all tribes have fertility rates twice as high as the general U.S. rate. There is also a high rate of alcoholism among Native American people. Therefore, it is not surprising that the rate of alcohol-related birth defects is higher among Native Americans, although there are marked intertribal differences in the rates of incidence.

Drinking alcohol during pregnancy can be dangerous to a developing baby. Alcohol passes freely from the mother's body to the baby's body and affects the developing systems of the unborn baby. The more a pregnant mother drinks, the greater the chances of harm to the unborn child. Children whose mothers drink frequently or heavily during pregnancy may be born with fetal alcohol syndrome (**FAS**). There are certain characteristics that constitute a diagnosis of FAS. If a child shows one or more signs in each of the following three categories, a diagnosis of FAS is likely: (1) prenatal or postnatal growth retardation; (2) central nervous system involvement, such as mental retardation or delayed development; and (3) characteristic cranial and facial abnormalities. There are many more children who have been affected by alcohol *in utero* but who lack the full set of characteristics that define FAS. These babies may be at higher risk because they are too small at birth, or they may have some but not all of the features of FAS. These problems, when attributable to alcohol, are called fetal alcohol effects (**FAE**).

Module II.7

Module II.7—Handout #4 *(continued)*

What can be done about alcohol- and other drug-related birth defects?

Many organizations, tribes, and states have developed fetal alcohol syndrome prevention programs.

Currently, the Indian Health Service is increasing community awareness about the dangers of maternal alcohol and other drug use and encouraging clinical staff to emphasize screening and education to prevent these birth defects.

Such prevention programs can serve a two-fold purpose. In addition to preventing alcohol- and other drug-related birth defects in newborns, the programs can be a starting point for talking in general about alcohol and other drugs in Native American communities.

According to Dr. Phil May of the University of New Mexico, Native Americans are eager for more information on how they can assure that their children are born healthy.

"In my experience spanning five years and over 400 presentations by myself and three colleagues, it has become obvious that the topic of fetal alcohol syndrome is universally well received among Indian groups," Dr. May says. "Our experience has shown that Indian groups of all ages are interested, motivated and stimulated to action by this topic. It is a much more effective starting point to ongoing education and exchange of information about alcohol and drugs than any other specific topic."

What about alcohol and other drug abuse treatment for Native Americans? We've heard that the usual treatment methods do not work for Native Americans.

It is not known which treatment approaches are most effective with different patients. According to Frank L. Iber of the Veterans Administration, it appears that the most effective programs are "run by persons of the same background who by lifetime experiences have the kind of understanding that is difficult to teach."

Unfortunately, there is a sense of futility felt by many Native American communities—as well as individuals—that alcoholism is inevitable and possibly untreatable. Therefore, one of the main messages of the Office of Substance Abuse Prevention (OSAP) is that alcohol and other drug problems are both preventable and treatable. OSAP also focuses attention on attempts that Native American people are making to free themselves of afflictions due to alcohol.

There is a resurgence of interest in traditional culture in Native American communities today, and this has resulted in treatment approaches that involve traditional healers, such as medicine men and women.

Office of Substance Abuse Prevention. (1988). *Alcohol and other drug problems are a major concern of Native American communities.* (Document #M53292). Rockville, MD: Author.

Module II.7—Handout #5

NATIONAL INSTITUTE ON DRUG ABUSE: MAJOR DRUG ABUSE SURVEYS WITH DATA ON MINORITY POPULATIONS

Data Base	Collection Frequency	Sample Size	Description
National High School Senior Survey	Annually: 1975 to present	16,000–17,000	Drug use, attitudes, availability, and perceptions of harm. (W/B)*
National Household Survey on Drug Abuse	1985 data on Hispanics and Blacks	8,038 total	Epidemiologic survey of use and consequences of 13 drugs or classes (includes alcohol and cigarettes). (RE)**
Drug Abuse Warning Network (DAWN)	Annually: 1972 to present	About 150,000 episodes annually	Ongoing drug abuse surveillance of emergency rooms and medical examiner cases from selected cities and a national panel (RE)
National Alcoholism and Drug Abuse Treatment Units (NADATUS)	Annually: 1977 to 1982; 1984 and 1987	About 12,000 units for 1987	Survey of treatment services and resources, directory of drug abuse and alcohol units, and program availability of special services for minorities. (W/B/H/O)
Client-Oriented Data Acquisition Process (CODAP)	Annually: 1975–1985	About 100,000 in the nation	Treatment prevalence, data on client treatment of drug abuse, 1975–1981 samples were national, 1982–1985 samples were of volunteer states. (W/B/H/O)
Treatment Outcome Prospective Study (TOPS)	1979–1981	1,300–2,400 follow-up sample yearly; 11,750 total intakes from 1979–1981	Longitudinal study of drug abuse clients in treatment. (RE)

*Groups in the data base can be specified as (W) White, (B) Black, (H) Hispanic, (O) Other.
**RE = Race/ethnicity specified; e.g., specific Hispanic group and American Indians also can be specified.

Module II.7

Module II.7—Handout #6

RESOURCES OF DATA ON THE HOMELESS

Clearinghouse on Homelessness among
Mentally Ill People (CHAMP)
8630 Fenton Street, Suite 300
Silver Spring, MD 20910
(301) 588-5484

Homelessness Exchange
Community Information Exchange
1120 G Street, NW, Suite 900
Washington, DC 20005
(202) 628-2990/2981

National Coalition for the Homeless
1439 Rhode Island Avenue, NW
Washington, DC 20005
(202) 659-3310

NYC/National Coalition for the Homeless
105 East 22nd Street
New York, NY 10010
(212) 460-8110

National Volunteer Hotline
Operated by the Community for Creative Non-Violence
425 Second Street, NW
Washington, DC 20001
1-800-HELP-664

New York Coalition for the Homeless
90 State Street
Albany, NY 12207
(518) 436-5612

Westchester Coalition for the Homeless
201 Palisades Avenue, Suite 103
Yonkers, NY 10703
(914) 476-0008

Legislative Alert System
National Coalition for the Homeless
(212) 460-8110

For an appointment or to support a bill:
Call Senators and Representatives at (202) 244-3121

Instructor's Guide

RECOMMENDED TEACHING STRATEGIES AND SAMPLE ASSIGNMENTS

RECOMMENDED TEACHING STRATEGIES

- Clinical placement in drug and alcohol treatment centers and community agencies
- Lecture
- Small group discussion
- Attitude assessment
- Seminars
- Role-playing to sensitize providers.
    1. Role-playing to increase cultural sensitivity in students working with ethnic minorities:
        a. Provide specific profiles of individuals in ethnic minority groups in order to minimize stereotyping.
    2. Role-playing to increase general sensitivity:
        a. HIV-positive client who is an active substance abuser.
        b. Homeless client.
- Attendance at Twelve-Step meeting, Women for Sobriety group, to increase understanding of self-help experience.
- Field trips to city shelter system, therapeutic communities, community drop-in centers, halfway houses, grass-roots, and lay/professional organizations.
- Map out and diagram comprehensive community resources.
- Develop networking charts and interrelated agencies, including the functions of each.

SAMPLE ASSIGNMENTS

Role-Play Exercise I—Joseph Ramirez

CASE VIGNETTE

Joseph Ramirez is 28 years old. He is unmarried, a high school graduate and, for the past 10 months, has been employed as a bank teller. He lives in a multi-generational household

Module II.7

in a well-kept working class neighborhood. The house is owned by his parents, who have many neighborhood friends of Hispanic background. The Ramirez family espouses strong religious values and a commitment to improving their socioeconomic status through education and "honest work."

The nurse first meets Joseph upon his admission to an emergency room. He is one of several young men involved in an automobile accident. All of the occupants and the driver have been drinking alcohol. Although Joseph's injuries are minor, the incident appears to have a strong emotional impact on him. He sits isolated from his comrades, appears withdrawn and tearful.

Role-Play—Nurse's Script

Your task in this role-play is to:

1. Assess the severity and intensity of Mr. Ramirez' alcohol use.
2. Identify client factors associated with his cultural background.
3. Assess risk factors which might affect his alcohol-using patterns.
4. Provide direct nursing care to this client by:
   a. Attending to immediate needs.
   b. Educating him about consequences of this incident.
   c. Setting goals, in collaboration with the client.
   d. Establishing a baseline for preventive intervention, commensurate with his current level of alcohol use.
   e. Refer and/or provide for follow-up.

Role-Play Exercise II—Starhawk Jones

CASE VIGNETTE

Starhawk Jones is a 42-year-old Native American who functions as a car mechanic on a reservation. He has drunk heavily on a daily basis for the past three years and rarely leaves the reservation. He is markedly reticent around strangers and has become increasingly sad and hopeless lately. He believes that his father's spirit is unable to rest peacefully because a new sewage system is being built near the burial grounds. He often walks many miles rather than risk further disruption to the ground by driving his truck. His sister brought Starhawk to the health clinic because she found him crying and unkempt last week. He has not been to his job for 10 days and his boss is threatening to fire him.

Role-Play—Nurse's Script

Your task in role-play is to:

1. Assess health deviations associated with alcohol problems in this Native American man.
2. Identify client needs related to health deviations in association with alcoholic drinking.

Instructor's Guide

3. Utilize institutional and community resources in delivering direct care to this client.
4. Provide direct nursing care to this client; e.g., by:
   a. Helping him identify areas he can control.
   b. Assisting him in setting realistic goals for himself.
   c. Teaching him methods of assertiveness and effective communication.
   d. Providing frequent contact with this client, realizing that he will rarely initiate contact with a white, female authority figure whom he fears.

Role-Play Exercise III—Bonnie Jackson

CASE VIGNETTE

Bonnie Jackson is a 34-year-old black woman who supports her heroin addiction by prostitution. She has been living a "junkie" lifestyle for about five years but longs to get sober, marry, and settle down to have a child. Bonnie insists that all of her clients wear condoms; however, this was not always her policy and she tries never to be desperate enough for a fix that she gets careless. After her morning "wake up," Bonnie hustles unless she happens to "go on the nod." She never frequents shooting galleries but is unsure about whether her regular boyfriend has, or at least shared needles, in the past. Bonnie claims that she has never personally shared her works. She kicked her habit twice in the past year by going "cold turkey" and neither wants nor trusts the help of professionals.

Role-Play—Nurse's Script

Your task in this role-play is to:

1. Assess the pattern of drug and alcohol use in relation to social and cultural traditions, as well as lifestyle in this minority, female, IV drug user.
2. Identify multiple health risks which interact to create problems secondary to drug addiction in this client and her significant other.
3. Determine the client's awareness of resources that she might find helpful.
4. Intervene with this client; e.g., by:
   a. Offering unconditional positive acceptance of her.
   b. Assisting her in exploring and accepting the positive and negative aspects of herself.
   c. Reinforcing the importance of safer sex practices, especially the use of condoms with all partners.

SENSITIVITY EXERCISE

Imagine You Are Homeless . . .

Imagine you are a 33-year-old woman with three children. Your apartment burned down six months ago. You and your children had been living with your sister in her cramped apartment until she had another baby, and there simply was not enough room for everyone.

Module II.7

You sleep in your car at night. During the day, you walk the streets with your children trying to find an apartment you can afford. Finally, you go to the department of social services to try to find shelter for the night and are told that your children may have to be placed in foster care if a place cannot be found for all of you. Knowing that the foster care system in this city is unreliable and sometimes unsafe, you agree to spend the first night in an overcrowded warehouse-type shelter, where you end up sleeping on the floor.

You and your children have no privacy here. Many of the children and adults have colds and you hear that tuberculosis has been an increasing problem among the homeless. When the opportunity arises, you agree to move into one of the single-room occupancy hotels that the city is using to house homeless families "temporarily." That temporary shelter becomes your home for 13 months.

The temporary shelter consists of one 10 × 10 foot room. You have no kitchen, no refrigerator, no stove or cooking facilities. There is one bed for you and your three children.

You pull the mattress off the bed at night to make room for all of you to sleep and then pull the sheets off the bed in the day to eat on the floor.

You use running water to keep your baby's milk cool and you do the dishes in the tub where you bathe and store things.

There is no place for your children to play, no place to sit, no place to do homework. When they try to play in the hall, they are approached by drug dealers and sometimes even by pimps.

This is what life is like for you and your children. Imagine the gradual dissipation of your own and your children's self-esteem and the isolation and depression that eventually overwhelm you. Imagine having a future without space, without privacy, without hope.

(Source of vignette: Berne, A., Dato, C., Mason, D., & Rafferty, M. (1990). A nursing model for addressing the health needs of homeless families. *Image, 22*(1), 11.)

1. Imagine the 33-year-old woman with a name: Mary, Carmelita, Cyndra, Olga, Kathleen.

2. Does the picture in your mind change with the knowledge that this woman is a drug abuser? An alcoholic? A deeply religious abstainer?

3. Discuss the critical issues facing this woman and the complications wrought by the high risk of substance abuse which is inherent in this population.

4. Discuss the major constraints confronting health care providers who have access to this population.

5. Look to the future. What do you see for this woman in the next five years? In 10 years? What do you see for her three children?

OTHER SAMPLE ASSIGNMENTS

Identify one program for the homeless in your community.

1. Describe the program in terms of the population and the exact nature of the services it provides.

2. What physical facilities are utilized by the program? Describe the facility in terms of its appropriateness and adequacy for the goals of the program.

3. How does this program contribute to the health care needs of the homeless relative to phenomena of concern to nurses?

Instructor's Guide

4. Discuss preventive interventions appropriate to the population and how these interventions might be implemented.

5. Interview a participant in this program. In what ways is life different for this person? What components does this person feel remain as serious problems?

Interview a nurse working with the homeless population.

1. How do alcoholism and substance abuse impact on the potential for change in the health status of these people?

2. What knowledge and skills are most valuable in implementing effective interventions with the homeless population?

Module II.7

TEST QUESTIONS AND ANSWERS

TEST QUESTIONS

1. Which of the following are true of female drinking habits?
    1. Females may begin later in life but progress to problem drinking faster.
    2. Alcohol abuse results in more rapid physical damage in females than in males.
    3. Heavy drinking among women has increased in recent years.
    4. Female alcoholics are harder to treat than male alcoholics.
    a. 1, 2, & 3
    b. 1, 2, & 4
    c. 2 & 4
    d. 1 & 2

2. Nurses who care for ethnic minority substance abusers need to take into account the clients' culture in order to better understand:
    a. the clients' ways of thinking, feeling, and responding.
    b. why clients use drugs excessively.
    c. dietary practices necessary to maintain good health.
    d. the clients' objective symptomatology.

3. In setting up a plan of care for Ms. Lopez, a 64-year-old Spanish speaking woman, which treatment would be most beneficial considering her cultural background?
    a. Individual therapy.
    b. "Family" counseling with her significant peers.
    c. Assertiveness training.
    d. Antidepressants.

4. The incidence of alcohol and drug use in ethnic groups can best be described as:
    a. more prevalent in lower socioeconomic classes.
    b. about equal among males and females.
    c. less prevalent because of religious beliefs.
    d. highly variable among women in these groups.

5. The link between substance abuse and AIDS is resulting in an increased incidence of AIDS for:
    a. male intravenous drug users.
    b. male homosexuals and their sexual partners.

Instructor's Guide

   c. intravenous drug users and their sexual partners.

   d. infants born of seropositive mothers.

6. Factors which support the prevalence of alcoholism in homeless populations are considered to be primarily:

   a. related to the health care delivery system.

   b. biologic in origin.

   c. related to social services.

   d. linked with seropositive status.

7. Widespread dependence on alcohol in Native American populations is:

   a. due to physiological vulnerability.

   b. caused by stress between dominant and minority cultures.

   c. problematic in both men and women in respective Indian nations.

   d. the primary cause of unemployment in this population.

8. Which statement best describes alcohol and other drug use among African-Americans?

   a. Dominant religions prohibit use of alcohol and drugs.

   b. Use patterns vary according to cultural traditions.

   c. African-Americans of Caribbean descent are the largest groups of marijuana users.

   d. Drug use is central to the practice of folk medicine.

9. While overall alcohol consumption is similar for African-Americans and Caucasians, African-Americans experience higher rates of:

   a. peripheral neuropathy.

   b. cancer.

   c. vehicular homicide.

   d. brain tumors.

10. Which factor appears to correlate most closely with drug use by Hispanic women?

    a. Childbearing status.

    b. Marital status.

    c. Traditional cultural values.

    d. Traditional religious beliefs.

Module II.7

ANSWER KEY

1. a
2. a
3. b
4. d
5. c
6. c
7. c
8. b
9. b
10. c

BIBLIOGRAPHY

MODULE II.7 DRUG AND ALCOHOL PROBLEMS IN SPECIAL POPULATIONS

American Nurses' Association, Drug and Alcohol Nurses Association, & National Nurses' Society on Addictions. (1987). *The care of clients with addictions: Dimensions of nursing practice.* Kansas City, MO: American Nurses' Association.

American Nurses' Association & National Nurses Society on Addictions. (1988). *Standards of addictions nursing practice with selected diagnoses and criteria.* Kansas City, MO: American Nurses' Association.

Atkins, B. J., Klein, M. A., & Mosley, B. (1987). Black adolescents' attitudes toward the use of alcohol and other drugs. *International Journal of Addictions, 22*(12), 1201–1211.

Beauvais, F., Oetting, E. R., & Edwards, R. W. (1985). Trends in drug use of Indian adolescents living on reservations: 1975–1983. *American Journal of Drug and Alcohol Abuse, 11*(3–4), 209–229.

Beckman, L. J., & Bradsley, P. (1981). The perceived determinants and consequences of alcohol consumption among young women heavy drinkers. *International Journal of Addictions, 16*(1), 75–88.

Berne, A., Dato, C., Mason, D., & Rafferty, M. (1990). A nursing model for addressing the health needs of homeless families. *Image, 22,* 11.

Blume, S. (1986). Women and alcohol: A review. *Journal of the American Medical Association, 256*(11), 1467–1469.

Bowker, L. H. (1977). *Drug use among women young and old.* San Francisco, CA: R & E Research Associates.

Bradstock, K., Forman, M. R., Binkin, N. J., Gentry, E. M., et al. (1988). Alcohol use and health behavior lifestyles among U.S. women: The behavioral risk factor surveys. *Addictive Behaviors, 13*(1), 61–71.

Breakey, W. R. (1987). Treating the homeless. *Alcohol Health and Research World, 11*(3), 42–47, 90.

Brickner, P. W., Scharer, L. K., & Cananan, B. (Eds.). (1985). *Health care of homeless people.* New York: Springer.

Brunswick, A., & Messeri, P. (1984). Causal factors in onset of adolescents' cigarette smoking: A prospective study of urban black youth. *Advances in Alcohol & Substance Abuse, 3*(1–2), 35–52.

Module II.7

Bry, B. (1983). Substance abuse in women: Etiology and prevention. *Issues in Mental Health Nursing, 5*(1–4), 153–172.

Caetano, R. (1987). Alcohol use and depression among U.S. Hispanics. *British Journal of Addictions, 82*(11), 1245–1251.

Celentano, D. D., & McQueen, E. C. (1980). Substance abuse by women: A review of the epidemiologic literature. *Chronic Disease, 33,* 383–394.

Celentano, D. D., & McQueen, D. V. (1984). Alcohol consumption patterns among women in Baltimore. *Journal of Studies on Alcohol, 45,* 355–358.

Centers for Disease Control. (1989, September). *HIV/AIDS surveillance report.* Atlanta, GA: Author.

Dawkins, M. P. (1980). *Alcohol and the black community.* Saratoga, CA: Century Twenty-One.

Delgado, M. (1988). Alcoholism treatment and Hispanic youth. *Journal of Drug Issues, 18*(1), 59–68.

DiCicco-Bloom, B., Space, S., & Zahourek, R. P. (1986). The homebound alcoholic. *American Journal of Nursing, 86*(2), 167–169.

Doshan, T., & Bursch, C. (1982). Women and substance abuse: Critical issues in treatment and health. *Journal of Drug Education, 12*(3), 229–239.

Estep, R. (1987). Influence of the family on the use of alcohol and prescription depressants by women. *Journal of Psychoactive Drugs, 19*(2), 171–179.

Faltz, B. G., & Madover, S. (1988). Treatment of substance abuse in patients with HIV infection. *Advances in Alcohol and Substance Abuse, 7*(2), 143–157.

Fischer, P. J., & Breakey, W. R. (1987). Profile of the Baltimore homeless with alcohol problems. *Alcohol Health and Research World, 11*(3), 36–37, 61.

Gelberg, L., Linn, L. S., & Leake, B. D. (1986). Mental health, alcohol and drug use and criminal history among homeless adults. *American Journal of Psychiatry, 145*(2), 191–196.

Gilbert, M., & Alcocoer, A. (1988). Alcohol use and Hispanic youth: An overview. *Journal of Drug Issues, 18*(1), 33–48.

Glick, R., & Moore, J. (Eds.). (1990). *Drugs in Hispanic communities.* New Brunswick, NJ: Rutgers University Press.

Guinan, M. E., & Hardy, A. (1987). Epidemiology of AIDS in women in the United States. *Journal of the American Medical Association, 257,* 2039–2042.

Harper, F. D. (1976). *Alcohol abuse and black Americans.* Alexandria, VA: Douglas.

Institute of Medicine. (1990). *Broadening the base of treatment for alcohol problems.* Washington, DC: National Academy Press.

Kagle, J. D. (1987). Secondary prevention of substance abuse. *Social Work, 32*(5), 446–448.

Kandel, L. L., & North, S. (1982). Sex roles, sexuality and the recovering woman alcoholic: Program issues. *Journal of Psychoactive Drugs, 14,* 163–166.

Kelly, J. A., et al. (1988, March/April). A women's concern. *International Nursing Review*, *35*(2), 55.

Lancaster, J. (1988). Substance abuse. In M. Stanhope & J. Lancaster (Eds.), *Community health nursing*. St. Louis, MO: C. V. Mosby.

Lawson, G. W., & Lawson, A. W. (1989). *Alcoholism and substance abuse in special populations*. Rockville, MD: Aspen.

Lee, L. J. (1983). Reducing black adolescents' drug use: Family revisited. In R. Israelowitz & M. Singer (Eds.), *Adolescent substance abuse: A guide to prevention and treatment* (pp. 57–69). New York: Plenum.

Manson, S. M. (Ed.). (1982). *New directions in prevention among American Indian and Alaskan Native communities*. Portland, OR: Oregon Health Sciences University.

McGoldrick, M., Pearce, J., & Giordano, J. (Eds.). (1980). *Ethnicity and family therapy*. New York: Guilford.

Moore, M. H., & Gernstein, D. K. (Eds.). (1981). *Alcohol and public policy: Beyond the shadow of prohibition*. Washington, DC: National Academy Press.

Morales, A. (1984). Substance abuse and Mexican-American youth: An overview. *Journal of Drug Issues*, *14*(2), 297–311.

Naegle, M. A. (1988). Substance abuse among women: Prevalence, patterns and treatment issues. *Issues in Mental Health*, 9, 2.

National Coalition for the Homeless. (1990). *Portrait of the homeless*. Washington, DC: Author.

National Institute on Drug Abuse. (1986). *Drug abuse statistics: 1985 population estimates*. Rockville, MD: National Clearinghouse for Alcohol and Drug Information.

National Institute on Drug Abuse. (1986). *Heroin statistics: 1985 population estimates*. Rockville, MD: National Clearinghouse for Alcohol and Drug Information.

National Institute of Drug Abuse. (1987). *National drug and alcoholism treatment unit survey: Final report (NDATUS)*. Rockville, MD: Author.

National Institute on Drug Abuse. (1986). *NIDA's activities in the areas of AIDS and IV drug use: 1985 population estimates*. Rockville, MD: National Clearinghouse for Alcohol and Drug Information.

National Institute on Drug Abuse. (1988). *Drug Abuse Warning Network (DAWN) annual data series*, *1*(8). Rockville, MD: Author.

National Institute on Drug Abuse. (1989). *National household survey on drug abuse: 1988 population estimates*. Rockville, MD: National Clearinghouse for Alcohol and Drug Information.

New York City Department of Health. (1990, August 3). *AIDS surveillance report*. New York: Author.

Office of Substance Abuse Prevention. (1988). Alcohol and other Drug Problems Are a Major Concern in Native American Communities. (Document #M53292) Rockville, MD: Author.

Module II.7

Okwumabua, J. O., & Duryea, E. J. (1987). Age of onset, periods of risk and patterns of progression in drug use among American Indian high school students. *International Journal of Addictions, 22*(12), 1269–1276.

Penniman, L. J., & Agnew, J. (1988). Women and alcohol. In C. Wright (Ed.), *Rehabilitation of the alcoholic* (pp. 171–180). Philadelphia, PA: Handey & Belfus, Inc.

Reed, B. G. (1985). Drug misuse and dependency in women: The meaning of being considered a special population or minority group. *International Journal of the Addictions, 20*(1), 13–62.

Reed, B. G. (1987). Developing women-sensitive drug dependence treatment services: Why so difficult? *Journal of Psychoactive Drugs, 19*(2), 151–164.

Robert-Gurnoff, M. (1986). Prevalence of antibodies to HTLV-I, II and III in intravenous drug abusers from an AIDS endemic region. *Journal of the American Medical Association, 255*(22), 3133–3137.

Ropers, R. H. (1987). Homelessness as a health risk. *Alcohol Health and Research World, 11*(3), 38–41, 89.

Schinke, S. P., Botvin, G., & Trimble, J. E. (1988). Preventing substance abuse among American Indian adolescents: A bicultural competence skills approach. *Journal of Counseling Psychology, 35*(1), 87–90.

Smith, J. M. (1990). Using a community survey to determine health action priorities. *The Provider, 15*(10), 134–138.

Stall, R. (1988). Prevention of HIV infection associated with drug and alcohol abuse. *Advances in Alcohol and Abuse, 7*(2), 73–87.

Stimmel, B. (1987). AIDS, alcohol and heroin: A particularly deadly combination. *Advances in Alcohol and Substance Abuse, 6*(3), 1–5.

U.S. Department of Health and Human Services. (1990a, January). *Secretary's seventh special report to the U.S. Congress on alcohol and health.* Washington, DC: Author.

U.S. Department of Health and Human Services. (1990b). *Citizen's alcohol and other drug prevention directory: Resources for getting involved* (DHHS Publication No. (ADM) 90-1657). Rockville, MD: U.S. Public Health Service.

Vener, A. M., Kreyoka, L. R., & Climio, J. J. (1980). Drug use and health characteristics in non-institutionalized Mexican-American elderly. *Journal of Drug Education, 10,* 343–353.

Watts, T. D., & Wright, R., Jr. (Eds.). (1983). *Black alcoholism: Toward a comprehensive understanding.* Springfield, IL: Charles C. Thomas.

Williams, J., & Bates, W. (1970). Some characteristics of female narcotic addicts. *International Journal of Addictions, 5*(2), 245–256.

Wilsnack, S. C., Klassen, A. D., Schor, B. E., & Wilsnack, R. (1991). Predicting onset and chronicity of women's problem drinking: A five-year longitudinal analysis. *American Journal of Public Health, 81*(3), 305–317.

Wilsnack, S., Wilsnack, R., & Klassen, A. (1987, Winter). Drinking and drinking problems among women in a U.S. national survey. *Alcohol Health and Research World,* 3–12.

Wilsnack, S., Klassen, C., & Wilsnack, R. W. (1984). Drinking and reproductive dysfunction among women in a national survey. *Alcoholism: Clinical and Experimental Research, 8,* 451–458.

Wilsnack, S., & Beckman, L. (1984). *Alcohol problems in women.* New York: Guilford.

Wolper, B., & Scheiner, Z. (1981). *Family therapy approaches and drug dependent women.* (Treatment Research Monograph). Rockville, MD: National Institute on Drug Abuse.

Wright, R., & Watts, T. D. (1988). Alcohol and minority youth. *Journal of Drug Issues, 18*(1), 1–7.

Young, T. J. (1987). Inhalant use among American Indian youth. *Child Psychiatry and Human Development, 18*(1), 36–46.

MODULE II.8
NURSING CARE OF
DRUG AND ALCOHOL PROBLEMS
IN SPECIAL POPULATIONS

Aileen H. Clucas, MSN, RN, CCDN
Vivian P. J. Clarke, EdD, CHES
Consultant

Madeline A. Naegle, PhD, RN, FAAN
Project Director
Janet S. D'Arcangelo, MA, RN, C
Project Coordinator

Project SAEN
SUBSTANCE ABUSE
EDUCATION IN NURSING

CONTENT OUTLINE

I. Assessing Drug and Alcohol Use in Specific Populations
    A. Cultural Groups/Ethnic Minorities
    B. Intravenous Drug Users
    C. Women
    D. Homeless

II. Identification of Health Care Needs in Special Populations
    A. Defining Alcohol and Drug Specific Health Needs
    B. Factors Influencing Clients and Group Behavior in Relation to Health Care Problems
    C. Nursing Diagnoses of Drug and Alcohol Problems

III. Implementation of Nursing Intervention
    A. Community Factors Which Influence Care Delivery
    B. Prevention of Alcohol- and Drug-Related Problems
    C. Care Delivery to Specific Groups
    D. Evaluation of Care Provision in Response to Special Population Needs

Module II.8

CONTENTS

I. ASSESSING DRUG AND ALCOHOL USE IN SPECIFIC POPULATIONS

A. Cultural Groups/Ethnic Minorities

1. Ethnic minorities are often stereotyped or associated with stereotypical behaviors.
2. Ethnic minorities are heterogenous populations.
3. Ethnic minorities may be stratified according to:
   a. Degree of acculturation. For example, African-Americans may:
      (1) Have assimilated white cultural values.
      (2) Adopt some African-American and some Caucasian values.
      (3) Be culturally immersed in Black culture.
      (4) Hold values considered traditional to this country.
   b. Degree of cultural "dissonance" as traditional roles/values are breaking down.
      (1) Ethnic groups moving to an urban environment where children learn English more easily may adopt the American value system, causing strain on family systems; e.g., Mexicans from rural environment.
   c. Socioeconomic status.
      (1) Fewer employment opportunities and/or unemployment as major life stressors contribute to alcohol/drug use and/or drug trafficking.
   d. Education and literacy.
      (1) Few treatment centers have bilingual staff.
      (2) Some treatment centers require literacy or English language capability.
      (3) Expectations regarding acculturation may compromise accessibility of treatment.
   e. Region of origin.
      (1) National origins.
      (2) Urban.
      (3) Rural.
4. Most providers are not sensitive to ethnicity as a major dynamic in treatment.
5. Cultural/ethnic background and value systems pattern thinking, filter perceptions, and influence behavior. Alcohol and drug use are influenced by many factors, including:
   a. Self-reported first use.
   b. Choice of substances used and abused.
   c. Patterns of abuse.
   d. Treatment.
   e. Perceptions of treatment.

Drug and Alcohol Problems in Special Populations

5. Nurses and treatment providers must be aware of the ways in which personal values create a filtering system.
6. Racism, prejudicial treatment, and discrimination must be acknowledged as realities.
7. Psychosocial assessment must include:
    a. Cultural/ethnic background.
    b. Cultural supports, strengths or lack thereof:
        (1) Kinship systems.
        (2) Religious and spiritual belief systems.
    c. Comprehensive physical assessment and mental status exam.
    d. References to common health consequences in ethnic minorities.
8. Self-assessment.
    a. The health provider must understand her/his own attitudes and biases.
    b. Assumptions about commonalities between provider and client may offend the client.

B. Intravenous Drug Users

1. Assess the current status of patient. Formulate treatment and referral plans.
    a. Acute intoxication vs. less immediately life threatening medical consequences.
    b. Motivation for treatment:
        (1) Level of denial.
        (2) Patient/client perception of problem.
        (3) Patient/client agenda may be just for medical treatment and release.
2. Drugs used.
    a. Concurrent alcohol, pill, inhalant use.
    b. Frequency.
    c. Amount.
    d. History of use.
3. History of treatment.
    a. Detoxifications, number, associated conditions, outcomes.
    b. Methadone maintenance programs.
    c. Therapeutic communities.
    d. Involvement in self-help; e.g., Twelve-Step Programs.
    e. Other.
4. Periods of abstinence.
    a. Timing and efforts which maintained abstinence.
    b. Relapses, "trigger" items.

5. HIV status.
    a. Test status.
    b. Patient/client's interest in being tested.
    c. Counseling.
6. Current life stressors.
    a. Relationships.
    b. Work-related/unemployment.
    c. Home/environmental.
    d. Other significant life events.
    e. Socioeconomic factors.
7. Sources of support.
    a. Family, extended family, friends.
    b. Kinship systems.
    c. Religious affiliations.
    d. Community organizations.
8. History and physical assessment; special attention to:
    a. Needle tracks.
    b. Skin ulcers/cellulitis.
    c. History of hepatitis, bacterial endocarditis, sepsis, etc.
9. Sexual history.
    a. Sexual preference.
    b. Number of partners.
    c. Sexual practices.
    d. Safer sex practices.
    e. Reproductive history.
    f. Drug use associated with sex.

C. **Women**

1. Health care providers should demonstrate sensitivity to the stigmatic social position and low self-esteem in female alcoholics and drug abusers.
2. Assess possible concurrent sedative abuse, both prescription and OTC drugs.
3. Assessment should include:
    a. Differential diagnosis for other psychiatric disturbances.
    b. History of treatment of other disorders.
4. Hormonal variations influencing abuse patterns.
    a. Menstrual cycle variation.
    b. Premenstrual syndrome.
    c. Therapeutic interventions for menopause or dysfunctions.

Drug and Alcohol Problems in Special Populations

5. Comprehensive sexual history; special emphasis on:
   a. History of incest, rape, sexual abuse as source of shame and anger.
   b. History of unsafe sexual behavior.
      (1) Risk for HIV.
      (2) AIDS often presents differently in women.
         (a) Cervical dysplasia.
         (b) Pelvic inflammatory disease.
         (c) Yeast infections.
         (d) Venereal warts.
         (e) Other sexually transmitted diseases.
   c. History of sexual dysfunction in women can be a predictor of subsequent alcohol/drug abuse.
6. Current stressors.
   a. Use patterns of partner(s), family members.
   b. Parenting obligations.
      (1) Child care.
      (2) Parenting problems, including neglect or abuse:
         (a) Active.
         (b) Passive.
      (3) Custody issues, including fear of losing custody.
   c. Socioeconomic stressors.
      (1) Source of income.
      (2) Employment.
      (3) Factors related to stability of income and dependence on others.
7. Physical assessment. Special considerations.
   a. Sexual/reproductive history.
   b. Physical consequences are "telescoped" in women. End organ damage occurs more quickly and more severely in women.
8. Resources and support.
   a. Alternative sources for child care.
      (1) Spouse.
      (2) Partner.
      (3) Family.
      (4) Extended family.
      (5) Kinship systems.
   b. Support from church and other community organizations.

D. Homeless

1. Housing
   a. Access to safe shelter.
   b. Living on streets.

2. Client priorities of needs.
3. Concurrent psychiatric symptoms.
4. Degree of social isolation.
5. Patterns of alcohol/drug abuse; e.g., "bottle gangs" vs. lone use.
6. Vocational skills assessment.
7. Sources of sober support.
    a. Twelve-Step self-help programs.
    b. Community drop-in centers, shelter, meal programs.
    c. Religious organizations.
8. Homeless women:
    a. Are more easily victimized.
    b. Have fewer available services.
9. Identify client's perceptions of barriers to treatment. Explore ways in which perceived barriers can be reduced or eliminated.
    a. Access to safe housing.
    b. Assistance in utilizing social services.
    c. Knowledge of treatment centers.
10. Assess client strengths. Explore healthy survival mechanisms which client has demonstrated as source of internal support.
11. Physical exam and assessment should be comprehensive and include:
    a. Tuberculosis past history, present signs/symptoms.
    b. Pulmonary disease.
    c. HIV related signs/symptoms.
    d. Evidence of malnutrition.
    e. Dermatological conditions.
    f. Exposure-related conditions.
    g. Cirrhosis.

II. IDENTIFICATION OF HEALTH CARE NEEDS IN SPECIAL POPULATIONS

A. Defining Alcohol and Drug Specific Health Needs

1. Alcohol.
    a. Nutritional needs related to:
        (1) Poor diet.
        (2) Malabsorption of nutrients.
    b. Prevention of complications related to end organ damage.
        (1) Allow for tissue repair through abstinence.

Drug and Alcohol Problems in Special Populations

- (2) Exercise care when giving any medications to individual who has severe liver damage.
- c. Prevention of complications from alcohol withdrawal (see Module II.5).
2. Cocaine/Crack.
   - a. Nutritional: Undernutrition and malnutrition secondary to appetite suppressant drug effects.
   - b. Compulsive use: Need for health testing regarding cravings for drug, which will decrease over time if not acted upon.
   - c. Sexual expression: Sexual compulsivity will often emerge and lead to relapse of cocaine/crack use unless teaching of patient/client supports change of compulsive patterns.
3. Health teaching on HIV infection.
   - a. Explore issues of testing with patients.
   - b. Teach safer sex techniques.
   - c. Discuss sexual practices and sexual partners.
4. Health risks of intravenous (IV) drug use.
   - a. HIV infection.
     - (1) Explore testing with patient.
     - (2) Provide information on cleaning of works.
     - (3) Review health practices, and nutritional and safety issues.
   - b. AIDS.

B. Factors Influencing Clients and Group Behavior in Relation to Health Care Problems

1. Multifactorial.
   - a. Interface of individual and group.
     - (1) Perceptions of problem.
       - (a) Cultural determinants.
       - (b) Educational level influences problem definition and definition of priorities.
       - (c) Socioeconomic status determines health care priorities.
     - (2) Perceptions of treatment.
       - (a) Culturally determined.
       - (b) Influenced by educational level and socioeconomic factors.
   - b. Barriers to treatment.
     - (1) Access to treatment resources is limited.
       - (a) Waiting lists.
       - (b) Insurance and documentation.
       - (c) Limited treatment services for women; no provisions for child care.

(d) Limited treatment resources for medicaid patients/indigent.

(e) Few treatment centers for pregnant women.

(2) Negative experiences with health care system and health care providers may interfere with seeking treatment.

(3) Psychological barriers.

(a) Shame.

(b) Low self-esteem.

(c) Feelings of hopelessness.

(d) Fatalistic attitude.

(e) Denial; individual and group.

C. Nursing Diagnoses of Drug and Alcohol Problems

(Source: National Nurses Society on Addictions. (1989). *Nursing care planning with the addicted client: Volumes I and II.* Skokie, IL: Midwest Education Association, Inc. Please refer to texts for more complete listings.)

1. Common nursing diagnoses for the client who is chemically dependent.
   a. Sociocultural isolation.
   b. Ineffective individual coping.
   c. Spiritual distress.
   d. Altered family processes.
   e. Self-care deficits.
   f. Impaired communication.

2. Common nursing diagnoses for the older client who is an alcoholic.
   a. Sensory-perceptual alteration.
   b. Hopelessness.
   c. Alteration in self-concept.
   d. Ineffective individual coping.

3. Common nursing diagnoses for the homeless, schizophrenic alcoholic.
   a. Sensory-perceptual alteration related to alcohol withdrawal and acute psychotic symptoms.
   b. Alteration in thought processes related to overwhelming anxiety.
   c. Self-care deficit related to perceptual impairment and loss of contact with reality.
   d. Social isolation related to suspiciousness and inadequate home maintenance skills.

III. IMPLEMENTATION OF NURSING INTERVENTION

A. Community Factors Which Influence Care Delivery

1. Geographical environment.

Drug and Alcohol Problems in Special Populations

   a. Determined by sociological/demographic factors.
   b. Influences number and type of health care resources within community:
      (1) Accessibility.
      (2) Comprehensiveness of services.
   c. Influences drug seeking behaviors.
      (1) Accessibility of drugs.
      (2) Poverty and stress may support continued drug use.
2. Organizational systems in community infrastructure.
   a. Health care resources.
      (1) Hospitals.
      (2) Clinics.
      (3) Detoxification wards.
      (4) Drug rehabilitation units.
      (5) Out-patient treatment facilities.
   b. Integration (or lack thereof) of health care resources.
3. Community culture.
   a. Perceptions, beliefs, and expectations.
   b. Influenced by cultural background of individuals/groups.
   c. Influences communities' perceptions, beliefs, and expectations concerning health care.
   d. Within the community culture will be drug subcultures.
      (1) Alcohol subculture.
         (a) Bars.
         (b) Store-fronts.
         (c) "Bottle gangs."
      (2) Intravenous drug subculture: Shooting galleries.
      (3) Crack subculture: Crack houses.
      (4) Drug-dealing subculture.
4. Neighborhoods in which people function on a daily basis.
   a. Health care resources available.
   b. Sources of neighborhood sober support.
      (1) Church organizations.
      (2) Women in Sobriety.
      (3) Alcoholics Anonymous (AA), Narcotics Anonymous (NA), Cocaine Anonymous (CA) meetings.
   c. Local drug culture is supported or opposed.
      (1) Block associations to prevent drug use.
      (2) Voluntary law enforcement.
      (3) Proximity and involvement of police.

Module II.8

5. People whom the individual sees and interacts with on a daily basis.
    a. Shared belief systems and behaviors.
    b. Support of drug seeking behaviors, moderation, or abstinence.

B. **Prevention of Alcohol- and Drug-Related Problems: The Approach Must Integrate Resources**

1. Education.
    a. School systems.
    b. Media.
    c. Public education.
2. Socioeconomic factors.
    a. Availability of housing.
    b. Employment opportunities.
3. Access to treatment.
    a. Availability of all levels of care.
    b. Reduce barriers to access.
4. Comprehensive treatment.
    a. Include vocational skills training.
    b. Social skills training.
    c. Child care when necessary.
    d. Assertiveness training, especially for women.
5. Community support of recovery.
    a. Housing for substance abusers who are in treatment or who have completed treatment.
    b. Job opportunities.
    c. Positive, supportive attitude.
    d. Church and neighborhood sober support infrastructure.

C. **Care Delivery to Specific Groups**

1. Little research clarifies which specific culturally sensitive treatment strategies are most effective.
2. Treatment centers should have multilingual, racially mixed staff.
3. Staff should be trained in:
    a. Cultural diversity
        (1) Spiritual and religious belief systems and how they impact on health problem identification, perception, and treatment.
            (a) African-Americans.
            (b) Hispanic Americans.
            (c) Native Americans.

Drug and Alcohol Problems in Special Populations

- (2) Definition of family and its cultural importance should be part of staff education.
  - (a) Extended family.
  - (b) Systems of kinship.
- (3) Impact of values of dominant society on traditional values, roles, and cultural beliefs.
  - (a) On individual.
  - (b) On family.
  - (c) On community.

b. Special needs of:
  - (1) Women.
    - (a) Treatment of incest/sexual and physical abuse.
    - (b) Treatment of psychological problems.
    - (c) Education of sexual and sex-role issues and difficulties.
    - (d) Provision of child care, support services, and social resources.
  - (2) Homeless.
  - (3) Intravenous drug users.

3. Staff development includes supervising/support in working through countertransferential issues associated with specific groups and how these issues interfere with treatment.
  a. Racism.
  b. Negative attitudes.
   - (1) Intravenous substance abuser.
   - (2) Seropositive patient.
   - (3) Child-bearing drug dependent women.

D. Evaluation of Care Provision in Response to Special Population Needs

1. Alcohol- and drug-related hospital admissions.
2. Admissions to treatment centers.
   a. Detoxification facilities.
   b. Acute treatment centers.
      - (1) Alcohol rehabilitation.
      - (2) Drug treatment centers.
   c. Out-patient programs.
      - (1) Alcoholism programs.
      - (2) Methadone maintenance.
   d. Residential long-term care.
      - (1) Therapeutic communities.

Module II.8

3. Drug- and/or alcohol-related arrests.
    a. Domestic violence.
    b. Child abuse/neglect.
    c. Property crime.
    d. Hustling; pimping.
    e. Dealing.
4. School dropouts.
5. Runaway youth.
6. Poverty levels.
7. Opportunities for employment.
8. Efforts directed toward supporting:
    a. Drug subcultures.
    b. Recovery.
9. Program planning that reflects cultural- and gender-related differences and needs.

MODULE II.8
NURSING CARE OF
DRUG AND ALCOHOL PROBLEMS
IN SPECIAL POPULATIONS

INSTRUCTOR'S GUIDE

Aileen H. Clucas, MSN, RN, CCDN
Vivian P. J. Clarke, EdD, CHES
Consultant

Madeline A. Naegle, PhD, RN, FAAN
Project Director
Janet S. D'Arcangelo, MA, RN, C
Project Coordinator

Project SAEN
SUBSTANCE ABUSE
EDUCATION IN NURSING

CONTENTS

Component	Page
Module Description	620
Time Frame	620
Placement	620
Learner Objectives	621
Recommended Readings	622
Faculty Readings	622
Student Readings	622
Recommended Audiovisual and Other Resources	623
Overhead Masters	626
Handout Masters	647
Recommended Teaching Strategies and Sample Assignments	654
Test Questions and Answers	656
Bibliography	659

Module II.8

MODULE DESCRIPTION

This module promotes the development of students' abilities to deliver nursing care to special groups with atypical needs and high prevalence of drug- and alcohol-related problems. Assessment of groups with drug- and alcohol-related health deviations who reside in institutions and communities will be central to learning. Nursing interventions based on nursing diagnoses will be formulated and evaluated with consideration of lifestyle and health-related factors which impact upon these groups.

TIME FRAME

3 hours

PLACEMENT

Community Health, Nursing Care of the Adolescent, Psychiatric-Mental Health Nursing, Adult Health

Instructor's Guide

LEARNER OBJECTIVES

Upon successful completion of this module, the learner will:

1. Describe health deviations associated with drug and alcohol problems in specific populations.
2. Identify client needs related to health deviations in association with drugs and alcohol.
3. Formulate nursing diagnoses in response to needs of individuals and groups with health deviations.
4. Provide direct nursing care to clients and groups in relation to drugs and alcohol.
5. Utilize institutional and community resources in the delivery of direct client care.
6. Recognize policies and trends within the health care delivery system which influence nursing care.
7. Evaluate nursing interventions in response to drug- and alcohol-related health deviations manifested in certain special populations.

Module II.8

RECOMMENDED READINGS

FACULTY READINGS

Breakey, W. R. (1987). Treating the homeless. *Alcohol Health and Research World, 11*(3), 42–47, 90.

Delgado, M. (1988). Alcoholism treatment and Hispanic youth. *Journal of Drug Issues, 18*(1), 59–68.

DiMatteo, T. E., & Cesarini, R. M. (1986). Responding to the treatment needs of chemically dependent women. *Journal of Counseling and Development, 64,* 452–453.

Faltz, B. G., & Madover, S. (1988). Treatment of substance abuse in patients with HIV infection. *Advances in Alcohol and Substance Abuse, 7*(2), 143–157.

STUDENT READINGS

Anderson, F. D. (1986). Portal-systemic encephalopathy in the chronic alcoholic. *Critical Care Quarterly, 8*(4), 40–52.

DiCicco-Bloom, B., Space, S., & Zahourek, R. P. (1986). The homebound alcoholic. *American Journal of Nursing, 86*(2), 167–169.

Lee, L. J. (1983). Reducing black adolescents' drug use: Family revisited. In R. Israelowitz & M. Singer (Eds.), *Adolescent substance abuse: A guide to prevention and treatment* (pp. 57–69). New York: Plenum Press.

Reed, B. (1985). Drug misuse and dependency in women: The meaning of being considered a special population or minority group. *International Journal of the Addictions, 20*(1), 13–62.

Stimmel, B. (1987). AIDS, alcohol and heroin: A particularly deadly combination. *Advances in Alcohol and Substance Abuse, 6*(3), 1–5.

Instructor's Guide

RECOMMENDED AUDIOVISUAL AND OTHER RESOURCES

AUDIOVISUAL RESOURCES

1. **Beyond Black and White**

   This video, dramatizing the psychological and sociological origins of prejudice against minorities and women, reveals that for some of its victims, prejudice frequently results in alcohol or drug abuse, and for some, in criminal behavior. Dramatic vignettes present positive, believable behavior models, and encourage the utilization of programs designed to provide career opportunities for young adult minorities and women. Available from New York State Council on Alcoholism, Film Library, 155 Washington Avenue, Albany, New York 12210. Telephone: (518) 432-8281 or 1-800-252-2557.

2. **The Bottom Line: Women and Alcohol**

   Women alcoholics, social drinkers, treatment people, and a researcher candidly describe on camera the problems faced by women in an era of increased opportunity and motivation. This video explores some difficulties and survival techniques developed by modern women with respect to alcohol use and abuse. It is for general audiences. 20 minutes. Available from Addiction Research Foundation, 33 Russell Street, Toronto, Canada M5S2S1. Purchase ($160).

3. **Female Alcoholism**

   Alcoholism among women is a growing problem. This program examines the changing stereotype of the female alcoholic, as well as analyzing some case histories of recovered alcoholic women. It explains the dangers of drinking during pregnancy, the effect of the fetal alcohol syndrome on newborns and the emotional effect on children of being raised by an alcoholic mother. The program also explains why women are reluctant to seek help—and suggests ways to overcome this reluctance. 19 minutes. Available from Films for the Humanities and Sciences, P.O. Box 2053, Princeton, New Jersey 08543. Telephone: 1-800-257-5126. # BD-1366, purchase ($199).

4. **The Honour of All**

   This three-part docudrama captures the amazing, real-life story of the Alkali Indian Band's heroic struggle to overcome its widespread alcoholism. The people

Module II.8

who lived it tell the story in their own words and portray themselves in these videos that recreate the Band's gradual slide into alcoholism, beginning in 1940. The deterioration of this community from British Columbia is shown and how, in 1971, tribal member Phyllis Chelsea's recovery helped inspire the Band to attain a 95% sobriety rate within 14 years. These videos offer Native Americans an inspiring example of how their peers could and did recover from the alcoholism that was destroying their community and their culture.

Part One recreates the story of the Band's struggle to overcome and conquer its alcoholism. It dramatically portrays the painfully slow, often lonely, but ultimately rewarding road back to sobriety. 56 minutes.

Part Two outlines the community development process that occurred at Alkali Lake, British Columbia, as the Band moved from alcoholism to sobriety. Various members of the Band discuss what it was like, what happened, and what it's like now. 43 minutes.

Part Three expands on the general theme of community development and personal growth begun in Parts One and Two. 26 minutes.

Available from Hazelden Educational Materials, Pleasant Valley Road, Box 176, Center City, Minnesota 55012-0176. Telephone: 1-800-328-3000. Part One ($150), Part Two ($100), Part Three ($100).

5. Junkie

Explores the many faces of women's addiction, detailing not only the belief systems which sustain addictions but also the support systems which can free addicts to live healthy lives. Created out of the life experiences of company members of At the Foot of the Mountain Theater, all of whom are recovering addicts, the film explores addiction to alcohol, food, speed, work, sex, violence, marijuana, and romantic love. Each woman is forced to confront her own loneliness and fear as her personal story is dramatized and examined. Unable to sustain their denial, the women urge one another to let go of the controlling behavior and delusions which keep them trapped and find a spiritual path of healing. 60 minutes. **Available from Hazelden Educational Materials, Pleasant Valley Road, Box 176, Center City, Minnesota 55012-0176. Telephone: 1-800-328-3000.** 16mm film only, rental ($100) or purchase ($850).

6. Women and Their Use of Mood-Altering Drugs: The Immigrant Experience

This tape presents some of the stresses that immigrants, particularly women, may have to face in adjusting to a new society. The program shows some of the short- and long-term effects of using minor tranquilizers as a way of coping. A consumer's approach to medical care is presented, stressing the importance of informed consent. 16 minutes. **Available from Addiction Research Foundation, 33 Russell Street, Toronto, Canada M5S2S1.** Purchase ($150).

Instructor's Guide

7. A Thin Line: Recognizing Cultural Differences and Working with Black Chemically Dependent Clients

Produced by the Institute on Black Chemical Abuse in 1989, this film focuses on training counselors to work more effectively with African American clients in treatment. **Available from Institute on Black Chemical Abuse, 2614 Nicollet Avenue South, Minneapolis, Minnesota 55408. Telephone (612) 871-7878.** Contact David Grant or Sandy Vadnais. ($175 plus $3 shipping and handling.)

8. Long Road Home

This 1977 film portrays the development of a drinking problem in a young African American family man named Willie. The origins of his drinking and its impact on his family life are described, as are the improvements resulting from his successful treatment. Intended mainly for rural populations, the film attempts to show the special character and problems of rural African American culture. 20 minutes. Contact Elizabeth Peters. **Available from the South Carolina Commission on Alcohol and Drug Abuse, 3700 Forest Drive, Suite 300, Columbia, South Carolina 29204. Telephone (803) 734-9559.** Purchase ($250) or rental ($30).

9. Straight Talk

This first-person story describes drug addiction as a desperate attempt to feel like the king of the mountain. Former addict Roland Abner's straight talk describes what life is like when centered on drugs. He states emphatically that the wretchedness of addiction is not exclusive to the poor or downtrodden. Narcotics is an equal opportunity destroyer, he says. For teenage and adult audiences and healthcare professionals. 24 minutes. **Available from AIMS Media, 6901 Woodley Avenue, Van Nuys, California 91406-4878. Telephone (800) 367-2467.** Purchase (film, $475; video $395) or rental ($75).

10. Highlights: Expert Advisory Roundtable on African-American Issues

Morehouse College of Medicine, August 31–September 1, 1989. A panel of African-American experts, psychologists, health care professionals, and policymakers explores issues relevant to African-American families and communities in a videotape produced by the Office for Substance Abuse Prevention. This video is available as part of the audiovisual free-loan program operated by the National Clearinghouse for Alcohol and Drug Information (NCADI). **Available from NCADI, P.O. Box 2345, Rockville, Maryland 20852. Telephone 1-800-SAY-NO-TO (DRUGS).**

Module II.8

OVERHEAD MASTERS

MODULE II.8 NURSING CARE OF DRUG AND ALCOHOL PROBLEMS IN SPECIAL POPULATIONS

1. Cultural Stumbling Blocks
2. Core Issues Influencing Both Client and Care Provider
3. Effects of Cultural Influences
4. Facilitating Communication by Diminishing Language Barriers
5. Community Factors which Influence Health Care Delivery
6. Problems in Management of the Low Socioeconomic Status Patient
7. Additional Barriers to Treatment
8. Special Assessment Needs—Women
9. Special Assessment Needs—Homeless
10. Special Assessment Needs—Intravenous Drug Users

Instructor's Guide

Module II.8—Overhead #1

CULTURAL STUMBLING BLOCKS

Stereotyping:

Assuming conformity to a major pattern; based on limited information, generalizations from subgroups; overlooking the possibility of cultural change and variability.

Prejudice:

A hostile attitude toward individuals simply because they belong to a minority group.

Discrimination:

The differential treatment of individuals because they belong to a minority group.

Racism:

A mixed form of prejudice (attitude) and discrimination (behavior) directed at ethnic groups other than one's own.

Cultural Blindness:

A process by which a person ignores cultural differences and proceeds as if these did not exist.

Culture Shock:

A process in which the individual is stunned by cultural differences and even immobilized until he or she is able to work through his or her feelings related to the vastly different nature of the alien culture. Most likely to occur in response to behavior in a different culture that is disapproved of or forbidden in one's own.

From: Boyle, J., & Andrews, M. (1989). *Transcultural concepts in nursing care* (pp. 52–53). Glenview, IL: Scott, Foresman, & Co.

Module II.8—Overhead #2

CORE ISSUES INFLUENCING BOTH CLIENT AND CARE PROVIDER

- Stereotyping of ethnic minorities is common.
- Assumptions about commonalities offend the client.
- Ethnicity is a major dynamic in treatment.
- Ethnicity influences personal value systems.
- Consciously and unconsciously, personal value systems:
    - Pattern thinking.
    - Filter perception.
    - Influence behavior.
- Racism, prejudicial treatment, and discrimination must be acknowledged as realities.

Module II.8—Overhead #3

EFFECTS OF CULTURAL INFLUENCES

Cultural background and value systems ⟶ pattern thinking + filter perception + influence behavior
    Relative to alcohol and drug use, these three effects influence:

- Self-reported first use.
- Choice of substances used and abused.
- Patterns of abuse.
- Treatments.
- Perceptions of treatment.

Module II.8—Overhead #4

FACILITATING COMMUNICATION BY DIMINISHING LANGUAGE BARRIERS

Barriers.

- School vs. idiomatic English, particularly when describing symptoms.
- Multiple accents.
- Differences in street names for substances, distribution networks, and other jargon associated with drug culture.

Crossing language barriers.

- Speaking slowly.
- Avoiding slang.
- Providing printed material.
- Confirming verbal information by use of pictures, diagrams, and demonstrations.

Module II.8—Overhead #5

COMMUNITY FACTORS WHICH INFLUENCE HEALTH CARE DELIVERY

1. Geographical environment: influences number, accessibility, type of services.
2. Other organizational systems in community infrastructure, existence or lack of hospitals, clinics, etc.
3. Community culture.
4. Neighborhoods.
5. Individuals with whom client interacts on a daily basis.

Module II.8—Overhead #6

PROBLEMS IN MANAGEMENT OF THE LOW SOCIOECONOMIC STATUS PATIENT

1. Estrangement and distrust in therapeutic relationships.

   (Experiential differences → inability to identify with one another → fear)

   - Within patient.
   - Within nurse.

2. Low resources.
   - Lack of funds for treatment precludes certain services.
   - Lack of basic literacy, schooling, and job skills with which to establish new resources.
   - Lack of opportunities for establishing ego strength, identity, and self-respect to overcome feelings of despair and powerlessness to effect real changes.
   - Debilitating results stemming from prior experience with treatment, either for self, loved ones, or acquaintances.
   - Lack of family or social supports having resources to share.

3. Traditional care plans, utilizing such patient resources as money, employment, marketable skills, or support of family members, are often inappropriate for clients from resource-negative backgrounds.

Module II.8—Overhead #7

ADDITIONAL BARRIERS TO TREATMENT

1. Access to resources.
   - Waiting lists.
   - Insurance.
   - Documentation.
   - Limited services meeting special needs, such as day care for mothers in treatment, shelter for homeless in treatment, transportation, and multilingual staff.
2. Prior negative experience with health care system and health care providers.
3. Psychological barriers.
   - Shame.
   - Low self-esteem.
   - Hopelessness.
   - Fatalistic attitude.
   - Denial.

Module II.8—Overhead #8

SPECIAL ASSESSMENT NEEDS—WOMEN

1. Assess level of denial.
2. Screen for concurrent psychopathology, especially affective disorders.
3. Assess patterns between substance use and menstrual cycle.
4. Explore child-bearing status, child care, and other parenting issues.
5. Involve spouse.
6. Explore psychological issues such as assertiveness, role conflict, and sexuality.

Module II.8—Overhead #9

SPECIAL ASSESSMENT NEEDS—HOMELESS

1. Housing.
2. Client priorities of needs.
3. Concurrent psychopathology.
4. Patterns of substance abuse.
5. Degree of social isolation.
6. Availability of sober social supports.
7. Vocational skills.
8. Client perceptions of barriers to treatment.
9. Client strengths.
10. Gender specific needs.
11. Vocational skills.
12. History and physical assessment with special attention to communicable diseases and conditions associated with exposure, malnutrition, and neglect.

Module II.8—Overhead #10

SPECIAL ASSESSMENT NEEDS—INTRAVENOUS DRUG USERS

1. Current status, especially relative to severity, and motivation for treatment.

2. Specific drugs, poly-drugs used, with special attention to frequency.

3. History of treatment and periods of abstinence.

4. HIV status.

5. Current life stressors.

6. Sources of support.

7. History and physical assessment, with special attention to conditions secondary to drug use (skin conditions, medical consequences).

8. Sexual history.

Instructor's Guide

HANDOUT MASTERS

MODULE II.8 NURSING CARE OF DRUG AND ALCOHOL PROBLEMS IN SPECIAL POPULATIONS

1. Cultural Stumbling Blocks
2. Nursing Strategies that Minimize Transcultural Conflicts
3. Strategies to Facilitate Collection of Problem Specific-Cultural Data
4. Issues in Nursing Care Planning with Substance Abusing Women
5. Example of Applications of Nursing Diagnosis: Potential for Infection—Biological
6. Example of Applications of Nursing Diagnosis: Alteration in Self-Concept Related to Personal Identity—Psychosocial

Module II.8—Handout #1

CULTURAL STUMBLING BLOCKS

Stereotyping:

Assuming conformity to a major pattern; based on limited information, generalizations from subgroups, overlooking the possibility of cultural change and variability.

Prejudice:

A hostile attitude toward individuals simply because they belong to a minority group.

Discrimination:

The differential treatment of individuals because they belong to a minority group.

Racism:

A mixed form of prejudice (attitude) and discrimination (behavior) directed at ethnic groups other than one's own.

Cultural Blindness:

A process by which a person ignores cultural differences and proceeds as if these did not exist.

Culture Shock:

A process in which the individual is stunned by cultural differences and even immobilized until he or she is able to work through his or her feelings related to the vastly different nature of the alien culture. Most likely to occur in response to behavior in a different culture that is disapproved of or forbidden in one's own.

From: Boyle, J., & Andrews, M. (1989). *Transcultural concepts in nursing care* (pp. 52–53). Glenview, IL: Scott, Foresman, & Co.

Instructor's Guide

Module II.8—Handout #2

NURSING STRATEGIES THAT MINIMIZE TRANSCULTURAL CONFLICTS

1. Delivery of holistic patient care that emphasizes the interrelationships among person, environment (culture), health, and nursing.

2. Facilitation of the nurse-client relationship through the development of special resources, such as bilingual nurses, translators, and bicultural nurses.

3. Establishment of norms allowing family involvement in healing processes.

4. Identification and knowledge about nontraditional community resources, such as local herbalists or specialty stores.

5. Referral to folk and popular healers when appropriate.

6. Use of in-service programs to further explain community-specific health practices.

7. Promotion of cultural pluralism as a concept in the education of nursing students.

Module II.8—Handout #3

STRATEGIES TO FACILITATE COLLECTION OF PROBLEM-SPECIFIC CULTURAL DATA

It is important to identify the major values, beliefs, and behaviors as they influence and relate to alcohol and substance abuse within the client's specific culture.

Elicit the client's subjective reasons for seeking the health professional and ideas about the problem, as well as the client's previous and anticipated treatment. The following questions may be helpful:

1. What do you think has caused your problem (drug/substance abuse)?
2. Why do you think it started when it did?
3. What does your sickness (addiction) do to you? How does it work?
4. How severe is your addiction?
5. What kind of treatment do you think you should receive?
6. What are the most important results you hope to achieve?
7. What are the chief problems that your substance abuse has caused you?
8. What do you fear about your addiction? What do you think might happen if you don't get treatment for it?

From: Tripp-Reimer, T., Brink, P. J., & Saunders, J. (1991). Cultural assessment: Content and process. In B. W. Spradley (Ed.), *Readings in community health nursing* (4th ed., pp. 503–511). Philadelphia: Lippincott.

Instructor's Guide

Module II.8—Handout #4

ISSUES IN NURSING CARE PLANNING WITH SUBSTANCE ABUSING WOMEN

1. The etiology of substance abuse in women differs from that in men.

2. Women have a high degree of denial; significant others may be unaware of how seriously ill the woman is, or may refuse to recognize her problem.

3. Screening for primary affective disorders should be done.

4. Be alert for correlations between drinking levels and menstrual, midcycle, and premenstrual periodicity patterns.

5. Role clarification is a critical issue for women.

6. Involve the spouse in therapy. Women are often financially and psychologically dependent on spouses. Improved communication and marital understanding are couples issues.

7. Individual therapy issues may be assertiveness training and anger management.

8. Help regarding career development for those women seeking a more independent life outside their marriage, so as to enable them to increase self gratification and achieve their own goals instead of achieving vicariously through their husbands.

9. A female therapist may provide a trusting and supportive relationship as well as being a role model.

10. A supportive, helpful, and understanding male therapist may provide a corrective emotional experience for the woman's perception of men.

From: Lawson, G., & Lawson, A. (1989). *Alcoholism and substance abuse in special populations* (pp. 21–23). Rockville, MD: Aspen.
Zimberg, S. (1982). Special approaches for sub-populations of alcoholics. In *The clinical management of alcoholism* (pp. 157–176). New York: Brunner/Mazel Publishers.

Module II.8

Module II.8—Handout #5

EXAMPLE OF APPLICATIONS OF NURSING DIAGNOSIS: POTENTIAL FOR INFECTION—BIOLOGICAL

Defining Characteristics

- Alteration of skin integrity.
- Practice of unsafe sex.
- History of intravenous drug use.

Process Criteria—The nurse:

- Assesses skin integrity and provides independent and collaborative nursing interventions to prevent infection and promote healing, such as hygiene and hydration.
- Teaches safe sex practices, including use of condoms.
- Refers to community resources as appropriate.
- Assesses nutritional status and collaborates with clients, significant others and the dietitian to develop an appropriate dietary plan.

Outcome Criteria—The individual:

- Verbalizes an understanding of the relationship between the identified abuse or addiction pattern (lifestyle) and potential risk of infection.
- Demonstrates freedom from infection.

Instructor's Guide

Module II.8—Handout #6

EXAMPLE OF APPLICATIONS OF NURSING DIAGNOSIS: ALTERATION IN SELF-CONCEPT RELATED TO PERSONAL IDENTITY—PSYCHOSOCIAL

Defining Characteristics

- Fluctuating feelings about self.
- Negative self-concept.
- Exploitative behavior with others (manipulation).

Process Criteria—The nurse:

- Offers unconditional positive acceptance of the individual.
- Conveys the importance of individual responsibility.
- Encourages the appropriate use of support groups.
- Assists the individual in exploring, accepting, and owning positive and negative aspects of self.

Outcome Criteria—The individual:

- Makes positive statements regarding self-concept.
- Chooses an interaction style that promotes health for self and significant others.

Module II.8

RECOMMENDED TEACHING STRATEGIES AND SAMPLE ASSIGNMENTS

RECOMMENDED TEACHING STRATEGIES

- Clinical placement in drug and alcohol treatment centers and community agencies
- Lecture
- Small group discussions
- Attitude assessment
- Role-playing/micro-teaching
- Seminars

SAMPLE ASSIGNMENTS

Class Activities

1. Have students scan nationally focused newspaper (e.g., *The New York Times* or any newspaper with substantial national coverage) and read articles on:
   a. Native American issues.
      (1) Majority of Supreme Court decisions on Native American issues are on land rights, sovereignty, or environmental issues.
      (2) Fishing and hunting rights are often challenged by dominant culture and receive national attention.
   b. Racial issues.
   c. Discrimination issues.
   d. Issues of poverty.
2. Open group discussion on the above; and:
   a. Native Americans are still battling the dominant culture for property rights, including land that is held sacred; and the legacy that oppression leaves.
   b. Racism and discrimination are forces in our society that continue to exist.
   c. The problems of lower incomes, fewer job opportunities, and less access to housing.
   d. Stressors will interface in the use of alcohol and other drugs in many ways.

Instructor's Guide

3. Have students experience some exposure to alcohol and other drug subcultures.
   a. Arrange one-day placement in shelter system, or a public detoxification ward.
   b. Arrange one-day placement with agency that actually goes to shooting gallery and/or crack house to offer health promotion techniques such as:
      (1) Distribution of clean needles and bleach.
      (2) Distribution of condoms.
4. Plan field trips to city shelter system, therapeutic communities, community drop-in centers, halfway houses, grass roots and lay/professional organizations, to acquaint students with resources.
5. Make a listing and diagram of services supplied by specific agencies in the community.
6. Develop networking charts and interrelated agencies.

CASE VIGNETTE

Bonnie Jackson

Bonnie is a 34-year-old black woman who supports her heroin addiction by prostitution. She has been living a "junkie" lifestyle for about five years but longs to get sober, marry, and settle down to have a child. Bonnie insists that all of her clients wear condoms. However, this was not always her policy and she tries never to be desperate enough for a fix that she gets careless. After her morning "wake up," Bonnie hustles unless she happens to "go on the nod." She never frequents shooting galleries but is unsure about whether her regular boyfriend has visited them, or has at least shared needles, in the past. Bonnie claims that she has never personally shared her works. She kicked her habit twice in the past year by going "cold turkey" and neither wants nor trusts the help of professionals.

Role-Play—Nurse's Script

Your task in this role-play is to:

1. Assess the pattern of drug and alcohol use in relation to social and cultural traditions, as well as lifestyle, in this ethnic minority, female, intravenous drug user.
2. Identify multiple health risks which interact to create problems secondary to drug addiction in this client and her significant other.
3. Determine the client's awareness of resources that she might find helpful.
4. Intervene with this client; e.g., by:
   a. Offering unconditional positive acceptance of her.
   b. Assisting her in exploring and accepting the positive and negative aspects of herself.
   c. Reinforce the importance of safe sex practices, especially the use of condoms with all partners.

Module II.8

TEST QUESTIONS AND ANSWERS

TEST QUESTIONS

1. Methadone maintenance is a treatment recommendation for many IV drug users. This practice is controversial mainly because it:
   a. is just as expensive as heroin.
   b. interferes with the client's motivation to change.
   c. is a synthetic opiate substance.
   d. maintains the client's dependence on another drug.

2. Before administering Methadone, the nurse should:
   a. check the dietary intake.
   b. collect a urine specimen.
   c. draw blood.
   d. take vital signs.

3. When a client enters a rehabilitation program for heroin abuse, the nurse should be concerned with:
   1. the stage of physical withdrawal.
   2. the denial of the disease.
   3. avoidance of responsibility.
   4. knowledge deficits.
      a. 1, 3, & 4
      b. 2 & 3
      c. 2, 3, & 4
      d. all of the above

4. Drug use takes place in a social context. The nurse provider should:
   a. learn the client's native language.
   b. assess the client's cultural practices.
   c. assess predominant ethnic values important to the client.
   d. only treat the client in the family setting.

5. Victoria, a 20-year-old model, is admitted to the surgical service after an appendectomy. On the first postoperative day, the following nursing observations are made: V. does not seem to be relieved by her prescribed medication of meperidine 25 mg IM q 4 h prn. Within 15 minutes of receiving an injection, she asked a different nurse for her pain medicine. There are recent needle marks and scars on her left

Instructor's Guide

arm. Although she denies drug use, a tentative medical diagnosis of opiate withdrawal is made. Nurses should observe V. for behaviors related to opiate withdrawal, including:

  a. lacrimation, constricted pupils, or hypotension.
  b. lacrimation, rhinorrhea, dilated pupils, and hypotension.
  c. lacrimation, constipation, and constricted pupils.
  d. somnolence, constipation, and hypertension.

6. Victoria's failure to attain pain relief from the meperidine injections indicates that she is experiencing the phenomenon known as:

  a. psychological addiction.
  b. physical addiction.
  c. tolerance.
  d. habituation.

7. You conduct a team conference to plan nursing care for Victoria. One staff member says, "I don't know why we waste time on that little junkie princess. We all know she'll be back into drugs as soon as she gets back to her glamorous job." Your best initial response would be:

  a. "Since you have such strong feelings, I'll assign someone else to V."
  b. "I know it's difficult, but we're obligated to take care of her."
  c. "I guess you feel guilty because she overdosed on your shift."
  d. "It's important for us to share our feelings about caring for a frustrating client like V."

8. Victoria recovers from her drug overdose. The nursing care plan must be revised to focus on a long-term approach to her drug abuse. An appropriate long-term nursing goal would be for the patient to:

  a. before discharge, verbalize her intention to abstain from drugs.
  b. after discharge, attend a drug treatment program at least once a week.
  c. after discharge, find new friends.
  d. after discharge, use a less harmful drug, such as marijuana.

9. The needs of homeless men and women experiencing substance abuse problems:

  a. are difficult to meet because of many associated social and economic problems.
  b. are essentially the same as those of domiciled individuals.
  c. are undetected due to problems with screening and consistent contact.
  d. are usually limited to alcohol abuse.

10. Problems which impact on effective treatment of substance abuse problems in women include:

  a. the severity of addiction in women.
  b. treatment approaches which are based on the needs of male abusers.
  c. failure to address family issues.
  d. women's high relapse rate.

Module II.8

ANSWER KEY

1. d
2. b
3. c
4. b
5. b
6. c
7. d
8. b
9. d
10. b

Instructor's Guide

BIBLIOGRAPHY

MODULE II.8 NURSING CARE OF DRUG AND ALCOHOL PROBLEMS IN SPECIAL POPULATIONS

American Nurses' Association, Drug and Alcohol Nurses Association, & National Nurses' Society on Addictions. (1987). *The care of clients with addictions: Dimensions of nursing practice.* Kansas City, MO: American Nurses' Association.

American Nurses' Association & National Nurses Society on Addictions. (1988). *Standards of addictions nursing practice with selected diagnoses and criteria.* Kansas City, MO: American Nurses' Association.

American Public Health Association. (1990). Hispanics' health and nutrition examination survey, 1982–1984. *American Journal of Public Health, 80*(Suppl.), 1–70.

Atkins, B. J., Klein, M. A., & Mosley, B. (1987). Black adolescents' attitudes toward the use of alcohol and other drugs. *International Journal of Addictions, 22*(12), 1201–1211.

Beauvais, F., Oetting, E. R., & Edwards, R. W. (1985). Trends in drug use of Indian adolescents living on reservations: 1975–1983. *American Journal of Drug and Alcohol Abuse, 11*(3–4), 209–229.

Beckman, L. J., & Bradsley, P. (1981). The perceived determinants and consequences of alcohol consumption among young women heavy drinkers. *International Journal of Addictions, 16*(1), 75–88.

Bergmark, A., Oscarsson, L., & Binion, A. (1988). Rationales for the use of alcohol, marijuana and other drugs by eighth grader Native American and Anglo youth. *International Journal of Addictions, 23*(1), 47–64.

Berne, A. S., Dato, C., Mason, D., & Rafferty, M. (1990, Spring). A nursing model for addressing the health needs of homeless families. *Image, 22*(1), 8–13.

Blume, S. (1986). Women and alcohol: A review. *Journal of the American Medical Association, 256*(11), 1467–1469.

Boyd-Franklin, N., & Shevoda, N. (1990). A multi-systems approach to the treatment of a Black, inner-city family with a schizophrenic mother. *American Journal of Orthopsychiatry, 60*(2), 186–195.

Boyle, J., & Andrews, M. (1989). *Transcultural concepts in nursing care* (pp. 52–53). Glenview, IL: Scott, Foresman, & Co.

Bradstock, K., Forman, M. R., Binkin, N. J., Gentry, E. M., et al. (1988). Alcohol use and health behavior lifestyles among U.S. women: The behavioral risk factor surveys. *Addictive Behaviors, 13*(1), 61–71.

Breakey, W. R. (1987). Treating the homeless. *Alcohol Health and Research World, 11* (3), 42–47, 90.

Brickner, P. W., Scharer, L. K., & Cananan, B. (Eds.). (1985). *Health care of homeless people*. New York: Springer.

Brunswick, A., & Messeri, P. (1984). Causal factors in onset of adolescents' cigarette smoking: A prospective study of urban black youth. *Advances in Alcohol and Substance Abuse, 3*(1–2), 35–52.

Bry, B. (1983). Substance abuse in women: Etiology and prevention. *Issues in Mental Health Nursing, 5*(1–4), 153–172.

Caetano, R. (1987). Alcohol use and depression among U.S. Hispanics. *British Journal of Addictions, 82*(11), 1245–1251.

Celentano, D. D., & McQueen, E. (1980). Substance abuse by women: A review of the epidemiologic literature. *Chronic Disease, 33*, 383–394.

Celentano, D. D., & McQueen, E. (1984). Alcohol consumption patterns among women in Baltimore. *Journal of Studies on Alcohol, 45*, 355–358.

Charette, L., Tate, D. L., & Wilson, A. (1990). Alcohol consumption and menstrual distress in women at higher and lower risk for alcoholism. *Alcoholism: Clinical and Experimental Research, 14*(2), 152–157.

Closser, M. H. (1991). Benzodiazepines and the elderly. *Journal of Substance Abuse Treatment, 8*, 35–41.

Dawkins, M. P. (1980). *Alcohol and the black community*. Saratoga, CA: Century Twenty-One.

Delgado, M. (1988). Alcoholism treatment and Hispanic youth. *Journal of Drug Issues, 18*(1), 59–68.

DiCicco-Bloom, B., Space, S., & Zahourek, R. P. (1986). The homebound alcoholic. *American Journal of Nursing, 86*(2), 167–169.

Doshan, T., & Bursch, C. (1982). Women and substance abuse: Critical issues in treatment and health. *Journal of Drug Education, 12*(3), 229–239.

Estep, R. (1987). Influence of the family on the use of alcohol and prescription depressants by women. *Journal of Psychoactive Drugs, 19*(2), 171–179.

Faltz, B. G., & Madover, S. (1988). Treatment of substance abuse in patients with HIV infection. *Advances in Alcohol and Substance Abuse, 7*(2), 143–157.

Fischer, P. J., & Breakey, W. R. (1987). Profile of the Baltimore homeless with alcohol problems. *Alcohol Health and Research World, 11*(3), 36–37.

Flores-Ortiz, Y., & Bernal, G. (1989). Contextual family therapy of an addiction with Latinas. *Journal of Psychotherapy and the Family, 6*(1–2), 123–142.

Frezza, M., Di Padova, D., Pozzato, G., Terpin, M., Baraona, E., & Lieber, C. S. (1990). The role of decreased gastric alcohol dehydrogenase activity and first-pass metabolism. *New England Journal of Medicine, 322* (2), 95–99.

Gelberg, L., Linn, L. S., & Leake, B. D. (1986). Mental health, alcohol and drug use, and criminal history among homeless adults. *American Journal of Psychiatry, 145*(2), 191–196.

Gilbert, M., & Alcocoer, A. (1988). Alcohol use and Hispanic youth: An overview. *Journal of Drug Issues, 18*(1), 33–48.

Glick, R., & Moore, J. (Eds.). (1990). *Drugs in Hispanic communities.* New Brunswick, NJ: Rutgers University Press.

Guinan, M. E., & Hardy, A. (1987). Epidemiology of AIDS in women in the United States. *Journal of the American Medical Association, 257,* 2039–2042.

Hall, J. M., & Stevens, P. (1988). AIDS: A guide to suicide assessment. *Archives of Psychiatric Nursing, 1*(2), 115–120.

Harper, F. D. (1976). *Alcohol abuse and black Americans.* Alexandria, VA: Douglas.

Houseman, C., & Pheifer, W. (1988). Potential for unresolved grief in survivors of persons with AIDS. *Archives of Psychiatric Nursing, II*(5), 296–300.

Institute of Medicine. (1990. *Broadening the base of treatment for alcohol problems.* Washington, DC: National Academy Press.

Jacobsen, R. (1986). Female alcoholics: A controlled CT brain scan and clinical study. *British Journal of Addictions, 81,* 661–669.

Kagle, J. D. (1987). Secondary prevention of substance abuse. *Social Work, 32*(5), 446–448.

Kendall, J., Gloersen, B., Gray, P., McConnell, S., Turner, J., & West, J. (1989). Doing well with AIDS: Three case illustrations. *Archives of Psychiatric Nursing, III*(3), 159–165.

Lancaster, J. (1988). Substance abuse. In M. Stanhope & J. Lancaster (Eds.), *Community health nursing,* 2nd Edition (pp. 682–702). St. Louis, MO: C. V. Mosby.

Lawson, G. W., & Lawson, A. W. (1989). *Alcoholism and substance abuse in special populations.* Rockville, MD: Aspen.

Lee, L. J. (1983). Reducing black adolescents' drug use: Family revisited. In R. Israelowitz & M. Singer (Eds.), *Adolescent substance abuse: A guide to prevention and treatment* (pp. 57–69).

Mandel, L., & North, S. (1982). Sex roles, sexuality and the recovering woman alcoholic. *Program Issues, 14*(1–2), 163–166.

Manson, S. M., Beals, J., Dick, R. W., & Duclas, C. (1989). Risk factors for suicide among Indian adolescents at a boarding school. *Public Health Reports, 104*(6), 609–614.

Manson, S. M. (Ed.). (1982). *New directions in prevention among American Indian and Alaskan Native communities.* Portland, OR: Oregon Health Sciences University.

McGoldrick, M., Pearce, J. K., & Giordano, J. (Eds.). (1980). *Ethnicity and family therapy.* New York: Guilford Press.

Miller, B., Downs, W., & Gondoli, B. (1989). Delinquency, childhood violence and the development of alcoholism in women. *Crime and Delinquency (Special issue: Women and crime), 35*(1), 94–108.

Moore, J., & Devitt, M. (1989). The paradox of deliverance in addicted Mexican American mothers. *Gender and Society, 3*(1), 53–70.

Moore, M. H., & Gernstein, D. K. (Eds.). (1981). *Alcohol and public policy: Beyond the shadow of prohibition.* Washington, DC: National Academy Press.

Morales, A. (1984). Substance abuse and Mexican-American youth: An overview. *Journal of Drug Issues, 14*(2), 297–311.

Naegle, M. A. (1988). Substance abuse among women: Prevalence, patterns and treatment issues. *Issues in Mental Health, 9,* 2.

National Nurses Society on Addiction. (1989). *Nursing care planning with the addicted client: Volumes I and II.* Skokie, IL: Midwest Education Association, Inc.

Okwumabua, J. O., & Duryea, E. J. (1987). Age of onset, periods of risk and patterns of progression in drug use among American Indian high school students. *International Journal of Addiction, 22*(12), 1269–1276.

Penniman, J. L., & Agnew, J. (1988). Women and alcohol. In C. Wright (Ed.), *Rehabilitation of the alcoholic.* Philadelphia: Hanley & Belfus, Inc.

Reed, B. G. (1987). Developing women-sensitive drug dependence treatment services: Why so difficult? *Journal of Psychoactive Drugs, 19*(2), 151–164.

Robert-Gurnoff, M. (1986). Prevalence of antibodies to HTLV–I, II and III in intravenous drug abusers from an AIDS endemic region. *Journal of the American Medical Association, 255*(22), 3133–3137.

Roper, R. H. (1987). Homelessness as a health risk. *Alcohol Health and Research World, 11*(3), 38–41, 89.

Roth, P. (1991). *Alcohol and drugs are women's issues, Volume Two: The model program guide.* Metuchen, NJ: Scarecrow Press, Inc.

Schinke, S. P., Botvin, G., & Trimble, J. E. (1988). Preventing substance abuse among American Indian adolescents: A bicultural competence skills approach. *Journal of Counseling Psychology, 35*(1), 87–90.

Stall, R. (1988). Prevention of HIV infection associated with drug and alcohol abuse. *Advances in Alcohol and Abuse, 7*(2), 73–87.

Stimmel, B. (1987). AIDS, alcohol and heroin: A particularly deadly combination. *Advances in Alcohol and Substance Abuse, 6*(3), 1–5.

Tripp-Reimer, T., Brink, P. I., & Saunders, J. (1991). Cultural assessment: Content and process. In B. W. Spradley (Ed.), *Readings in community health nursing* (4th ed. pp. 503–511). Philadelphia: Lippincott.

U.S. Department of Health and Human Services. (1990, January). *Secretary's seventh special report to the U.S. Congress on alcohol and health.* Rockville, MD: Author.

U.S. Department of Health and Human Services. (1990). *Citizen's alcohol and other drug prevention directory: Resources for getting involved* (DHHS Publication No. (ADM) 90-1657). Rockville, MD: Author.

Van Wormer, K. (1989). Co-dependency: Implications for women and therapy. *Women & Therapy, 8*(4), 51–63.

Vener, A. M., Kreyoka, L. R., & Climio, J. J. (1980). Drug use and health characteristics in non-institutionalized Mexican-American elderly. *Journal of Drug Education, 10,* 343–353.

Watts, T. D., & Wright, R., Jr. (Eds.). (1983). *Black alcoholism: Toward a comprehensive understanding.* Springfield, IL: Charles C. Thomas.

Weinreb, L., & Bassuk, E. (1990). Substance abuse: A growing problem among homeless families. *Family and Community Health, 13*(1), 55–64.

Williams, A. (1986). Primary care of parenteral substance abuse. *Nurse Practitioner, 11*(6).

Wilsnack, S., Wilsnack, R., & Klassen, A. (1984, Winter). Drinking and drinking problems among women in a U.S. national survey. *Alcohol Health and Research World,* 3–12.

Wilsnack, S., Klassen, C., & Wilsnack, R. W. (1984). Drinking and reproductive dysfunction among women in a national survey. *Alcoholism: Clinical and Experimental Research, 8,* 451–458.

Wilsnack, S., & Beckman, L. (1984). *Alcohol problems in women.* New York: Guilford.

Winokur, G., & Corzell, W. (1989). Familial alcoholism in primary unipolar major depressive disorder. *American Journal of Psychiatry, 148*(2), 184–188.

Wolper, B., & Scheiner, Z. (1981). *Family therapy approaches and drug dependent women.* (Treatment research monograph). Rockville, MD: National Institute on Drug Abuse.

Wright, R., & Watts, T. D. (1988). Alcohol and minority youth. *Journal of Drug Issues, 18*(1), 1–7.

Young, T. J. (1987). Inhalant use among American Indian youth. *Child Psychiatry and Human Development, 18*(1), 36–46.

Zimberg, S. (1982). Special approaches for sub-populations of alcoholics. In *The clinical management of alcoholism* (pp. 157–176). New York: Brunner/Mazel Publishers.